Behavioral and Developmental Pediatrics

A Handbook for Primary Care

Behavioral and Developmental Pediatrics

A Handbook for Primary Care

Edited by

Steven Parker, M.D.

Associate Professor of Pediatrics, Boston University School of Medicine; Director, Division of Developmental and Behavioral Pediatrics, Boston City Hospital, Boston

Barry Zuckerman, M.D.

Professor and Chairman, Department of Pediatrics, Boston University School of Medicine; Chief, Department of Pediatrics, Boston City Hospital, Boston

Foreword by
Joel J. Alpert, M.D.

Professor of Pediatrics and Public Health, Former Chairman of Pediatrics, Boston University School of Medicine, Boston

Little, Brown and Company
Boston   New York   Toronto   London

Library of Congress Cataloging-in-Publication Data

Behavioral and developmental pediatrics : a handbook for primary care
/ edited by Steven Parker, Barry Zuckerman.
    p. cm.
  Includes bibliographical references and index.
  ISBN 0-316-69090-2
  1. Pediatrics—Psychological aspects—Handbooks, manuals, etc.
  2. Behavior disorders in children—Handbooks, manuals, etc.
  3. Child development deviations—Handbooks, manuals, etc.
  I. Parker, Steven. II. Zuckerman, Barry S.
  [DNLM: 1. Child Development Disorders—diagnosis—handbooks.
  2. Child Development Disorders—therapy—handbooks. 3. Child
  Behavior Disorders—therapy—handbooks. 4. Child Behavior
  Disorders—diagnosis—handbooks. WS 39 B419 1994]
  RJ47.5.B37 1994
  618.92'89—dc20
  DNLM/DLC
  for Library of Congress   94-17875
                                                                      CIP

Printed in the United States of America
ICP

10 9 8 7 6 5

Editorial: Nancy E. Chorpenning, Kristin Odmark
Production Editor: Cathleen Cote
Production Services: Julie Sullivan
Cover Designer: Nina Garfinkle

Contents

Contributing Authors

Marilyn Augustyn, M.D.

Fellow in Developmental and Behavioral Pediatrics, Boston University School of Medicine; Department of Pediatrics, Boston City Hospital, Boston
30. Fears

Abraham Joseph Avni-Singer, M.D.

Fellow, Department of Pediatrics, Yale University School of Medicine, New Haven, Connecticut
39. Hospitalization

Howard Bauchner, M.D.

Associate Professor of Pediatrics, Boston University School of Medicine; Director, Division of General Pediatrics, Boston City Hospital, Boston
49. Pain

Gayle Belin-Frost, M.A., C.C.C.-SLP

Clinical Supervisor and Lecturer in Communication Sciences, University of Vermont, Burlington, Vermont
62. Stuttering

Jane Bernzweig, Ph.D.

Assistant Research Psychologist, Department of Pediatrics, University of California, San Francisco, School of Medicine, San Francisco
2. Talking with Children

James A. Blackman, M.D., M.P.H.

Professor of Pediatrics, University of Virginia School of Medicine; Director of Research, University of Virginia Kluge Children's Rehabilitation Center, Charlottesville, Virginia
51. Prematurity: Follow-Up

Peter A. Blasco, M.D.

Associate Professor of Pediatrics, University of Minnesota Medical School—Minneapolis; Director of Training, Center for Children with Chronic Illness and Disability, University of Minnesota Health Sciences Center, Minneapolis
45. Motor Delays

W. Thomas Boyce, M.D.

Professor of Pediatrics, University of California, San Francisco, School of Medicine; Director, Division of Behavioral and Developmental Pediatrics, The Medical Center at the University of California, San Francisco, San Francisco
12. Coping with Stressful Transitions

Robert J. Boyle, M.D.

Associate Professor of Pediatrics, University of Virginia School of Medicine; Director, Neonatal Follow-up Clinic, University of Virginia Health Sciences Center, Charlottesville, Virginia
51. Prematurity: Follow-Up

T. Berry Brazelton, M.D.

Professor Emeritus of Pediatrics, Harvard Medical School; Children's Hospital, Boston
3. Touchpoints for Anticipatory Guidance in the First Three Years

Robert B. Brooks, Ph.D.

Assistant Professor of Psychology, Harvard Medical School, Boston; Director, Department of Psychology, McLean Hospital, Belmont, Massachusetts
57. Self-Esteem

John C. Carey, M.D.

Professor of Pediatrics, University of Utah School of Medicine; Chief, Division of Genetics, University of Utah Health Sciences Center, Salt Lake City
26. The Dysmorphic Child

Jonathan M. Cheek, Ph.D.

Professor of Psychology, Wellesley College, Wellesley, Massachusetts
60. Shyness

Edward R. Christophersen, M.D.

Professor of Pediatrics, University of Missouri—Kansas City School of Medicine; Chief, Section of Behavioral Pediatrics, Children's Mercy Hospital, Kansas City, Missouri
11. Behavioral Management: Theory and Practice

Susan Coates, Ph.D.

Clinical Associate Professor of Medical Psychology, Department of Psychiatry, Columbia University College of Physicians and Surgeons; Director, Childhood Gender Identity Clinic, St. Luke's–Roosevelt Hospital Center, New York
35. Gender Identity Issues

Donald J. Cohen, M.D.

Professor, Child Study Center, Yale University School of Medicine; Director, Department of Child Psychiatry, Yale–New Haven Hospital, New Haven, Connecticut
68. Tics and Tourette's Syndrome

James Coplan, M.D.

Associate Professor of Pediatrics, State University of New York Health Science Center at Syracuse College of Medicine; Chief, Division of Child Development, Department of Pediatrics, State University Hospital, Syracuse, New York
41. Language Delays
Appendix E. Early Language
*   Milestone Scale*

David L. Coulter, M.D.

Associate Professor of Pediatrics and Neurology, Boston University School of Medicine; Director, Division of Pediatric Neurology, Boston City Hospital, Boston
44. Mental Retardation: The
*   Diagnostic Workup*

Howard Dubowitz, M.D.

Associate Professor of Pediatrics, University of Maryland School of Medicine; Director, Child Protection Program, University of Maryland Hospital, Baltimore
79. Foster Care

Paul H. Dworkin, M.D.

Professor and Head of General Pediatrics, University of Connecticut School of Medicine, Farmington; Director and Chairman, Department of Pediatrics, Saint Francis Hospital and Medical Center, Hartford, Connecticut
55. School Failure

Ilgi Ertem, M.D.

Fellow in Pediatrics, Yale University School of Medicine, New Haven, Connecticut
42. Masturbation

Bryan W. C. Forsyth, M.B., Ch.B.

Associate Professor, Pediatrics and Child Study Center, Yale University; Attending Physician, Department of Pediatrics, Yale–New Haven Hospital, New Haven, Connecticut
89. Vulnerable Children

Linda Forsythe, M.D.

Instructor of Psychiatry, Harvard Medical School; Staff Physician, Child Psychiatry Service, Massachusetts General Hospital, Boston
23. Depression

Sharon W. Foster, Ph.D.

Associate Professor of Pediatrics, University of Wisconsin Medical School; Clinical Associate Professor, General Pediatric and Teenage Clinic, University of Wisconsin Hospital and Clinics, Madison, Wisconsin
77. Divorce

Deborah Frank, M.D.	Associate Professor of Pediatrics, Boston University School of Medicine; Assistant Professor of Public Health, Boston University School of Public Health; Director, Growth and Development Program, Boston City Hospital, Boston 29. *Failure to Thrive*
Tamar Gershon, M.D.	Clinical Instructor of Pediatrics, University of California, San Francisco, School of Medicine; Department of Pediatrics, San Francisco General Hospital, San Francisco 80. *Lesbian and Gay Parents*
Frances Page Glascoe, Ph.D.	Assistant Professor of Pediatrics, Division of Child Development, Vanderbilt University School of Medicine; Educational Specialist, Department of Pediatrics, Vanderbilt University Medical Center, Nashville, Tennessee 7. *Developmental Screening*
Stuart Goldman, M.D.	Instructor of Psychiatry, Harvard Medical School; Director of Psychiatric Education, Department of Psychiatry, Children's Hospital, Boston 24. *Disruptive Behavior: Lying, Stealing, and Aggression*
Linda Grant, M.D., M.P.H.	Associate Clinical Professor of Pediatrics, Boston University School of Medicine; Staff Physician, Department of Adolescent Medicine, Boston City Hospital, Boston 58. *Sex and the Adolescent*
Stanley I. Greenspan, M.D.	Clinical Professor of Psychiatry and Behavioral Sciences and Pediatrics, George Washington University School of Medicine and Health Sciences; Academic Faculty, Children's National Medical Center, Washington 9. *Monitoring Social and Emotional Development of Young Children*
Jessie R. Groothuis, M.D.	Associate Professor of Pediatrics, University of Colorado School of Medicine; Director, Neonatal High Risk Follow-up Program, The Children's Hospital, Denver 88. *Twins*
Betsy McAlister Groves, M.S.W., L.I.C.S.W.	Assistant Clinical Professor of Pediatrics, Boston University School of Medicine; Director, Child Witness to Violence Project, Boston City Hospital, Boston 72. *Witness to Violence*

Barry Guitar, Ph.D.	Professor and Chairman of Communication Sciences, University of Vermont, Burlington, Vermont *62. Stuttering*
Karen Hacker, M.D.	Assistant Clinical Professor of Medicine and Pediatrics, Boston University School of Medicine; Director of Adolescent and School Services, Division of Public Health, Department of Health and Hospitals, Boston *63. Substance Abuse in Adolescence*
Randi Hagerman, M.D.	Professor of Pediatrics, University of Colorado School of Medicine; Associate Director, Child Development Unit, Children's Hospital, Denver *33. Fragile X Syndrome*
Lawrence Hammer, M.D.	Associate Professor of Pediatrics, Stanford University School of Medicine, Stanford; Director, Division of General Pediatrics, Lucile Salter Packard Children's Hospital, Palo Alto, California *48. Obesity*
Gordon Harper, M.D.	Assistant Professor of Psychiatry, Harvard Medical School; Director, Inpatient Psychiatry, Children's Hospital, Boston *52. Psychosomatic Illness*
Alexander H. Hoon, M.D., M.P.H.	Assistant Professor of Pediatrics, Johns Hopkins University School of Medicine; Director, Neurodevelopmental Clinic, Kennedy Kreiger Institute, Baltimore *20. Cerebral Palsy*
Barbara Howard, M.D.	Clinical Assistant Professor of Pediatrics, Duke University School of Medicine; Faculty, Child Development Unit, Duke University Medical Center, Durham, North Carolina *10. Managing Behavior Problems in an Office Practice* *17. Biting*
Susan Jay, M.D.	Professor of Pediatrics, Loyola University of Chicago Stritch School of Medicine; Director, Department of Adolescent Medicine, Loyola University Medical Center, Maywood, Illinois *47. The Noncompliant Adolescent*
Michael Jellinek, M.D.	Associate Professor of Psychiatry, Harvard Medical School; Chief, Child Psychiatry Service, Massachusetts General Hospital, Boston *23. Depression*

Alain Joffe, M.D., M.P.H.	Associate Professor of Pediatrics, Johns Hopkins University School of Medicine; Director, Department of Adolescent Medicine, Johns Hopkins Hospital, Baltimore *14. Anorexia Nervosa and Bulimia*
Herbert M. Joseph, Jr., Ph.D.	Clinical Instructor in Psychiatry, Boston University School of Medicine; Director of Psychology and Center for Multicultural Training in Psychology, Boston City Hospital, Boston *76. Cultural Responses to Behavioral Problems*
Theodore Kastner, M.D.	Associate Professor of Clinical Pediatrics, Columbia University College of Physicians and Surgeons, New York; Director, Center for Human Development, Morristown Memorial Hospital, Morristown, New Jersey *43. Mental Retardation: Behavioral Problems*
Kathi J. Kemper, M.D., M.P.H.	Clinical Associate Professor of Pediatrics, University of Washington School of Medicine; Associate Director for Research, Department of Family Medicine, Swedish Hospital Medical Center, Seattle *8. Psychosocial Screening* *82. Parental Drug, Alcohol, and Cigarette Addiction*
Teresa M. Kohlenberg, M.D.	Assistant Professor of Pediatrics, Boston University School of Medicine; Director, Teen-Tot Clinic, Boston City Hospital, Boston *76. Cultural Responses to Behavioral Problems* *86. Teen Mothers*
Barbara Korsch, M.D.	Professor of Pediatrics, University of Southern California School of Medicine; Attending Pediatrician, Department of General Pediatrics, Children's Hospital of Los Angeles, Los Angeles *1. Talking with Parents* *4. Difficult Encounters with Parents*
John M. Leventhal, M.D.	Professor of Pediatrics, Child Study Center, Yale University School of Medicine; Attending Physician, Department of Pediatrics, Yale–New Haven Hospital, New Haven, Connecticut *39. Hospitalization* *42. Masturbation*

Melvin D. Levine, M.D.

Professor of Pediatrics, University of North Carolina at Chapel Hill School of Medicine; Director, Clinical Center for the Study of Development and Learning, Chapel Hill, North Carolina
70. Unpopular Children

Catherine C. Lewis, Ph.D.

Adjunct Associate Professor of Pediatrics and Psychiatry, University of California, San Francisco, School of Medicine; Director of Formative Research, Developmental Studies Center, Oakland, California
2. Talking with Children

Melvin Lewis, M.B.B.S., D.Ch.

Professor of Pediatrics and Psychiatry, Child Study Center, Yale University School of Medicine; Attending Physician, Departments of Child Psychiatry and Pediatrics, Yale–New Haven Hospital, New Haven, Connecticut
78. Dying Children

Deborah Madansky, M.D.

Associate Professor of Pediatrics and Psychiatry, University of Massachusetts Medical School; Medical Director, Child Advocacy Team, University of Massachusetts Medical Center, Worcester, Massachusetts
59. Sexual Abuse

Rebecca McCauley, Ph.D.

Associate Professor of Communication Sciences, University of Vermont, Burlington, Vermont
15. Articulation Disorders

Barbara A. Morse, Ph.D.

Assistant Research Professor of Psychiatry, Boston University School of Medicine, Boston; Program Director, Fetal Alcohol Education Program, Boston University School of Medicine, Brookline, Massachusetts
32. Fetal Alcohol Syndrome

Robert Needlman, M.D.

Assistant Professor of Pediatrics, Case Western Reserve University School of Medicine; Director, Continuity Clinic, Department of Pediatrics, Rainbow Babies and Childrens Hospital, Cleveland
65. Temper Tantrums
83. Sibling Rivalry

Kathleen Nelson, M.D.

Professor of Pediatrics, University of Alabama School of Medicine; Director, Division of General Pediatrics, The Children's Hospital of Alabama, Birmingham, Alabama
31. Feeding Problems

Eli Newberger, M.D.

Director, Family Development Program, Children's Hospital, Boston
50. Physical Abuse

Karen Norberg, M.D.

Assistant Professor of Pediatrics, Boston University School of Medicine; Attending Psychiatrist, Boston City Hospital, Boston
64. Suicide

Karen Olness, M.D.

Professor of Pediatrics, Family Medicine, and International Health, Case Western Reserve University School of Medicine; Director, Department of International Child Health, Rainbow Babies and Childrens Hospital, Cleveland
13. Self-Regulation Therapy

Lucy Osborn, M.D.

Professor of Pediatrics, University of Utah School of Medicine; Associate Vice President, University of Utah Health Sciences Center, Salt Lake City
81. Parental Depression

Judith S. Palfrey, M.D.

Associate Professor of Pediatrics, Harvard Medical School; Chief, Division of General Pediatrics, Children's Hospital, Boston
56. School Readiness

Frederick B. Palmer, M.D.

Shainberg Professor of Pediatrics, University of Tennessee, Memphis, College of Medicine; Director, Boling Center for Developmental Disabilities, Memphis, Tennessee
20. Cerebral Palsy

Robert Pantell, M.D.

Professor of Pediatrics, University of California, San Francisco, School of Medicine; Director, Division of General Pediatrics, The Medical Center at the University of California, San Francisco
2. Talking with Children

Steven Parker, M.D.

Associate Professor of Pediatrics, Boston University School of Medicine; Director, Division of Developmental and Behavioral Pediatrics, Boston City Hospital, Boston
22. Colic
69. Toilet Training

John M. Pascoe, M.D., M.P.H.

Associate Professor of Pediatrics, University of Wisconsin Medical School; Head, Division of General Pediatrics and Adolescent Medicine, University of Wisconsin Hospital and Clinics, Madison, Wisconsin
77. Divorce

Ellen C. Perrin, M.D.

Professor of Pediatrics, University of Massachusetts Medical School; Staff Physician, Department of Pediatrics, University of Massachusetts Medical Center, Worcester
6. *Behavioral Screening*
21. *Chronic Conditions*

Nicole Prudent, M.D., M.P.H.

Assistant Professor of Pediatrics, Boston University School of Medicine; Primary Care Pediatrician, Departments of Pediatrics and Adolescent Medicine, Boston City Hospital, Boston
76. *Cultural Responses to Behavioral Problems*

Siegfried M. Pueschel, M.D., Ph.D., M.P.H.

Professor of Pediatrics, Brown University School of Medicine; Director, Child Development Center, Rhode Island Hospital, Providence, Rhode Island
25. *Down Syndrome*

Leonard Rappaport, M.D.

Assistant Professor of Pediatrics, Harvard Medical School; Associate Chief, Division of General Pediatrics, Children's Hospital, Boston
28. *Enuresis*
53. *Recurrent Abdominal Pain*

Gary Remafedi, M.D., M.P.H.

Assistant Professor of Pediatrics, University of Minnesota Medical School—Minneapolis; Director, Youth and AIDS Project, University of Minnesota Health Sciences Center, Minneapolis
34. *Gay, Lesbian, and Bisexual Youth*

Vesta Richardson, M.D.

Assistant Professor of Pediatrics, Boston University School of Medicine; Director, Inpatient Unit, Department of Pediatrics, Boston City Hospital, Boston
76. *Cultural Responses to Behavioral Problems*

Vaughn Rickert, Psy.D.

Associate Professor of Pediatrics, University of Arkansas for Medical Sciences College of Medicine; Associate Director, Section of Pediatric Psychology, Arkansas Children's Hospital, Little Rock, Arkansas
47. *The Noncompliant Adolescent*

Nancy Roizen, M.D.

Assistant Professor of Clinical Pediatrics, University of Chicago Pritzker School of Medicine; Chief, Section of Developmental Pediatrics, Wyler Children's Hospital, Chicago
73. *Adoption*

N. Paul Rosman, M.D.

Professor of Pediatrics and Neurology, Tufts University School of Medicine; Chief, Division of Pediatric Neurology, Floating Hospital for Children at New England Medical Center, Boston
16. Autism

Larry Scahill, M.S.N., M.P.H.

Associate Research Scientist, Child Study Center, Yale University School of Medicine, New Haven, Connecticut
68. Tics and Tourette's Syndrome

Neil Schechter, M.D.

Professor of Pediatrics and Head, Division of Developmental and Behavioral Pediatrics, University of Connecticut School of Medicine, Farmington; Director, Section of Developmental and Behavioral Pediatrics, Saint Francis Hospital and Medical Center, Hartford, Connecticut
36. The Gifted Child

Albert P. Scheiner, M.D.

Professor of Pediatrics, University of Massachusetts Medical School; Vice Chairman, Department of Pediatrics, University of Massachusetts Medical Center, Worcester, Massachusetts
18. Blindness

Hilde S. Schlesinger, M.D.

Professor Emerita of Psychiatry, University of California, San Francisco, School of Medicine, San Francisco
38. Hearing Loss

Barton D. Schmitt, M.D.

Professor of Pediatrics, University of Colorado School of Medicine; Director, General Pediatric Consultative Services, The Children's Hospital, Denver
54. School Avoidance

David J. Schonfeld, M.D.

Assistant Professor of Pediatrics, Child Study Center, Yale University School of Medicine; Director, Behavioral Pediatrics Clinic, The Children's Hospital at Yale–New Haven, New Haven, Connecticut
78. Dying Children

Clifford W. Sells

Fellow in Adolescent Medicine, Pediatrics, University of Minnesota Medical School—Minneapolis; Attending Physician, Adolescent Health Program, University of Minnesota Hospitals and Clinic, Minneapolis
34. Gay, Lesbian, and Bisexual Youth

Jack P. Shonkoff, M.D.

Professor of Pediatrics, University of Massachusetts Medical School; Chief, Division of Developmental and Behavioral Pediatrics, University of Massachusetts Medical Center, Worcester, Massachusetts
5. Helping Families Deal with Bad News

Benjamin S. Siegel, M.D.

Professor of Pediatrics and Psychiatry, Boston University School of Medicine; Senior Pediatrician, Primary Care Program, Boston City Hospital, Boston
74. Bereavement and Loss

Martin Stein, M.D.

Professor of Pediatrics, University of California, San Diego, School of Medicine, La Jolla; Attending Pediatrician, UCSD Medical Center, San Diego
37. Headaches

Victor C. Strasburger, M.D.

Associate Professor of Pediatrics, University of New Mexico School of Medicine; Chief, Division of Adolescent Medicine, Department of Pediatrics, University of New Mexico Hospital, Albuquerque
87. Television

Peter Stringham, M.D.

Instructor of Pediatrics, Boston University School of Medicine; Staff Physician, Department of Pediatrics, East Boston Neighborhood Health Center, Boston
71. Violent Youth

J. Lane Tanner, M.D.

Assistant Clinical Professor of Pediatrics, University of California, San Francisco, School of Medicine; Assistant Director, Division of Behavioral and Developmental Pediatrics, The Medical Center at the University of California, San Francisco; San Francisco
84. Single Parents

Stanley Turecki, M.D.

Assistant Clinical Professor of Psychiatry, Mount Sinai School of Medicine of the City University of New York; Attending Psychiatrist, Lenox Hill Hospital, New York
66. Temperamentally Difficult Children

Kerline Vassell, M.D.

Fellow in Developmental and Behavioral Pediatrics, Boston University School of Medicine; Department of Pediatrics, Boston City Hospital, Boston
67. Thumb Sucking

Emily B. Visher, Ph.D.

Instructor, California School of Professional Psychology, Alameda, California
85. Stepfamilies

John S. Visher, M.D.

Lecturer Emeritus in Psychiatry, Stanford University School of Medicine, Stanford, California
85. Stepfamilies

Kevin Walsh, Ph.D.

Director of Research, Center for Human Development, Morristown Memorial Hospital, Morristown, New Jersey
43. Mental Retardation: Behavioral Problems

Lyn Weiner, M.P.H.

Associate Professor of Public Health, Boston University School of Medicine, Boston; Executive Director, Fetal Alcohol Education Program, Boston University School of Medicine, Brookline, Massachusetts
32. Fetal Alcohol Syndrome

Esther Wender, M.D.

Clinical Professor of Pediatrics, Albert Einstein College of Medicine of Yeshiva University, Bronx; Program Director, Child Health Services, Westchester County Department of Health, Hawthorne, New York
40. Hyperactivity

Sabrina Wolfe, Ph.D.

Associate Director, Childhood Gender Identity Clinic, St. Luke's–Roosevelt Hospital Center, New York
35. Gender Identity Issues

Yvette E. Yatchmink, M.D., Ph.D.

Assistant Professor of Pediatrics, Division of Developmental and Behavioral Pediatrics, University of Massachusetts Medical School; Director, Infant-Toddler Clinic, University of Massachusetts Medical Center, Worcester, Massachusetts
5. Helping Families Deal with Bad News

Barry Zuckerman, M.D.

Professor and Chairman, Department of Pediatrics, Boston University School of Medicine; Chief, Department of Pediatrics, Boston City Hospital, Boston
19. Breath Holding
27. Encopresis
46. Night Terrors and Nightmares
61. Sleep Problems

Meg Zweiback, R.N., M.P.H., C.P.N.P.

Associate Clinical Professor, Department of Family Health Care Nursing, University of California, San Francisco, School of Nursing, San Francisco
75. Child Care

Foreword

The field of pediatrics occasionally recognizes pressing issues for children and families late in the course of clinical events. Behavioral and developmental pediatrics is one such example—it is a field that has only recently moved into the pediatric mainstream, even though recognition came over 30 years ago when it was described as the "new morbidity." This handbook should herald the end of that outdated phrase. Behavioral and developmental issues are neither new, nor usually pathological. Rather, they occur in many normal children and are often preventable by appropriate pediatric anticipatory guidance.

It also is clear that behavioral and developmental issues will continue to play an ever increasing (and vexing) role in our clinical practice. Clinicians today are unlikely to see polio, but we will see children with attentional problems. We can immunize against bacterial meningitis, but how do we deal with drugs and violence? As most organ-specific diseases have become low prevalence events, behavioral and developmental problems have come to the fore of pediatric practice.

For these reasons, *Behavioral and Developmental Pediatrics: A Handbook for Primary Care* is greatly needed and long overdue. Doctors Parker and Zuckerman have edited a comprehensive and authoritative work for the busy primary care clinician. The contributors to this handbook have covered a wide array of important topics and provide the reader with clinically useful, relevant information presented in an efficient format. Today's practitioners will find much to use in the handbook, whether seeking concise and authoritative guidance, more detailed references, books and phone numbers of national organizations for parents, or just reliable counsel through the complex web of etiologies and treatments.

This handbook teaches us that there are no magic bullets in caring for children and families with behavioral and developmental problems, but there are proven therapies and interventions that can make a difference and belong in the practice of every clinician. To that end, Drs. Parker and Zuckerman have enhanced our ability to address these issues in the context of primary care and improve the well-being of the families and children we serve.

Joel J. Alpert, M.D.

To Ann, Hyman, Philip, and Karen Parker and to Anne, Leo, Elliot, Diana, Pamela, Jake, and Katherine Zuckerman. Our enduring interest in the well-being of children and our commitment to helping them through teaching and clinical care has been fueled by the nurturance and support we have received from our families. It is to them, with great love and thanks, that we dedicate this book.

Preface

Behavioral and developmental issues play a role in almost every pediatric encounter and are often among the most challenging diagnostic and therapeutic dilemmas facing the pediatric primary care clinician. Busy practices, significant time constraints, inadequate training, reluctance to delve into all but purely "medical" problems, and a lack of scientifically validated solutions—all result in the neglect of such issues by many clinicians.

Behavioral and Developmental Pediatrics: A Handbook for Primary Care evolved from our work as primary care clinicians and as educators in developmental and behavioral pediatrics for practitioners. We have learned that primary care clinicians are most effective when they can form therapeutic alliances with children and families; sensitively elicit information; understand the psychological, biological, and social roots of problems; and have ready concrete, practical, and effective treatment strategies.

This book is intended to strengthen these skills in primary care clinicians— pediatricians, family practitioners, nurse practitioners, physicians' assistants, pediatric nurses, and others who care for children. Chapters are written by experts in the field and provide the key information needed to effectively address specific problems. This book is *not* meant to provide encyclopedic, exhaustive information. Rather, we have asked experts to *distill* their experience and the extant scientific literature into a concise, user-friendly format that can be easily understood and applied by the busy clinician. For those desiring more extensive information, a bibliography at the end of each chapter refers to additional key articles or chapters.

Part I discusses the fundamentals of behavioral and developmental pediatrics. It is designed to enable the clinician to create a therapeutic atmosphere in primary care and covers such topics as forming a therapeutic alliance, interviewing, diagnosis, and management. This information informs and enriches the subsequent sections and adds depth and sophistication to the clinician's skills.

Parts II and III address issue-specific developmental and behavioral problems. Each chapter is presented in a similar format to enhance accessibility. Most chapters provide sample questions to facilitate the history-taking process by modeling sensitive ways to elicit the information. The descriptions of the problems are intended to provide sufficient information to allow the clinician to explain the relevant issues to parents and children in a way that demystifies the problem and enhances families' ability to deal with it. Additionally, we have provided useful developmental and behavioral questionnaires and screening instruments in the appendixes for the interested clinician.

We hope this book will help to promote excellence in the management of behavioral and developmental problems during primary care visits and enhance the clinician's satisfaction in addressing such issues. As the pace of social change has quickened, so too have threats to children's behavioral and developmental well-being multiplied in frequency and severity. It is often the health care provider who is in the best position to help families and children deal with these threats. As we approach the twenty-first century, it is clear that pediatric clinicians must become more efficient, sophisticated, and clever in addressing behavioral and developmental issues if families and children are to be well served. We hope *Behavioral and Developmental Pediatrics* will contribute to the achievement of that end.

We thank Margaret Stanhope-Lavoye and Jeanne McCarthy for their invaluable help in the preparation of this manuscript. Their attention to detail, organizational skills, support, and timely responsiveness at crunch time are greatly appreciated.

S.P.
B.Z.

The Fundamentals of Behavioral and Developmental Pediatrics

Establishing a
Therapeutic Alliance

Talking with Parents

Barbara Korsch

The therapeutic alliance is achieved in large measure during the interview. Rapport building, engaging the patient, eliciting psychosocial and personal aspects of the patient's experiences, supporting the parents in their roles as parents, including the child, grandparent, and other significant others—all of these are essential to establish a therapeutic relationship. Although there are no techniques that work for all patients or all clinicians, there are some basics that virtually always strengthen the therapeutic alliance (Table 1-1).

I. **Listening.** Letting the parent know that you are listening is basic. Body language—sitting down, looking at the parent, leaning forward, showing appropriate concern—is effective in conveying a listening attitude and does not require extra time in the interview. Responding to nonverbal expressions of parent affect is also essential. For example, if the mother's face falls when the clinician suggests the use of a pacifier for a colicky baby, the responsive clinician needs to inquire, "You do not seem to like that idea. Is there any special reason why you do not want your baby to use the pacifier?" He or she may find out that the mother had difficulty in weaning her first-born from the pacifier or that she finds pacifiers disgusting. When screening behavioral checklists have been used (see appendixes A and B), the parental responses can provide the topics for discussion.

II. **Facilitating the dialogue.** The parent's story should be facilitated by appropriate empathetic responses, such as, "Tell me more about that" or "I can see that it did not work out so well for you," or "That must be hard for you." The clinician should avoid interruptions, subject changes, and judgmental comments and not prematurely pursue other diagnostic hypotheses, which can derail the parent's narrative. Attentive listening during the opening of an interview promotes communication and rarely takes more than a couple of minutes. Yet it has also been shown that, on the average, physicians interrupt the patients within 18 seconds. The reason is conflicting agendas: patients want to tell their story, and clinicians want to pursue their decision making. There are other strategies to facilitate a diagnosis:

A. **Elicit the reasons for the parent's concerns early in the interview.** "What worried you especially when you brought John in to see us today? . . . Why did that worry you?"

B. **Elicit the parent's expectations for the visit and acknowledge them.** "What had you hoped we might be able to do for your child today? What would you like to have us explain to you today?" These inquiries may reveal unrealistic expectations for specific therapies or magical cures. At other times, such questions make the clinician's job simple; it may be that all the family wants is reassurance. Once the parent's expectations have been acknowledged, the clinician, the parents, and the child can set an agenda for the visit, which synthesizes the parent's and medical issues. It is only after this opening—after listening attentively to the parent—that the clinician can afford to pursue his or her line of questions and fact finding. The first phase of the interaction has taken care of urgent concerns, relaxed the parent, and made her or him realize that the clinician is interested. The parent will now be a better historian and partner in the task-oriented portion of the interview.

C. **Guide but do not dominate the discourse.** General questions allow parents to broach subjects of interest to them. For child health supervision visits, clinicians can use simple questions: "How are things going?" "What are some new things the baby is doing?" "How do things work out at bedtime?" "What is the hardest

Table 1-1. How to enhance the therapeutic alliance

Process Steps	Sample comments

Greet
   Introduce self
   Set agenda jointly	

Listen
   Allow pauses
   Maintain eye contact	

Facilitate
   Do not judge
   Do not interrupt
	"Tell me more about that."

Elicit and acknowledge parent's concerns	"What worries you most at this time?" "You thought the high fever might bring on a seizure?"
Elicit and acknowledge parent's expectations	"What are you hoping we'll do for her today?"
Involve the child	
Be family centered	
Guide (not dominate) discourse	
Elicit the parent's solutions	"What have you tried so far?"
Make treatment decisions jointly	"Do you think you'll be able to give him the medicine 4 times a day?"
Make closure and agenda setting explicit	

part of taking care of him now?" "What is most enjoyable about taking care of him?" "Is the baby's father (or mother) able to give you any help?"

III. Using common courtesy. All the amenities of nonmedical human interaction must also be observed. Even clinicians who usually have good manners will, in the task-oriented medical encounter, omit greetings, introductions, and courtesies (such as knocking on the door before entering the examining room or explaining the reasons for keeping someone waiting). These courtesies should include a few appropriate remarks acknowledging the parent as a person, such as, "You sure have your hands full today," to the parent who comes with several children and all the attending paraphernalia, or, "I bet you are impatient with us for having kept you waiting so long. I had to deal with an emergency upstairs."

IV. Talking with the child. Early in the visit an appropriate approach must be made to the child, especially important when the social distance between practitioner and family is great or when communication is difficult because of the parent's anxiety, suspicion, or hostility. The awareness of a mutual interest in helping the child creates a bond between parent and clinician. Throughout the interview, in spite of the necessary record keeping, the practitioner must maintain eye contact with the child and parent and watch for nonverbal signs of distress or disagreement or of reassurance and relief.

V. Dealing with acute illnesses. During an acute illness, the interview must be focused. As the parent tells the story of the illness, the practitioner can facilitate responsively: "So the fever has been high for almost 3 days now. . . . What are some of the other things you have noticed? . . . How did you handle that? . . . How did that work out? . . . What about feeding? . . . Sleep? . . . Any other changes?"

If the parents have used home remedies, it is essential not to make judgmental statements. If the treatment was harmless and the parent feels it was effective (even when the practitioner would not have chosen it), it is best to support the parent's approach.

On the other hand, if a parent has attempted an intervention that is potentially harmful (e.g., giving aspirin for a viral infection), the clinician should not use this moment to give the alarming warnings (e.g., about Reye's syndrome). Yet the family needs to be informed. Our approach is: "I am glad she is feeling better, but I need to give you some new information. Aspirin has been around a long time, and it has given relief to many patients. However, we have learned that aspirin can have side effects that involve severe liver damage and can be very serious, although rare. Your baby is obviously fine, but I feel strongly that from now on you should avoid aspirin and use acetaminophen instead."

After the episode is over and the parent is less likely to be overwhelmed by guilt and anxieties, more complete and forceful information can be given. Alternatives and additional treatments can be suggested without undermining the parent's self-confidence and self-esteem.

To avoid embarrassment and fractures of the clinician-parent alliance, at all times the clinician should ask, "How have you handled that? . . . What have you been doing or giving her so far?" before launching into medical advice. Whenever possible, the parent's own solution should be supported. When developing other approaches, it is best to involve the parent—for example, "Do you think you could manage to give the breathing treatment every 3 hours for a few days?" or "Have you thought of trying to keep her off milk for a few days?" A therapeutic plan has to be a joint venture. Rarely should it be imposed without parental input.

VI. Redirecting the interview. The clinician needs to keep control of the interview, even while being supportive and accepting. When the discussion gets off track, the clinician needs to redirect the discourse—for instance, "We must sit down and discuss that on another occasion after he is over this illness," or "There is some other information I need right now so we can decide about the treatment for this illness." If the parent makes an unreasonable request, such as, "You will give him a shot of penicillin today, won't you?" the clinician can back off and state, "I do not know whether that will be necessary today. We will talk about that after I have examined your son."

VII. Counseling and reassurance. Advice giving and counseling the patient and family can be a continuing process. Some concerns may be addressed at the first mention. For example, if the mother says, "He still wakes up once in the night and calls for me," the clinician may reassure promptly that this is not unusual at his age: "He misses you in the dark alone in his bedroom. Just comfort him, but do not start a night bottle again." Other concerns may best be allayed during the physical examination: "The arches of the foot normally do not develop before the child has been weight bearing for a while." Other topics require a discussion at the end of the visit or even at another scheduled conference time: "I can see you are having real difficulty in setting limits for his behavior at this time. We need to take some time to see what we can work out to help him accept your discipline and to make your life a little easier."

VIII. Closure

A. Summarize the relevant points the parent has raised and information he or she has given toward the end of the encounter.

B. Offer other educational materials, such as handouts, but individualize them by underlining certain specific issues or relating them to the parent's concerns.

C. Invite questions from caregivers, family, and child. Even when there is no time for full responses, they can be included in jointly setting the agenda for subsequent visits and follow-up health care.

Bibliography

Beckman H, Frankel R. The effect of physician behavior on the collection of data. *Ann Intern Med* 101:692–696, 1984.

Korsch BM, Aley EF. Pediatric interviewing techniques. *Cur Prob Pediat* 3:33–42, 1973.

Mishler EG. *The Discourse of Medicine: Dialectics of Medical Interviews.* Norwood NJ: Ablex, 1984.

Stewart M, Roter D (eds). *Communicating with Medical Patients.* London: Sage, 1989.

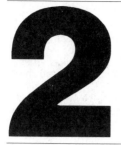

Talking with Children

Jane Bernzweig,
Robert Pantell, and
Catherine C. Lewis

I. Problems with clinician-patient communication. The typical pediatric visit lasts less than 15 minutes. In such a brief encounter, it can be difficult to establish rapport and to communicate medical information effectively to children and parents. A rushed clinician sends signals that he or she does not welcome parents' and children's expressions of their worries and concerns. Additionally, failing to establish rapport with a family establishes a barrier that teaches that health care is delivered in an authoritarian fashion, with little to no give and take. Under these circumstances, many parents and children will not bring up issues that are troubling them. Studies have shown that there is not a significant correlation between the amount of time of a primary care visit and patients' satisfaction with that visit; rather, the high *quality* of an interaction can supersede the limited *quantity*.

Even when clinicians establish good rapport with parents, they often leave children out of substantive communication, such as discussions about the diagnosis and the management of their illness. Even the best intentioned and highly skilled clinician may experience communication barriers with children because of limitations in children's abilities to understand information and the clinician's difficulty in communicating information at the appropriate developmental level. For example, an 11 year old, newly diagnosed with "diabetes," heard she was going to "die of betes." A 13 year old was frightened when his abdominal pain was diagnosed as "gas" because he had always heard that gas from a stove could be lethal. A 9 year old who was told that his lungs were like a balloon became terrified because he knew how easily balloons can pop.

II. Communication goals of the pediatric visit. The primary goal of open communication is the establishment of a therapeutic alliance with children and parents. The benefits of such a therapeutic alliance have been well documented.

    A. In hospitalized children, special opportunities for preoperative communication with a health care provider can **reduce surgical morbidity and improve physiologic and behavioral outcomes.**

    B. Health education programs for children and their families are effective in **improving competence, decision making, and self-management skills,** leading to fewer emergency room visits and fewer days of hospitalization.

    C. Involving children more actively during office visits results in **improved coping with disease, fewer days of school missed, and better functional health status.**

III. Coping with the medical encounter. The therapeutic alliance can be strengthened when clinicians understand how children cope with the stress of a medical encounter. Coping is defined as emotional, cognitive, or behavioral efforts to alleviate stress and entails two categories: (1) direct efforts to modify the sources of a problem (e.g., overt behaviors such as the child's running away from the clinician or hiding in a parent's lap with the hope that the clinician will not see the child) and (2) internal strategies (such as the child's belief that he or she is not very sick or that the clinician is going to make him or her better). Table 2-1 discusses coping strategies used by children at different ages under varying amounts of stress.

IV. Establishing therapeutic communication.

    A. The TEACHER mnemonic. One useful strategy for developing a therapeutic alliance with children and their parents is to use the TEACHER method of communication (Table 2-2). We have proposed different ways to use the TEACHER mnemonic based on the Piagetian stages of cognitive development.

Table 2-1. Children's coping with stress at different ages

Under age 5 years
Use direct behavioral coping more than indirect strategies (e.g., running away, letting mother kiss a "boo-boo," putting a Band-aid on a cut to make it feel better)
Are more likely to deny feeling negative emotions than older children in stressful situations (e.g., a 5 year old with an injury from a fall may report feeling "fine" when asked)

Age 5–9 years
Use more sophisticated direct strategies than younger children (e.g., telling the doctor that the medicine tastes bad rather than hiding behind a parent when the clinician asks about the medicine)

Over age 9 years
Use more internal coping strategies, such as distraction and reframing a problem so that it does not seem so bad (e.g., an adolescent with diabetes reframes by reporting that her illness has advantages because it helps her to stay thin)
Distract themselves from painful situations by thinking about things they like to do. However, in highly stressful situations, may feel overwhelmed and regress to an earlier way of coping

Table 2-2. TEACHER: A method for enhancing communication with pediatric patients and their parents

T	Trust	Build trust and rapport with the child by asking nonthreatening questions not related to illness
E	Elicit	Elicit information from both parent and child regarding parental fears and concerns and the child's understanding of the reason for the visit
A	Agenda	Set an agenda early in the visit to help ensure that the parent's concerns are addressed
C	Control	Help the child feel control over the visit (e.g., knowing what will and will not happen), to help decrease fear and increase cooperation
H	Health plan	Establish a health plan with child and parent to meet the child's needs and limitations
E	Explain	Explain the health plan to the child in a way she or he can understand
R	Rehearse	Have the child rehearse the health plan as a way of assessing understanding; reinforce the child's jobs related to health care; explore any potential problems in the plan with the child and parent

1. **0–2 years old (sensorimotor stage).** At this stage of cognitive development, learning occurs through sensory experience. A soft tone of voice and gentle handling of the baby are very important. Infants and toddlers may want to hold and examine instruments, which will provide them with sensory stimulation.
    T: To establish *trust* with parents, clinicians should elicit their concerns and listen carefully to what they have to say. They should also be supportive of parents who may be under stress with the new baby.
    E: Careful *examination* of the baby and frequent comments about the child's condition will be reassuring to the parents. A soft tone of voice and gentle handling will help the baby to feel safe. In addition, making sure that injections are quick will prevent unnecessary stress.
    A: Setting an *agenda* for the visit with the parents lets them know what will

occur during the visit and provides time to address their concerns and develop the health plan.

2. **2–6 years old (preoperational stage).** Children may confuse cause and effect because they focus on the perceptual salience, not the logical content, of an event. For example, children may think that the sharp and pointed needle used for an injection will go right through them and put a hole in them. Children at this stage perceive illness and medical procedures as punishments for being "bad." Information for children at this age should be concrete and reassuring.
   T: Establishing *trust* with preschoolers involves using direct verbal praise and allowing the child to have some control over the visit (e.g., by listening with the stethoscope to the clinician's heart).
   E: Information may be *elicited* by playing with the child (e.g., using puppets). Information will also need to be elicited from the parents. Of particular interest are issues of safety and discipline.
   A: The clinician's *agenda* must include parental concerns.
   H: A *health plan* should be devised jointly with the parent, and the child's role in it should be rehearsed. It is important to include the child equally in all discussions.

3. **7–10 years old (concrete operational stage).** Children at this stage appear able to tolerate medical visits better, yet they are still very much focused on the concrete aspects of the situation. It is useful at this stage to begin to give them more control over their health and to anticipate their concerns—for example, "Sometimes kids have questions about getting an x ray done. Do you have any questions?"
   T: It is very important to enhance the confidence of the school-aged child. To establish *trust,* the clinician should show an interest in the child's life, perhaps by finding out from the child what he or she likes to do. Engage the child by, for example, commenting on a drawing done in the waiting room.
   E: The child can often supplement parental information. *Elicit* information from the child by asking simple and concrete questions. If the child responds positively to the questions, more can be asked. If the child shows signs of becoming upset, do not convey displeasure, simply move on to the parents.
   A: Make sure that both parent and child are involved not only in information gathering but in setting the *agenda* and establishing a health plan. It is important to communicate that both the parents' and child's opinions are valued. Model communication for the child, and establish particular tasks for the which the child will be responsible.
   C: Make sure that the child understands and agrees to these tasks, and rehearse them with the child. When a 7 year old asks the clinician whether getting blood drawn is going to hurt, the clinician's response should be straightforward and acknowledge that it will hurt a little bit. After the procedure is over, the clinician should ask the child whether the pain had been described accurately. Distraction techniques at this age often work well. For example, say to the child, "Yes, the shot will hurt a bit, but since you were here last, we got a batch of Waldo bandages, and you can pick two stickers out of our sticker bin." As children become older, the clinician can give them a business card and tell them to call when they need to. Rather than increasing telephone contacts, this symbolizes the child's growing role in health responsibility.

4. **11–17 years old (formal operational stage).** Children begin to be able to reflect on their own thought processes and to understand how the body works. It is important to respect the adolescent's growing independence and ability to make decisions. The clinician should solicit the adolescent's opinion, needs, and limitations before recommending a course of action.
   T: The clinician must acknowledge that the adolescent can assume much responsibility for his or her health care.
   E: Information should be elicited and conveyed in a nonjudgmental way. Showing respect for what the adolescent has to say gives him or her a sense of control. In this period of major change, it is good to look for change with questions such as, "How are your grades compared to last year?" Provide positive feedback. Unless the adolescent prefers, he or she should be exam-

ined alone, when parents are not in the room. Talking to the adolescent about risk-taking behavior (e.g., alcohol and drug use, as well as sexual behavior) is important, but so is a sensitivity to the adolescent's sense of privacy. For example, one might probe peer activity with indirect questions, such as, "Do any of your friends go out on the weekends and drink a lot?"

E: Make sure that the adolescent understands the health plan and feels comfortable trying it out.

Bibliography

Field TM, McCabe PM, Schneiderman N (eds). *Stress and Coping in Infancy and Childhood.* Hillside, NJ: Erlbaum, 1992.

Flavell JH. *The Developmental Psychology of Jean Piaget.* New York: Van Nostrand, 1963.

Kaplan SH, Greenfield S, Ware JE. Assessing the effects of physician-patient interactions on the outcomes of chronic disease. *Med Care* 27:S110, 1989.

Pantell RH, Lewis CC. Physician communication with pediatric patients: A theoretical and empirical analysis. *Adv Develop Behav Pediatr* 1986:65.

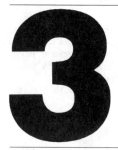

Touchpoints for Anticipatory Guidance in the First Three Years

T. Berry Brazelton

I. **Individual children and family systems.** The opportunity for primary care clinicians to play a role in preventing failures in child development is enormous. Their importance in optimizing each stage of a child's developmental progress—motor, cognitive, and emotional—is equal to their role in the prevention of disease and physical disorders.

Systems theory presents an optimistic approach to prevention. First, each member of the family system reacts to every stress incurred by that system (such as to the birth of a baby, as well as to each developmental step in that baby's development). Second, at each stress point, there is an opportunity for learning—learning to succeed or learning to fail. Clinicians who offer the necessary information and modeling for the parents to understand their baby's development and how to enhance it increase the capacity of the family to offer the baby an optimally nurturing environment. In this way the clinician can play a crucial role in the success of the family system as a whole and in the child's emerging developmental capacities.

Touchpoints are the times at which the impetus for change in the system is brought about by the child's development. Every developmental line progresses in spurts, only to level off and consolidate all that has just been learned. Just before each spurt in any line of development (motor, cognitive, or emotional), there is a short but predictable period of disorganization in the child that represents a period of reequilibration before the next spurt in development. During this time, the parents also are likely to feel disorganized and fear that the baby is regressing. For these reasons, parents are typically more open to counseling at such times. (The times of leveling off are easier, and parents are not as open to help at those times.)

Table 3-1 lists the touchpoints and their most salient clinical issues. These periods are predictable (one in pregnancy, seven in the first year, three in the second, and two in each subsequent year) and thus offer the ideal time for counseling families. Anticipatory guidance can help parents make the appropriate choices to facilitate the next developmental spurt. The child's success in development is experienced as the parents' success and the family as a system is fueled toward success.

A. Touchpoint 1: Prenatal period

1. **Concern about the future.** The first touchpoint is important in forming a relationship between the clinician and the parents-to-be. Meeting with parents in the seventh month of pregnancy and sharing their concerns will create a trusting relationship before the baby arrives. This visit need not demand more than 10–15 minutes but because it occurs at a time when parents' concerns about the new baby are at a peak, it is especially powerful. For example, all parents worry about whether they will be able to nurture the new baby. They dream of two babies: the perfect one (with the behavior and appearance of a 3 month old) and an impaired one (who is damaged and dissimilar to any baby from their past experience). The dread of an impaired baby, matched with the parents' concern if they could ever nurture such a baby, elicits alarm and energy in the parents, which need to be channeled into constructive caregiving fantasies.

2. **Concern about the present.** Another major focus is the fetus's behavior. Parents wonder whether he is "too active" or "too quiet," or whether he is well formed or not. The clinician can share in the parents' dreams and fantasies and assure them of support in optimizing the baby's development (whichever baby they get). Clinician and parents have then established their relationship in this first touchpoint and are ready to work as a system.

Table 3-1. Touchpoints

Time period	Salient issues
Prenatal period	*Effects on siblings *Possible impairments of baby Preparation for birth (natural or anesthesia) Breast or bottle? Circumcision? Maternal health habits Family constellation
Postpartum	*Responsibility for infant *"Language" of behavior Feeding Reflexes Physical examination
2–3 wk	*Communication with the baby *Crying as night comes Parental exhaustion Postpartum blues Feeding Sleep and waking Fussy period Thumbsucking/pacifiers
2 mo	*Communication (smiling) *Temperament *Back to work Growth Feeding Spitting up Fussy period Sleeping and waking Motor skills Cognitive skills
4 mo	*Feeding (turning away from breast) *Sleep (learning to get to sleep independently) Increased interest in environment Vocalizing Nighttime sleep rituals Teething Reaching for objects Transfer of objects Learning expectancies Recognition of mother and father
6 mo	*Sudden burst in awareness of surroundings Stranger awareness first noted Temperament Motor skills, one-handed reach; trying to sit and support Sleeping Communication (smiling, vocalizing) Learning (peekaboos)

Table 3-1 (continued)

Time period	Salient issues
10 mo	*Discipline (teasing) *Sleeping (awakening when standing at crib) *Feeding (finger feeding, independence) Motor skills (stands with support; crawling; gets self to sit) Self-esteem Stranger awareness (object permanence, person permanence) Safety cleanup of baby's environment
12 mo	*Fears about being left *Negativism (understanding its importance) *Temper tantrums about to come Motor skills (trying to walk, standing alone) Sleep (awakening at night again) Feeding self and making choices Teething Language (two words) Learning (knows "mama," "dada") Discipline (when and how) Toilet training (to be postponed until age 2 yr) Biting, hitting, scratching coming (how to handle)
15 mo	*Feeding self entirely *Sleeping through night Discipline (for biting, etc.; spoiled child?) Motor skills (walking, climbing) Play Speech (several words) Toilet training (still postponed) Shifting attachments Temperament
18 mo	Discipline (clear, nonabusive) Feeding self entirely Sleeping through night Separation issues, especially strangers Motor skills (more and more complex) Learning and play (peers) Self-image, looking in mirror Imitation of each parent
2 yr	*Toilet training about to begin *Feeding self; balanced diet? Play and development, need for peers Language (words, phrase, short sentences) Sleep (awakening?, fears) Sexuality (imitates same-sex parent)
3 yr	*Peer relations *Habits (stuttering, nailbiting, etc.) *Sexual identity (imitating same sex) Meals (diet, self-feeding) Toilet training—leave to child Fears and phobias to balance aggression Imagination and fantasy play Cognitive development Speech development

*Issues that parents care most about.

B. **Touchpoint 2: Postpartum period.** It is useful to demonstrate the new baby's remarkable behavioral repertoire to the parents in the immediate period after birth. When a clinician shares the Neonatal Behavioral Assessment Scale (NBAS) with them, both mother and father can become significantly more sensitive to their baby's behavior. During the examination, they become aware of the clinician's interest in their baby and that he or she is seeing and understanding their new baby as an individual, with a remarkable capacity to respond to the world. In this shared interval, not only is their understanding of the new baby enhanced, but they are captured to return for the subsequent touchpoints. With the baby's behavior as a focus, their questions about breast or formula feeding and about their prospective handling of the baby's rhythms and responses can be addressed.

C. **Touchpoint 3: 2–3 weeks.** The clinician can note whether the mother has recovered from postpartum exhaustion and depression. The most important goal of the visit is to predict the upcoming fussy period at the end of the day. Most babies experience a period of irritable crying after the immature nervous system has handled environmental stimuli all day, and parents can learn to plan for it. The clinician who can explain the organizing value of the fussy time for the infant can help parents learn to reduce it significantly if they do not overload an already overwhelmed, immature nervous system.

D. **Touchpoint 4: 2 months.** This is a time for a reevaluation of the feeding, sleep, and fussing cycles, and also a time to share the exciting developments in the baby's awareness of her parents. By this age, a baby demonstrates by her behavior that she is exquisitely responsive to her parents in a face-to-face situation. In addition, she behaves differently with each parent. She has slow cycling of arms, legs, toes, fingers, eyes, and face with her mother, as if she anticipates a feeding or other caretaking. For her father, she has a wide-eyed "pounce look," with an anticipation of being played with. The clinician's comments on these patterns to parents will help them recognize the learning that has already gone on in their new baby; this awareness strengthens their feelings of responsibility and success and also strengthens their feeling of having a meaningful relationship with the clinician.

E. **Touchpoint 5: 4 months**

1. **Rapid cognitive and motor development.** At this visit, the clinician can predict an imminent burst in cognitive awareness of the environment. The baby may become difficult to feed as he looks around and listens to every sight and sound in the environment. He may begin to awaken again at night, even though he may have previously been sleeping through. Feeding and sleeping patterns may be disrupted. Coincident with the rapid burst in his awareness of his environment and strangers will be a burst in motor development. He starts to try to sit, loves to be stood up, reaches successfully with each hand, and plays with objects more effectively. When parents understand this period of relative disorganization as a natural precursor to the rapid development that will follow, they will not view the regressive behaviors as representing failure.

2. **Sleep issues.** The four month visit can be a time to discuss a preventive approach to sleeping problems. For example, it should be ascertained whether the baby independently knows how to get himself to sleep when he is put in bed at night. If he has learned to comfort himself with an independent pattern of putting himself to sleep (e.g., thumbsucking or clinging to his blanket), he can put himself back to sleep each time he has a nocturnal wakening.

3. **Feeding and parental caretaking styles.** This visit can give parents an awareness of their feelings about feeding refusals and affords a discussion of feeding from the standpoint of the baby's development. It also offers the clinician important insights into parental caretaking style and concerns, information that will be useful in the future as parents are guided through other touchpoints.

F. **Touchpoints 6, 7, and 8: 6, 10, and 12 months.** There are three more important touchpoints in the first year, each of which presents opportunities for discussing issues that will arise and for anticipating appropriate responses. When these topics are addressed in the context of a primary care visit, the parents will feel that the clinician is as concerned about the baby's psychological development as about his physical progress. By using touchpoints—the times at which families are most open to anticipatory guidance—the clinician can immeasurably enrich the confidence of the parents in themselves and their baby.

G. **Touchpoints beyond the first year.** Touchpoints continue throughout childhood, even adulthood. They follow a predictable map of development, as outlined in Table 3-1. The primary care clinician and parent can address each one as it arises. In this way the therapeutic alliance will continue to flourish. The child's issues will continue to be uppermost in everyone's mind, and the child will know that he or she has the support of all adults in his or her life.

Bibliography

For Parents
Brazelton TB. *Infants and Mothers.* New York: Delacorte, 1969.

Brazelton TB. *On Becoming a Family: The Growth of Attachment.* New York: Delacorte Press, 1981.

Brazelton TB. *Touchpoints: Your Child's Emotional and Psychological Development.* Reading MA: Addison-Wesley, 1992.

Brazelton TB, Cramer B. *The Earliest Relationships.* Reading MA: Addison-Wesley, 1990.

For Professionals
Brazelton TB, Vaughan VC. *The Family: Setting, Priorities.* New York: Science and Medical Publishing Co., 1979.

Dixon, SD, Stern MT. *Encounters with Children.* Chicago: Year book, 1987.

Hockelman R. *Primary Pediatric Care* (2nd ed). St. Louis MO: Mosby Year Book, 1992.

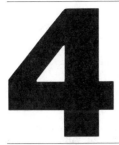

Difficult Encounters with Parents

Barbara Korsch

No honest clinician in pediatrics can claim to love all patients all of the time or to communicate well with everyone who appears in the practice. There are certain names on the day's schedule that make the practitioner's heart sink and feel fatigued in advance.

I. **Factors in difficult encounters.** The situations that trigger negative emotions are not the same for every practitioner. It is of fundamental importance for each practitioner to develop awareness and insight into his or her own individual sensitivities and idiosyncrasies in order to minimize counterproductive encounters and to develop strategies for assuring his or her own well-being.

A. **The clinician-parent relationship.** It is too easy to blame the parent: "The mother was a poor historian," or "She was ignorant, opinionated, and uncooperative." Unflattering labels are often used to take the onus and the blame off the clinician. If it were entirely the parent's "fault" that the medical encounter was difficult, there would be no way of mending the relationship. It is more productive for the clinician to realize that a ruptured relationship usually involves both sides. Knowledge, critical self-awareness, and an explicit focus of interest on the communication process and where it went wrong are helpful in this regard.

B. **Ambiguity.** Clinicians are trained to solve problems and finish tasks. They want diseases that can be named (labeling is one approach to mastery) and symptoms that can be cured. Yet patients' problems often defy simple solutions. A common reason for difficult encounters lies in the clinician's (or parents') discomfort with this ambiguity. Patients with symptoms that do not point to a known disease entity are annoying and frustrating.

C. **The overanxious parent.** In pediatrics, the parent who recites the child's complaints in an overanxious and overemotional manner is judged the equivalent of the hypochondriac in adult practice. He or she is equally unpopular and frequently given short shrift, although sympathetic listening to the concerns might reveal significant issues underlying the emotionality. Concluding that "it's the parent who is the problem" and not the child does not lead to problem recognition and sympathetic treatment.

D. **Slow treatment response.** Just as clinicians thrive on the instant gratification of a patient's getting well quickly, so too are they annoyed by patients who do not respond to treatment. Blaming the patient for a poor response to treatment (even unconsciously) impedes the collaboration with the family. The practitioner needs to join the family and patient in facing their common disappointments: "I know you had hoped to see him better by now. So did I. But we will have to be patient a little longer. We do know we are on the right track."

E. **Clinician limitations.** A frequent barrier to effective communication lies in the clinician's difficulty in accepting his or her own limitations. A parent who "shops" for medical care, who quotes other authorities ("When Johnny next door had the same thing, the doctor gave him penicillin and he was fine the next day"), who reads independently and forms strong opinions ("I always use a lot of vitamin C to stop his colds"), who challenges directly ("How many children have you raised doctor?" or "How many kids with this condition have you treated" or "How long have you been in practice?"): these are all unpopular parents. The reason, often, is that the health professional needs to feel that parents will accept *only his or her* authority. The idea that a parent might inquire elsewhere and that there are other valid (and sometimes better) ideas may seem unacceptable. But such paternalism is unjustified in all respects, especially in a therapeutic alliance between clinician and patient-family.

Failure to accept personal limitations in knowledge and competence may lead the practitioner to perceive patients as difficult. A simple, "You know, I have not really seen this particular combination of signs and symptoms before. I would like you to see Dr. X who has more experience in this line," may be an effective approach that relieves clinician stress and parental anxiety.

F. **Cultural differences.** The clinician's lack of knowledge about cultural factors that may provoke certain kinds of patient symptoms or behavior can also lead to irritation and impatience. For instance, resistance on the part of certain Latino families to have their daughter's perineum inspected might be interpreted as ignorance and resistance. The informed clinician understands that the mother's reluctance is not a personal reaction but is based on the cultural belief that privacy must be protected in young girls at all costs.

G. **Ambiguous boundaries.** Some parents are unwilling to assume any responsibility, thus putting everything onto the clinician's shoulders. ("Can you tell Margaret to stand up straight or she'll make her back crooked"? or "Oh! doctor, tell me what to do! You've got to help me." Having once become trapped in such a situation, the clinician will subsequently have to deal with a parent who continues to act helpless and expects him to solve every problem. This is a no-win situation with inevitable disappointment for the family. Instead, the clinician needs to support and mobilize the parents' resources and to help the family take ownership of their problems. Recognizing and setting clear boundaries about what the clinician is (and is not) able to do and establishing reasonable expectations for parent-patient responsibility is one of the essential principles of avoiding counterproductive clinician-parent communication.

H. **Judgmental attitudes.** Besides the need for power, authority, success, and the wish to please, there are other attributes of the clinician that constrain open communication. Some clinicians do not like fat children; others overreact to lack of cleanliness. Ways of dressing, sexual orientation, or mannerisms may trigger emotional reactions in clinicians of which they are not even aware.

I. **Overidentification.** Certain diagnoses (such as developmental disability, leukemia, blindness) may arouse feelings based on the clinician's personal experiences that negatively color the encounter. Overidentification, which is also a lack of boundary setting, is as counterproductive to the therapeutic alliance as is a lack of empathy.

J. **Systems problems.** Another barrier to good clinician-patient relationships lies in systems problems: lack of time; difficulty in obtaining relevant data; excess waiting time for families, which angers them before they even begin the encounter; pressures imposed by quality control and utilization review committees; fear of litigation; and the many other irritants in the health care system. When clinicians themselves feel abused by the system and helpless to overcome certain obstacles to optimal care, they are likely to transfer their frustrations to colleagues, families, and patients. Acknowledgment of the pressures for all involved and allowing mutual expression of frustration will often clear the air and lead to better cooperation (e.g., "I can understand that it annoys you that you are not seeing the same doctor today. It is difficult for me too because we could work things out better if I had all the information at hand. In the meantime, let's do the best we can").

K. **Time constraints.** Especially in busy practices, patients who take a lot of time are very irritating. Clearly, there are patients who suffer from such extreme psychosocial or emotional problems that they do not fit into the constraints of regular medical practice. Patients who arrive without appointments, bring in two children, or ask for advice for other family members need to be redirected with appropriate boundaries and limit setting. It will save the clinician time and frustration to learn to detect the truly pathologic personalities as early as possible so their care can be appropriately shared with mental health professionals or outside community agencies.

Instances of this type, however, are far less frequent than are those in which extra time is needed due to ineffective communication and the failure to recognize communication breakdown. When in the course of an encounter the clinician feels annoyed and impatient, repeating the same message with the sense that it is not getting across (e.g., "What you need is just a regular bedtime routine" to a mother who is struggling to survive in a chaotic and overwhelming family situation), he or she needs to consider: What is going wrong? Why am I angry? Why does this patient act so aggressively? Is there another approach I could try? What can I learn from this difficult encounter that could help this family?

II. Dealing with difficult encounters

A. Address the problem. Acknowledging that it is the *encounter* and not the parent that is difficult is the most important step. A number of techniques can be helpful,

1. **Confront the parent:** "You seem angry. Can you tell more about why?"

2. **Acknowledge the difficulty:** "I am having a problem here. I feel we are talking at cross-purposes. Let's see whether we can get off to a better start. What I really need to hear from you right now is . . ."

3. **Use the common concern over the child:** "Let's watch him walk together. Perhaps we'll observe the things that concern you about him, and then we can discuss plans."

4. **Offer a concrete sign of wanting to help.** For instance, if a parent is anxious about a sibling who will be getting out of school, allowing her to call a neighbor on the office telephone may turn things around. An extra diaper from the office supply or a quarter for the parking meter may make the point that the clinician does indeed want to help.

B. Expand the system. After setting boundaries for what can appropriately be dealt with, it may be time to expand the system.

1. **Include other other family members:** "Could you get your husband to come in or telephone me so we can include his ideas in our planning?"

2. **Call on other members of the health care team,** depending on the urgency and the main focus of the problem.

3. **Look to the community**—not necessarily to a health professional but perhaps to the family's clergy or other religious adviser. Sometimes the grandparent becomes a key figure.

C. Give it time. Many things cannot be dealt with on a single visit, and if the task cannot be completed to the parent's or the clinician's satisfaction, both will be frustrated. But if the clinician is able to deal at least partially with the problem and can explicitly defer some of the other concerns to a later occasion, harmony can be restored toward the end of the visit. Solutions may also be more likely after a certain amount of reflection and time has passed. Frequently the patients who annoy the clinician the most are those who require the most prompt follow-up.

Bibliography

Korsch BM. Do you know these patients? High risk pediatric encounters. *Pediatr Rev* 10:101–105. 1988.

Korsch BM, Gozzi EK, Francis V. Gaps in doctor-patient communication. I. Doctor-patient interaction and patient satisfaction. *Pediatrics* 42:855–871, 1968.

Quill TE. Recognizing and adjusting to barriers in doctor-patient communication. *Ann Intern Med* 111:51–57, 1989.

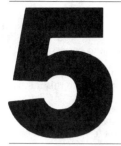

Helping Families Deal with Bad News

Jack P. Shonkoff and
Yvette E. Yatchmink

I. **Issues in delivering bad news.** Conveying difficult information—the diagnosis of a serious chronic illness, a significant developmental disability, or a fatal disease—is one of the most intellectually and emotionally challenging responsibilities a clinician faces. Helping families understand and come to terms with such knowledge can be a rewarding professional and personal experience.

  A. **The clinician-patient relationship.** The clinical challenge of sharing difficult information can be understood best within the broader context of the health care provider–patient relationship. Three essential features of that relationship are particularly critical:

  1. **All interactions must be open, honest, and built on a firm foundation of trust.** The practitioner must be comfortable with sharing all that he or she knows; the family must have confidence that nothing is being withheld.

  2. **All interactions must reflect a genuine sense of caring.** The need for professional objectivity and rational thinking should never be confused with the destructiveness of emotional detachment.

  3. **Supportive relationships cannot be developed instantaneously.** They must be nurtured and allowed to evolve over time.

  B. **Individual variations.** Studies of the process that individuals experience as they attempt to cope with stressful knowledge have postulated various stages of adaptation. Such models typically describe a sequential experience of shock, resistance, or denial, followed by sadness or anger, and ultimate accommodation and adaptation. Such frameworks can provide a general understanding of the process of adjustment to bad news, but individual differences among people must guide clinical behavior. Skilled clinicians are sensitive to such variation and have the intellectual and emotional flexibility to respond constructively. It is equally important, however, for practitioners to be aware of the extent to which their own individual values, personalities, and intellectual styles can affect their clinical approaches to difficult interactions with patients.

  C. **Self-awareness.** No clinician can deal with the communication of bad news in a helpful manner before confronting his or her own issues. Each professional must be aware of his or her own attitude toward chronic illnesses, significant disabling conditions, and the threat of death, and should be able to separate these feelings from those of the patient. Second, clinicians should have insight into their own tolerance for ambiguity and uncertainty, an issue that is embedded in much of the content of the news. Finally, all health care providers must be able to deal comfortably with a number of affective and cognitive boundaries. These include the capacity to share painful, intimate feelings in a way that is comforting and not burdensome for families and to acknowledge the limits of one's clinical powers without feeling personally responsible for the existence of the problem. As a skill that can be taught and refined with experience, the ability to share threatening or unpleasant information incorporates both the science and the art of clinical medicine.

II. **The process of delivering bad news.** Although the process of sharing difficult information cannot be programmed and must retain a significant degree of flexibility to meet individual needs and circumstances, the following framework may serve as a general clinical guide:

A. **Tell the family as soon as possible.** Studies of parents' reactions to hearing bad news about their child have demonstrated that most families would prefer to be told as soon as the health care provider suspects that there is a problem. Sensitive clinicians must feel comfortable sharing available information, even if it is incomplete and uncertain.

B. **Arrange for a private setting.** Difficult information should be shared in an environment that provides protection and security. A quiet setting that is free of distractions or interruptions will afford an opportunity for reflection and the provision of meaningful support. Bad news should never be transmitted over the telephone, in a hallway or crowded waiting room, or when strangers are present. Everyone involved should be seated. It must be clear that the family has the clinician's undivided attention.

C. **Ensure that key people are present.** Every effort should be made to ensure that both parents are present when difficult information about their child is conveyed. When appropriate, other important people (e.g., grandparents) may be present, at the discretion of the parents. The inclusion of more than one person provides an additional source of support and relieves one family member of the responsibility of transmitting information and answering questions for the others. If it is not possible to have all key people present when difficult information is first shared, a prompt follow-up visit should be offered.

D. **Personalize the discussion.** It is important for families to believe that the clinician who is sharing difficult news knows them and their child. Always refer to the child by name and acknowledge specifically his or her personal characteristics (both positive and worrisome).

E. **Get to the point.** Before sitting down with the family, the practitioner should identify the most important message to convey. When multiple issues are to be addressed, it is essential that the core message relate closely to the primary concerns that have prompted medical intervention. Recognizing the possibility that traumatic news may result in a self-protective "tuning out," the most salient information should be delivered at the beginning. Prior to initiating the conversation, the clinician might ask himself or herself: "What is the most important message for this family to understand?" Such information should then be provided briefly, directly, and sensitively.

F. **Stop, look, and listen.** Once the central message has been conveyed, the clinician should stop and wait for a reaction. The critical clinical challenge at this point is to assess the cognitive and emotional dimensions of the parents' verbal and nonverbal reactions. The experienced clinician will be prepared with an agenda for further discussion but will look to the family for guidance on the direction of the dialogue. A professional who is anxious has a tendency to talk too much at the beginning. Under such circumstances, it is particularly important to exert the self-discipline required to be brief, to stop, to listen, and to wait for guidance from the family on where to go next.

G. **Invite affect.** Multiple studies of parents' reactions to the experience of receiving bad news have underscored the importance of having an opportunity to discuss feelings. Because families vary dramatically in the extent to which they feel comfortable sharing their inner feelings, it is important that the clinician invite affective responses. Simple comments, such as, "How do you feel about what I have just shared with you?" or "I know that this is difficult to hear" send a signal that discussing feelings is part of the parent-professional relationship. The clinician should be prepared to allow and support a range of emotions, including tears, anger, and withdrawal. By conveying a sense of caring, kindness, and compassion and by remaining supportive whatever the realities, the sensitive health care provider offers a broad range of options that parents will pursue according to their own individual needs.

H. **Answer questions.** Sufficient time should be allocated for parents to ask questions. Some respond with a barrage of specific inquiries; others may ask very little, other than, "Why did this happen?" or "What can we do?" All questions must be answered directly and openly. When the answer is unclear, it is particularly important to distinguish between responses to questions that cannot be answered because of the limitations of the clinician's knowledge (e.g., "I don't know the answer to that question, but I will help you find out") and responses to questions that are essentially unanswerable (e.g., "It is difficult to say what your child will be like 5 years from now"). In the latter case, it is helpful to explain why the question cannot be answered and to discuss the process by which the health care provider and family together can try to reach a greater understanding, if not a definitive conclusion. It also may be useful during this part of the interaction to raise and answer questions that the parents do not identify (e.g., if the child's problem is in any way their fault), as well as to offer future opportunities to answer further questions after the information has been assimilated.

I. **Titrate the message.** One of the most important goals of the process of sharing bad news is to reach some closure (at least for this session) on a well-informed and balanced understanding of the child's problem. Some parents may react to the initial information with a sense of despondency and hopelessness. Others may seem not to hear the gravity of the situation. A skilled and sensitive clinician will listen to the parents and make a judgment about whether their assimilation of the information is overly pessimistic or excessively optimistic. In the former case, it is important to underscore a sense of hopefulness with specific examples of potential positive outcomes (e.g., "Your child will always continue to gain new skills"). In the latter case, it may be necessary to acknowledge the grounds for optimism but gently remind the family about the concerns and their probable sequelae (e.g., "Your child will always need special help in school"). As the clinician watches and listens to the parents, it is useful to ask oneself whether the family's perceptions are reasonably balanced, given the seriousness of the child's problem. No family should leave this session without any sense of hope.

J. **Discuss next steps.** The session should end with a concrete discussion regarding specific plans for further referrals, evaluations, and arrangements for appropriate therapeutic, educational, and supportive services. There should be no ambiguity with respect to the division of responsibilities between parent and professional regarding subsequent management and care. Individual differences are important to acknowledge. Some parents may want as much additional information as possible, others very little. Requests for second opinions should be honored and facilitated, and not interpreted as threatening. Follow-up plans should be negotiated collaboratively, and areas of agreement should be clear before the session is ended.

K. **Check whether the message has been heard.** As the meeting is terminated, it is important for the clinician to determine whether the family has heard and understood all of the important content. A useful technique is to ask the parents whether someone is waiting to hear about the results of this meeting. The clinician can then ask the parents what they will say and invite them to practice their response. This provides a useful opportunity to hear what the parents have retained from the discussion and to offer constructive assistance in "completing the story."

Bibliography

Cuddigan M, Hanson MB. *Growing Pains—Helping Children Deal with Everyday Problems Through Reading*. Bethesda MD: Association for the Care of Children's Health, 1988.

Drotar D et al. The adaptation of parents to the birth of an infant with a congenital malformation: A hypothetical model. *Pediatrics* 56:710–717, 1975.

Krahn GL, Hallum A, Klime C. Are there good ways to give "bad news"? *Pediatrics* 91:578–582, 1993.

Myers BA. The informing interview: Enabling parents to "hear" and cope with bad news. *Am J Dis Child* 137:572–577, 1983.

Nursey AD, Rohde JR, Farmer RDT. Ways of telling new parents about their child and his or her mental handicap: A comparison of doctors' and parents' views. *J Ment Def Res* 35:48–57, 1991.

Behavioral and Developmental Surveillance

Behavioral Screening

Ellen C. Perrin

I. **Need for systematic screening.** The scope of pediatric care has changed considerably over the past 50 years to include such elements as helping parents to understand their children's behavior, to distinguish annoying from problematic behavior, and to modify their parenting actions in the best interests of their children. The first step in this process is screening for and identifying parents' concerns about their children's behavior. The requirements for screening in general are that the condition under consideration be important, common, diagnosable, and treatable. Furthermore, its early recognition should lead to an improved outcome. Children's troublesome behavior, and their parents' concerns about it, meet these criteria.

II. **Approach to screening.** Information about children's behavior can be obtained from parents in a number of ways.

A. **Clinician questions.** A series of well-constructed questions in the course of the child health supervision visit (e.g., "What aspects of your child's behavior would you like to talk about?") may be adequate for some parents to describe their concerns. Other parents may benefit from more encouragement and specific direction to observe their children's behavior systematically and to describe it accurately. In this case, office handouts describing typical and worrisome behaviors at various ages can help parents to organize their observations, just as they do with regard to injury prevention or management of acute illnesses.

B. **Questionnaires.** An efficient means of obtaining information from parents *prior* to the office encounter may be desirable. A brief questionnaire, filled out in the waiting room, can help to initiate and to organize the discussion that will take place during the office visit. Such a checklist may provide a helpful mechanism to communicate concerns about children's behavior and development and about sensitive family issues. In one study, even when the completed checklist was not shown to the pediatrician, twice as many concerns were discussed during the subsequent health supervision visit than when parents had not completed the checklist. In asking parents to complete such a questionnaire, the primary care clinician communicates implicitly that children's behavior, development, and family life are integral to comprehensive health supervision. These checklists help to make parents' observations more systematic, to validate their concerns, and to provide a common language to help in describing children's behavior and parents' concerns.

This mechanism of learning about children's behavior and parents' concerns has been shown to be efficient as well. Completion of these questionnaires is acceptable to parents and takes no more than 10 minutes. Additional time spent in the health supervision visit itself has been found to be only 5 minutes. If serious or multiple concerns are revealed, many clinicians choose to arrange a subsequent appointment to address these concerns in depth.

III. **Types of screening questionnaires.** Previsit questionnaires or checklists may simply describe children's **typical behavior,** identify a **parent's concerns,** or screen for **potential child psychopathology.** It is not necessary to use a standardized questionnaire; clinicians should create checklists that reflect their own interests and practice style. These may include a wide range of topics, such as the child's usual diet, sleep, and elimination patterns; preventive health and safety practices; and questions about the child's developmental landmarks and usual behavior. Alternatively, a questionnaire may list potentially worrisome behaviors and family difficulties, in order to elicit parental concerns about them (Fig. 6-1).

Other questionnaires have been developed to screen for psychopathology. Among

Child's name _____ Date of Birth _____

Your relationship to child _____ Today's date _____

Child currently lives with: mother _____ father _____
                             another person (who?) _____

Do parents have any disagreements about the raising of this child? yes _____ no _____

Does anyone else care for the child on a regular basis?
                    relative _____ babysitter _____ child care center _____

Do you have concerns about this child care arrangement? yes _____ no _____

Are you concerned about your child with regard to any of the following issues?

sleeping	_____	problems at meals	_____
temper tantrums	_____	disobedience	_____
vision	_____	thumb sucking	_____
speech	_____	appetite	_____
general development	_____	hearing	_____
toilet training	_____	gets upset too easily	_____
shy, clinging	_____	wants too much attention	_____
activity level	_____	wetting the bed	_____
soiling	_____	feelings hurt easily	_____
sad or unhappy	_____	discipline methods	_____
relationships with		relationships with other children	_____
brothers and sisters	_____		

Do you have any other concerns about this child that you would like to discuss?

Have there been any important changes in your family recently?

child care arrangements	_____	new baby	_____
death or illness of a		marital problems, divorce	
family member	_____	or separation	_____
moving	_____	financial stresses	_____
other: _____			

Are there problems in the family related to alcohol or other drugs? yes _____ no _____

Do you have any concerns about your child's behavior
or progress at school or preschool?   yes _____ no _____

Are you ever afraid you might lose control and hurt your child? yes _____ no _____

In the past week how many days have you felt depressed? 0 _____ 1–2 _____
                                                    3–4 _____ 5–7 _____

In the past year have you had 2 weeks or more during which you felt
sad, blue, or depressed, or lost pleasure in things that you usually
cared about or enjoyed?   yes _____ no _____

Figure 6-1. Example of a previsit questionnaire

the most carefully investigated and widely published are the Preschool Children's Behavior Checklist (see Appendix A) and the Pediatric Symptom Checklist, a 35-item, true/false checklist that requires approximately 5 minutes to complete (see Appendix B).

IV. **Approaches to intervention.** The primary care clinician has many options once the parents' concerns about their children's behavior have been elicited.

A. **Listening attentively** to the parents' observations, supporting and validating them as legitimate concerns, and pointing out their significance in the sequence of children's behavioral development may help parents to understand the behavior from the point of view of the child. Such insight into the function of the troublesome behavior is often a helpful intervention in itself. Verbal or written advice about alternative ways to manage the behavior may help parents to provide more constructive guidance to their children. If the concerns are about behavior that is clearly within the range of normal variation, supportive comments such as, "Lots of children this age have problems like this," may be reassuring.

B. It may be helpful to arrange a subsequent meeting with both parents to explore the concerns further and to understand better the significance of the troublesome behavior. Such a meeting will enable the clinician to determine if the presenting concern represents a variation of normal development or is indicative of psychological or family dysfunction. After such a meeting, it may be appropriate to refer families directly to a colleague in the mental health disciplines.

C. Some clinicians with special interest, training, and expertise may prefer to offer **direct counseling.** Consultation with a mental health professional or a behavioral pediatrician can support such intervention. If there is serious dysfunction in either parent's family of origin, marital disturbance or abuse, psychopathology, or alcoholism, referral to a mental health professional is probably indicated.

Bibliography

Eisert DC, Sturner RA, Mabe PA. Questionnaires in behavioral pediatrics: Guidelines for selection and use. *J Dev Behav Pediatr* 12:42–50, 1991.

Jellinek MS et al. Pediatric Symptom Checklist: Screening school-age children for psychosocial dysfunction. *J Pediatr* 112:201–209, 1988.

Triggs EG, Perrin EC. Improving communication about behavior and development. *Clin Pediatr* 28:185–192, 1989.

Willoughby JA, Haggerty RJ. A simple behavior questionnaire for preschool children. *Pediatrics* 34:798–806, 1964 (December).

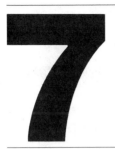

Developmental Screening

Frances Page Glascoe

I. **Detecting developmental problems.** The detection of children with developmental and behavioral or emotional disabilities typically depends on primary care clinicians—often the only professional with knowledge of development who are in constant contact with young children and their families. Developmental and behavioral problems can be difficult to identify because they may be subtle and because children may not cooperate with attempts at direct assessment. Additionally, many screening tests take longer to administer than the time usually allocated for well-child visits, some tests are inaccurate, and reimbursement for testing may be very limited. For these reasons, many clinicians rely not on screening tests but on clinical judgment. Unfortunately, studies show that the majority of children with developmental and behavioral or emotional problems are not detected in the absence of standardized screening tests.

II. **Using parents' concerns.** One way to improve early detection in the office is *developmental surveillance*, a technique that makes systematic use of clinical information and combines it, when needed, with standardized screening. The technique described in this chapter offers a high degree of accuracy without a great deal of time and expense and makes use of one readily available source of clinical information: parents' concerns.

Research shows that parents' concerns are extremely helpful in identifying children in need of assessment. Approximately 80% of children who fail screening tests have parents who are concerned about their speech-language, behavior, language, fine motor, or academic development. Parents, including those with less than a high school education or limited parenting experience, derive their concerns by comparing their children to others, an effective way of recognizing most problems in childhood.

Parents, however, are not always accurate; 20–25% do not raise concerns when they should, and many parents are concerned when they need not be. For these reasons, it is often misleading to rely exclusively on parents' concerns to identify children with problems. Nevertheless, parental concerns can be used as a prescreening test to reduce dramatically the number of children who require formal screening.

III. **Eliciting parents' concerns.** Parents' concerns can be elicited by the statement, "Please tell me any concerns about the way your child is learning, developing, and behaving." The use of the word *concerns* is important because parents may become anxious with more serious-sounding synonyms such as *worries* or *problems*. Pairing the words *learning* and *development* is also important because some parents are not familiar with the word *development*. The use of the word *behavior* is necessary for eliciting concerns about emotional well-being and self-control.

Because parents do not always think of development in the same way as professionals, it is necessary to repeat and rephrase the opening question. A standardized question is used to probe each developmental domain while avoiding unfamiliar terms (such as *expressive language, gross motor skills*): "Please tell me any concerns about the way your child is talking . . . making speech sounds . . . listening and understanding . . . getting along with others . . . behaving . . . using hands and fingers . . . arms and legs . . . taking care of himself or herself . . . learning school skills."

Responses to both questions are often quite clear and easy to categorize into the various developmental domains (e.g., "She can't talk plain," "He's shy"). However, even worried parents may try to downplay the concern: "Well, I was concerned about his talking, but he's doing better now" or "She seems a little slower than other kids, but I don't think it's really a problem." It is important to recognize these disclaimers

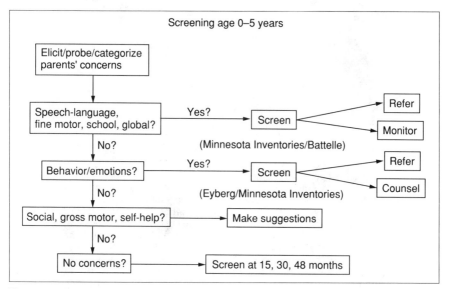

Figure 7-1. Decision-making process for developmental surveillance.

as a parental defense and say, "You're right. It may not be a problem, but I think we should explore it further."

IV. **Techniques for developmental and behavioral surveillance.** Figure 7-1 shows the entire process for eliciting parents' concerns and for making the decisions about when to administer formal screening tests.

A. **Elicit parents' concerns** and then follow with the probe question.

B. **Categorize parents' concerns** into the various developmental domains in order to consider each domain separately.

1. **Emotional/behavioral** concerns are raised by 35% of parents. Half the parents with such concerns have children with significant difficulties. Because the complaint can reflect more than just behavioral or emotional difficulties (e.g., parents who complain that their child "won't mind" may not have considered that the child does not hear or does not understand what she is asked to do), it is wise to administer a behavioral/emotional screen and a high-quality broad-band developmental screen (see Table 7-1 for a description of accurate, standardized screening measures). Screening tests, unlike checklists, allow clinicians to make an informed decision about whether to refer, and they minimize the vague, uncomfortable, and often inappropriate "wait and see" approach. When children fail screening tests, they are typically performing in the lowest 10% of their peers and clearly need a more careful evaluation. It is wise to review performance on screening measures to discern whether delays appear global (which suggest the need for a comprehensive evaluation) or specific (which suggest the need for more focused assessment, such as a speech-language evaluation). Parents whose children pass both measures should still be targeted for in-office counseling because their child's problems may be less severe but nonetheless worrisome. Specific items from the standardized screening tests can be used to focus suggestions.

2. **Concerns about speech-language** development are raised by 30% of all parents. Over half of the children whose parents noted speech-language difficulties failed developmental measures. A developmental screening test will help to discern which half needs referral and which half needs assurance. When children fail, an analysis of the errors will indicate what kinds of referrals are needed (see Chap. 41).

Table 7-1. Selected, accurate screening tests

Test	Description	Domains measured	Publication information
Battelle Developmental Inventory Screening Test (6 mo–8 yr)	Uses a combination of direct elicitation, parental description, and observation to provide cutoffs and age-equivalent scores for each developmental domain. Can be used to meet criteria for participation in early intervention programs. Takes about 30 min, longer with older patients. The receptive language subtest (5–7 items) can serve as an accurate prescreening test.	Gross/fine motor, personal, adaptive, expressive/ receptive language, cognitive	Riverside Publishing, 8420 Bryn Mawr Avenue, Chicago, Il 60631, (800) 767-8378
Screening level measures of the Child Development Inventory Minnesota Infant Development Inventory (0–15 mo) Early Child Development Inventory (15–36 mo) Preschool Development Inventory (36–72 mo)	Each of the three measures relies on parental report. Parents respond to 60 short statements on development and 20 items on behavior/ symptoms with yes-no answers. Can be administered over the telephone, completed in waiting rooms, or sent home prior to a second visit devoted to scoring and interpretation. Takes less than 10 min, longer if items administered directly.	Expressive/ receptive language, social, fine/ gross motor, preacademics, cognitive, behavior, symptoms	Behavior Science Systems, Inc., Box 580274, Minneapolis, MN 55440, (612) 929-6220
Eyberg Child Behavior Inventory (2–11 yr)	Relies on parental description by presenting 36 short statements of common behavior problems to which parents respond with yes-no answers. Helps refine referrals (e.g., mental health services versus behavioral intervention). Can be administered over the telephone, in interview, or completed independently by parents. Takes about 5 min.	Externalizing behaviors (problems with conduct, activity level, attention, aggression) and internalizing behaviors (depression, anxiety, adjustment)	From article by Eyberg S, *J Clin Child Psychology* 54:587–599, 1980

Note: There are many tests on the market, some substantially more accurate than others. The table lists a few of the more accurate measures.

Table 7-2. Recommended schedule and tools for formal screening

Age at visit	Screening method/tests
0–12 mo	Elicit parents' concerns*
15 mo	Administer Minnesota Infant Development Inventory/ Batelle Developmental Inventory
18–24 mo	Elicit parents' concerns*
30 mo	Administer Early Child Development Inventory or Eyberg Child Behavior Inventory/Batelle Developmental Inventory
36 mo	Elicit parents' concerns*
48 mo	Administer Preschool Development Inventory/Batelle Developmental Inventory
60–72 mo	Elicit parents' concerns*

*If significant concerns are mentioned, administer age-appropriate screening level measure from the Child Development Inventory/Eyberg Child Behavior Inventory.

3. **Concerns about social skills** and **self-help skills** have little relationship to true developmental problems. When these concerns are raised, screening is not needed; rather, parents need suggestions on such topics as how to help children get along with others or dress themselves independently. It is wise to maintain a library of handouts on various social, self-help, and other topics and dispense these to parents with concerns about nonsignificant problems. Several sources for handouts are listed in the chapter bibliography.

4. **Concerns about gross motor skills** are less common. If motor milestones and physical examinations are normal, concerns about gross motor skills often reflect concerns about social interactions. For example, a concern about poor athletic ability may be due to a child's lack of interest and talent in the sport. This complaint may reflect a conflict in the mutual interests of parent and child, not a developmental problem.

5. **Concerns about fine motor skills** can be worrisome. In these cases, parents are concerned about their child's lack of willingness to draw, color, cut, write, and so forth. Children's reluctance to engage in these activities may reduce their opportunity to learn preacademic skills. Complaints about fine motor skills tend to reflect true developmental problems and indicate the need to administer a screening test.

6. **When parents have global concerns** (e.g., "He's behind other kids," "She's slow," or "He can't do what other kids can do"), their children have a high probability of failing screening tests. Similarly, concerns about school skills (only in children age 4 years and older) also have a good chance of predicting true problems. In the presence of these concerns, the best response is to administer a screening test, counsel parents when children pass, and make referrals when children fail.

7. **What about children with problems whose parents' don't complain?** In order to identify these children, who comprise 20–25% of those with true problems, it is advisable to select several visits during the early childhood years in which to administer developmental screens for all children. The rationale for repeating screening several times is that children may develop normally early but then later fail to acquire needed skills. Table 7-2 shows suggested times and tools for screening at different ages.

Bibliography

For Parents

Computer Service

The Ambulatory Pediatric Association has an on-line computer service that physicians can access. It houses numerous handouts for parents on developmental and behavioral issues including speech-language development, social skills development, and discipline. These can be downloaded and personalized. Write to Jack Pascoe, M.D., MPH, APA Communications Director, Head Division of General Pediatrics and Adolescent Medicine, Department of Pediatrics, University of Wisconsin Medical School, 600 Highland Avenue, Madison, Wisconsin 53792. EMail: Pascoe@ VMS.MACC.Wisc.Edu (Internet); Pascoe@ WISCMACC (Bitnet).

For Professionals

Dworkin PH. British and American recommendations for developmental monitoring: The role of surveillance. *Pediatrics* 84:1000–1010, 1989.

Glascoe FP. Can clinical judgment detect children with speech-language problems? *Pediatrics* 87:317–322, 1991.

Glascoe FP, MacLean WE, Stone WL. The importance of parents' concerns about their child's behavior. *Clin Pediatr* 30:8–11, 1991.

Glascoe FP, Dworkin PH. Obstacles to developmental surveillance. *J Dev Behav Pediatr* 14:344–349, 1993.

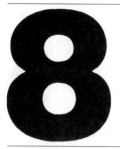

Psychosocial Screening

Kathi J. Kemper

Many children and families are faced with a complex array of psychosocial challenges, including poverty, crowding, homelessness, teenage pregnancy, divorce, racism, and violence. In addition, many parents are beset by alcohol, drug, and mental health problems and themselves may have been victims of neglect or abuse. Compounding these problems is the disintegration of traditional sources of support, stability, meaning, and hope for many families and communities.

Failure to recognize psychosocial problems can lead to inappropriate medical diagnostic testing, misuse of health care resources, and poor medical, developmental, and behavioral outcomes. Yet psychosocial problems have generally not been addressed systematically by primary care clinicians because many are uncomfortable talking about them, few clinically useful and valid screening instruments are available, resources for addressing families' needs are often scarce, and little research documents the effectiveness of many interventions.

This chapter will focus on screening for two common family psychosocial problems—parental history of abuse during childhood and current domestic violence—and two factors that may be protective—social support and resilience.

I. **Screening questionnaires.** Numerous studies have demonstrated that unless screening is done systematically, the vast majority of patients (families) with a condition will be missed. Clinicians are no better at guessing which patients are alcoholic or victims of violence than they are at detecting asymptomatic hypertension or hemoglobinopathies. Fortunately, it is possible to screen for many psychosocial factors quickly.

Systematic screening using self-administered questionnaires efficiently improves assessment of psychosocial factors. However, screening also carries risks: false positives, false negatives, and the consequences of labeling families as having psychosocial problems. Questionnaires need to be used in the context of history, observation, and physical examination; they cannot substitute for definitive diagnostic tests.

A. **Information elicited.** In our clinic, clinicians use a two-page questionnaire that can be completed by most English-speaking parents in less than 15 minutes. In addition to routine demographic (parental age, education, income, and marital status) and medical information (hospitalizations, medications, allergies, immunizations, and family medical history), it covers family health habits (seatbelts/car seat, smoking, drinking, drug use, and gun ownership and storage), domestic violence, parental history of childhood experiences (parental substance abuse, physical abuse, sexual abuse, and neglect), depression, social support, family planning, and interest in additional counseling or support groups. Questions have been selected to enhance sensitivity and reduce false negatives so that practitioners can confidently set aside areas with negative screens and focus on the positives. Because families and behaviors change, parents should update the questionnaires yearly.

B. **Parental response.** The vast majority of parents complete the questionnaire (even the items on substance abuse, income, and domestic violence). Although there is probably some denial about the existence or severity of psychosocial problems, in our urban clinic 50% of families have a positive screen in one or more areas, and suburban private practices have shown positivity rates of 30%. Parents who question the reason for certain items on the questionnaire are usually reassured when we emphasize the importance of understanding the child in the more comprehensive context of the family rather than just focusing on physical examinations and immunizations.

II. Screening for psychosocial problems

A. Parental history of abuse during childhood. Although many persons who were abused as children do not abuse their own offspring and others who had apparently "normal" childhoods do mistreat their children, research indicates an intergenerational cycle of abuse. The rate of child abuse among parents who were themselves abused as children is about six times higher than the base rate in the general population. A history of being physically abused as a child can also lead to mistaken notions about parenting, such as looking to the child for satisfaction of parental emotional needs, treating children as adults, and having overly high expectations for a child's performance. Generally persons who were more severely disciplined in childhood consider physical punishment as more appropriate than do those who report being less severely disciplined (especially if they believe that their treatment was deserved).

The question, "Have you ever been physically abused, neglected, or sexually abused?" has poor sensitivity for detecting a history of maltreatment. Screening that targets specific experiences has better sensitivity for detecting a history of abuse and identifying those who may benefit from additional counseling, parenting education or support. The following questions are used at our clinic:

As a child,
1. *How often did your parents ridicule you in front of friends or family?*
   Frequently   Often   Occasionally   Rarely   Never
2. *How often were you hit with an object such as a hairbrush, board, stick, wire or cord?*
   Frequently   Often   Occasionally   Rarely   Never
3. *How often were you thrown against walls or down stairs?*
   Frequently   Often   Occasionally   Rarely   Never
4. *Did your parents ever hurt you when they were out of control?*   *Yes   No*
5. *Do you feel you were physically abused?*   *Yes   No*
6. *Do you feel you were neglected?*   *Yes   No*
7. *Do you feel you were hurt in a sexual way?*   *Yes   No*
8. *Would you like more information about free parenting*   *Yes   No*
   programs, parent hotlines, or respite care?

While it is important to discuss effective discipline techniques with all parents, parents who have a positive screen for having been abused during childhood may require additional discussion about their experiences of discipline. Such families may benefit especially from parenting groups, parent education groups, or therapeutic day care settings in which appropriate teaching and discipline techniques are modeled.

B. Domestic violence. For families with a positive screen for domestic violence, it is important to evaluate the spectrum, extent, and pattern of violent interactions within the family. We use two questions to screen for domestic violence:

1. *In the past year, have you ever felt threatened in your home?*
2. *In the past year, has your partner or other family member pushed or shoved you, hit or punched you, kicked you, or threatened to hurt you?*

A risk assessment should determine immediate safety issues for the parent and children. The victim may need to make specific escape plans, including transportation, finances, and a safe place to live. It is important for clinicians to affirm that no person deserves physical abuse and that nothing that a parent did (or did not do) should result in physical violence. It is helpful for victims to know that they are not alone, to be informed about local resources, and to have their confidentiality affirmed. Most victims are especially fearful (with good reason) of what might happen if the batterer learns they have informed. It is also important to plan a follow-up visit and to be consistent in support of a domestic violence victim, even if the person does not take immediate action or returns to the batterer. Sometimes it is helpful to form an alliance with the victim around the child's safety and encourage the parent to make arrangements to escape the situation, not only for his or her own sake but also for the child's sake.

III. Screening for protective factors

A. Social support. Social support can be viewed as external confirmation that one is cared for, loved, esteemed, and a member of a social network. It is also a stable characteristic of the individual, reflecting the person's social skills and ability to seek out needed resources from the community. Functionally, social support serves as a mediator for other stressors; its absence has the least impact in the presence of few stressors and the most impact in the setting of multiple stressors.

Higher social support is associated with fewer perinatal complications, more positive maternal attitudes and behavior toward the infant, more secure infant-mother attachment, improved maternal responsiveness, decreased parenting stress, and a more stimulating home environment. Later, maternal social support is positively associated with parenting skills, such as being able to assume the child's perspective, providing a more stimulating home environment, and lower parent-child stress.

Low social support correlates with more punitive parental attitudes about discipline, a higher percentage of child abuse, and excessive use of the health care system.

The HMC Children's Clinic uses the three-item version of Sarason's Social Support Questionnaire:

1. *a. Who can you count on to be dependable when you need help? (just write their initials and relationship to you). [Provide space for up to nine supports.]*
   b. How satisfied are you with their support?
   very satisfied   fairly satisfied   little satisfied
   little dissatisfied   fairly dissatisfied   very dissatisfied
2. *a. Who accepts you totally, including your best and worst points? (just write their initials and relationship to you). [Provide space for up to nine supports.]*
   b. How satisfied are you with their support?
   very satisfied   fairly satisfied   little satisfied
   little dissatisfied   fairly dissatisfied   very dissatisfied
3. *a. Whom do you feel truly loves you deeply? (just write their initials and relationship to you). [Provide space for up to nine supports.]*
   b. How satisfied are you with their support?
   very satisfied   fairly satisfied   little satisfied
   little dissatisfied   fairly dissatisfied   very dissatisfied

A positive screen for low social support should trigger a discussion with the parent. Help should be offered in the form of support groups for families, frequent follow-up, and home visitors. Newer approaches to incorporating social support into the health care setting include group well-child visits.

B. **Resiliency.** Resiliency or hardiness refers to the child's ability to grow and develop in healthy ways despite the presence of hardship and stress. Such factors may be classified in three broad categories.

1. **Factors intrinsic to the child** include an easy-going and outgoing temperament, curiosity, healthy self-esteem, a sense that one is able to affect one's surroundings and experience (internal locus of control), good health, intelligence, being female, and a sense of hopefulness (the belief that change or novel situations represent an opportunity for mastery and challenge rather than eliciting a sense of helplessness).

2. **Family factors** that promote resilience include marital stability (or at least an alliance between the parents regarding parenting issues), parental sense of competence, family cohesiveness and supportiveness of its individual members, smaller family size (four or fewer children) with spacing of 2 years or more between siblings, close bonds of support between the child and at least one parent, structure and predictability in daily routines, and the availability of support from an adult outside the family (extended family, church, babysitters, teacher, coach).

   The following items are included in the questionnaire to tap family resilience:

   1. *How strong are your family's religious beliefs and practices?*
      Very strong   Moderately strong   A little
      Not important or not applicable

2. How often does your family eat meals together?
Never   Rarely   About once a week
Several times a week   Daily
3. What does your family do together for fun? _____

Several parental behaviors may be helpful in fostering resiliency in the child:
- A strong sense of family traditions, including family meetings, eating meals together, and bedtime routines.
- One-to-one time between parent and child, so that each child feels he or she is special to the parents.
- A time for each child to be heard by other family members on a regular basis (e.g., at mealtimes).
- Limits and boundaries, which often give children a sense of safety and security.
- Flexibility about daytime routines and rules when special circumstances arise.
- Encouragement for children to engage in social activities and fostering of peer relationships (e.g., through overnight parties and birthday parties) to encourage resilience.
- Adults outside the family to whom children can look for advice and counsel.

3. **Extrafamilial factors** (such as culture and community). Cultures that value children rely on the motto: "It takes a whole village to raise a child." Children and families with this kind of support are much more resilient than those whose cultures are more individualistic.

III. How to handle positive screens

A. **The primary care provider should not ignore information that families have revealed on the questionnaire.** If there is no time to review each question:

1. **Thank the parent**(s) for completing the questionnaire.

2. **Let the parent know how helpful it is for you as the child's clinician to know about the family.**

3. **Ask if the parent has any questions or would like clarification** about any item on the questionnaire.

4. **Ask if there is anything on the questionnaire that the parent would like to focus on** at this visit or any **resources/referrals** they would like now.

5. Assure the parent that **you will review the questionnaire carefully** and will **plan to cover other areas** at the next visit.

6. Inform the parent that **any area on the questionnaire is fair game for them to bring up at future visits.**

B. **After reviewing the questionnaire, pursue positive screens.** A structured diagnostic interview can be used or issues can be approached in a more open-ended fashion (e.g., "I notice that you marked the question on domestic violence as yes. Can you tell me more about that?" or "What was that like?" or "How do you feel about that?"). Open-ended questions allow the parent to tell his or her story. Follow up by asking what consequences this might have for the child. Asking parents to state their understanding about the impact of psychosocial issues is far more helpful than lecturing them about what you think the impact might be. Letting parents tell their story is therapeutic.

Ask the parent how he or she thinks the family might best address this issue. Affirm that he or she is not alone in facing problems. Acknowledge the person's courage and the healing inherent in facing and naming problems, support his or her problem-solving efforts, and offer continued support and the availability of additional resources. Follow up and follow through on your plans and stated concerns. Recognize that most behaviors and habits take years to develop and may take time to change.

IV. Clinical pearls and pitfalls

- If you do not take a temperature, you cannot find a fever. If you do not do psychosocial screening systematically, you are unlikely to uncover family factors affecting the child's health and behavior.

• Focus on risk factors that have substantial risk of morbidity and are modifiable. Evaluate conditions and resources that may be specific to your community.
• Administer the questionnaire to every family, even those you think are not at high risk.
• Be flexible. Be willing to change the questionnaire as new concerns or resources arise in your practice or community.
• Ask about specific experiences (e.g., "How often were you hit or punched?") rather than interpretations of those experiences (e.g., "Were you battered or abused?").
• Denial and minimizing are important parts of many parents' coping strategies. For example, a parent may acknowledge having been beaten or consistently ridiculed as a child but deny that he or she was abused because "everybody punished their kids that way" or "I deserved it" or "It wasn't that bad." It is not helpful to support this denial. Rather, explore the consequences and the alternatives that the parent might consider for his or her own child.
• Do not underestimate your own value by saying, "I can't help; there's nothing I can do." Listening in a caring way is therapeutic.
• When discussing psychosocial issues with a family, always note that:
—This family is not alone in facing such issues.
—Although negative family factors can adversely affect a child, recognition is the first step toward finding help. The family is helping the child when it acknowledges problems and seeks solutions.
—Affirm that resources are available to help.
—Acknowledge that this family has strengths.
• Focus on the positive. Compliment the family members on their strengths and what they're doing right.

Bibliography

For Parents

American Humane Association, Children's Division, (303) 792-9900.

Domestic Violence Hotline, (800) 562-6025.

Parents Anonymous, (800) 932-HOPE or local telephone listing.

Parents Without Partners, local telephone listing.

For Professionals

Kemper KJ. Self-administered questionnaire for psychosocial screening in pediatrics. *Pediatrics* 89:433–436, 1992.

Pellegrini DS. Psychosocial risk and protective factors in childhood. *J Dev Behav Pediatr* 11:201–209, 1990.

Werner EE. Children of the Garden Island. *Sci Am* April:106–111, 1989.

Zuckerman B. Family history: A special opportunity for psychosocial intervention. *Pediatrics* 87:740–741, 1991.

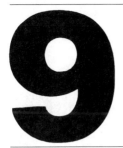

Monitoring Social and Emotional Development of Young Children

Stanley I. Greenspan

Recent advances in understanding how babies form relationships and interact have enabled us to formulate a sequence of socioemotional and interactive patterns that characterize healthy development.

The primary care clinician, following observation of the parent-child interaction and using the guidelines in this chapter, is in a position to identify early problems in an infant's socioemotional development, self-regulatory capacities, and parental caregiving. Such recognition is the first step to a treatment that can focus on helping parents to be more astute and sensitive observers and respondents to their infant's emerging sense of self.

I. **Clinical observations of unstructured parent-child interactions.** A 10–15-minute observation of an unstructured interaction between parent and child can provide rich clinical data on which to make a judgment concerning the child's socioemotional development. These interactions can be initiated by asking the caregiver to interact with the infant or child "just the way you like to play with and enjoy each other." If necessary, a series of semistructured interactive opportunities can be offered to the infant or child to help elicit core competencies (e.g., a developmentally appropriate toy or task).

The chapter appendix provides the themes and behaviors of normal socioemotional development at various ages, and can assist the clinician in monitoring healthy emotional growth and development, detecting lags, and identifying significant deviations and dysfunctions. More important, it enables the clinician to help parents understand and enjoy their children's emotional development and, if necessary, work with their children to overcome challenges.

II. **Exploration of self-regulatory development.** When an infant is described or observed having difficulty with an emotional milestone, the infant's self-regulatory capacity should be examined on a number of factors.

A. **Factors to explore**

1. The infant is **able to be calm** and not excessively irritable, clinging, active, or panicked.

2. The infant is **able to take an interest in sights, sounds, and people** and is not excessively withdrawn, apathetic, or unresponsive.

3. The infant is **able to focus his or her attention** and not be excessively distractible.

4. The infant **enjoys a range of sounds,** including high and low pitch, loud and soft, and different rhythms, and does not appear upset or confused by sounds.

5. The infant **enjoys various sights,** including reasonably bright lights, visual designs, facial gestures, moving objects, and does not appear upset or confused by various sights.

6. The infant **enjoys being touched,** bathed, and clothed and is not bothered by things touching his or her skin.

7. The infant **enjoys movement in space** (being held and moved up and down, side to side, etc.), does not get upset with movement, and does not crave excessive movement.

Table 9-1. Nonoptimal caregiving patterns

Overly stimulating

Withdrawn or unavailable

Lacking pleasure, enthusiasm, or zest

Random or chaotic in reading or responding to signals (e.g., vocalizes and interacts without regard for infant's signals, as in a pinching, poking, "rev-the-infant-up" type of caregiver)

Fragmented or insensitive to context (e.g., responds to one part of an infant's communication but misses the bigger picture, as when a caregiver is excessively upset and persistently hugs her active toddler who accidentally banged his leg while trying to run and who obviously wants to keep exploring the room and not be constrained)

Overly rigid and controlling; tries to get the infant to conform to rigid agenda (e.g., allows the toddler to play with a toy only one way)

Concrete in reading or responding to communication. Some parents are unable to tune into the symbolic level and instead keep communication at concrete behavioral and gestural levels (e.g., a child is pretending with a toy telephone that he will not talk to his mother; mother perceives this as a literal sign of rejection and refuses to "play anymore")

Illogical in reading or responding to infant's communication. Often the caregiver is so flooded with emotion that he or she misreads what is communicated (e.g., a 3-year-old child says, "I am scared of the monster, but I know it is just make-believe." The caregiver explains, "Monsters will never get in the room. Monsters can be nice, too, you know.")

Avoids selected emotional areas (e.g., in pretend play, parent always focuses on the child's interest in aggression but always ignores separation themes)

Unstable in the face of intense emotion (e.g., caregiver can support development only if emotions are not too intense; if emotions are strong, tends to become chaotic, unpredictable, withdrawn, or overly rigid)

---

8. The infant is **able to maintain motor tone** and carry out age-appropriate motor planning sequence (e.g., put fist in mouth, reach for object).

9. The infant **enjoys a range of age-appropriate foods** and is free of symptoms (e.g., abdominal pain, skin rash, irritability, or other symptoms) from most age-appropriate foods.

10. The infant **is comfortable and without symptoms around most routine household odors.**

B. **Interpretation.** If any of the responses is suboptimal, then **hyper- or hyposensitivity to environmental stimulation** should be considered. In such cases the infant may be especially sensitive to incoming sensory stimulation, such as touch (e.g., cries when wears flannel), sound (e.g., upset at loud noises), sight (e.g., avoids bright lights), smell (e.g., picky eater), or movement of his or her body in space. Other infants who are relatively insensitive barely respond to external stimuli and may crave excessive sight, sounds, and so forth. Some infants offer a mix of hyper- and hyposensitivities, making self-regulation even more difficult.

Others have difficulty in **processing, organizing** (making sense of), or **sequencing** incoming sensory information, such as sounds (e.g., ability of a 3 year old to follow two simple directions such as, "Take the glass and put it in the sink"), sights (e.g., copying a design), motor pattern (e.g., tying shoes), and spatial concepts (e.g., figuring out the geography of a new house).

III. **Observation of caregiver patterns.** The observation of the parent-child interaction must also focus on the caregiver's sensitivity to the infant's behavioral cues to determine the goodness of fit between the caregiving style and the infant's socioemotional development and self-regulatory abilities. Caregiver patterns can be observed to assess whether the parent is supporting or undermining the infant's mastery of his or her emotional milestones (Table 9-1 lists problematic caregiving patterns). Examples of appropriate caregiving include:

A. The caregiver tends to **comfort** the infant, especially when she or he is upset (e.g., by using relaxed, gentle, firm holding, rhythmic vocal or visual contact), rather than making the infant more tense (e.g., by being overly worried, tense, or anxious; or mechanical or anxiously over- or understimulating).

B. The caregiver tends to find **appropriate levels of stimulation** to interest the infant in the world (e.g., by being interesting, alert, and responsive; by providing appropriate levels of sound, sights, and touch; and by offering appropriate games and toys), rather than being hyperstimulating and intrusive (e.g., picking at and poking or shaking the infant excessively to gain his or her attention).

C. The caregiver tends to **engage the infant pleasurably** in a relationship (e.g., by looking, vocalizing, gentle touching), rather than ignoring the infant (e.g., by being depressed, aloof, preoccupied, withdrawn, indifferent).

D. The caregiver tends to read and respond to the infant's **emotional signals** and needs (e.g., by responding appropriately to the desire for closeness as well as the need to be assertive, explorative, and independent), rather than misreading signals or responding to only one emotional need (e.g., when caregiver hugs if the baby reaches out but hovers over baby and cannot encourage assertive exploration).

E. The caregiver tends to **encourage the infant to move forward in development** rather than to misread the infant's developmental needs by overprotecting, infantilizing, and/or punishing—for example:

    1. The caregiver helps the baby to crawl, vocalize, and gesture by actively responding to the infant's initiative and encouragement rather than over-anticipating the infant's needs and doing everything for him or her.

    2. The caregiver helps the toddler make the shift from proximal, physical dependency (e.g., being held) to feeling more secure while being independent (e.g., keeps in verbal and visual contact with toddler as he or she builds a tower on the other side of the room).

    3. The caregiver helps the 2–3-year-old child shift from motor discharge and gestural ways of relating to the use of ideas through encouraging pretend play and language around emotional themes (e.g., gets down on the floor and plays out dolls' hugging each other and then separating from each other).

    4. The caregiver helps the 3–4-year-old child take responsibility for behavior rather than "giving in all the time" or being overly punitive.

Appendix: Socioemotional Development of Infants and Children: Themes and Behaviors

---

3 Months: Regulation and Interest in the World

Developmental Goals
• Can be calm.
• Recovers from crying with comforting.
• Is able to be alert.
• Looks at one when talked to.
• Brightens up to appropriate experiences.

Clinical Observations
• Shows an interest in the world by looking at (brightening) or listening to (turning toward) sounds. Can attend to a visual or auditory stimulus for 3 or more seconds.
• Can remain calm and focused for 2 or more minutes at a time, as evidenced by looking around, sucking, cooperating in cuddling, or other age-appropriate activities.

5 Months: Forming Relationships (Attachments)

Developmental Goals
• Shows positive loving affect toward primary caregiver (and other key caregivers).
• Shows full range of emotions.

Clinical Observations
- Responds to social overtures with an emotional response of pleasure (e.g., smile, joyful vocalizations).
- Can display negative affect (e.g., frown, negative vocalizations, angry arm or leg movements).

9 Months: Intentional Two-Way Communication

Developmental Goals
- Interacts in a purposeful (i.e., intentional, reciprocal, cause-and-effect) manner.
- Initiates signals and responds purposefully to another person's signals.

Clinical Observations
- Responds to caregiver's gestures with intentional gestures of his or her own (e.g., when caregiver reaches out to pick up infant, infant may reach up with own arms; a flirtatious caregiver vocalization may beget a playful look and a series of vocalizations).
- Initiates intentional iterations (e.g., spontaneously reaches for caregiver's nose, hair, or mouth; uses hand movements to indicate wish for a certain toy or to be picked up).

13 Months: Developing a Complex Sense of Self

Developmental Goals
- Sequences a number of gestures together and responds consistently to caregiver's gestures, thereby forming chains of interaction (i.e., opens and closes a number of sequential circles of communication).
- Manifests a wide range of organized, socially meaningful behaviors and feelings dealing with warmth, pleasure, assertion, exploration, protest, and anger.

Clinical Observations
- Strings together three or more circles of communication (interactions) as part of a complex pattern of communication. Each unit or circle of communication begins with an infant behavior and ends with the infant's building on and responding to the caregiver response. For example, an infant looks and reaches for a toy (opening a circle of communication); caregiver points to the toy, gestures, and vocalizes, "This one?"; infant nods, makes a purposeful sound, and reaches further for toy (closing a circle of communication). As the infant explores the toy and exchanges vocalizations, motor gestures, or facial expressions with the caregiver, additional circles of communication are opened and closed.

18 Months: Increasingly Complex Sense of Self

Developmental Goals
- Comprehends, communicates, and elaborates sequences of interaction that convey basic emotional themes.

Clinical Observations
- Has the ability, with a responsive caregiver, to open and close 10 or more consecutive circles of communication (e.g., taking caregiver's hand and walking toward refrigerator, vocalizing, pointing, responding to caregiver's questioning gestures with more vocalizing and pointing; finally getting caregiver to refrigerator, getting caregiver to open door, and pointing to the desired food.)
- Imitates another person's behavior and then uses this newly learned behavior to convey an emotional theme (e.g., putting on daddy's hat and walking around the house with a big smile, clearly waiting for an admiring laugh).

24 Months: Representational Capacity of Emotional Ideas

Developmental Goals
- Creates mental representations of feelings and ideas that can be expressed symbolically (e.g., pretend play and words).

Clinical Observations

• Can construct, in collaboration with caregiver, simple pretend play patterns of at least one "idea" (e.g., dolls hugging or feeding the doll).
• Can use words or other symbolic means (e.g., selecting a series of pictures, creating a sequence of motor gestures) to communicate a need, wish, intention, or feeling (e.g., "want that"; "me toy"; "hungry!" "mad!").

30 Months: Greater Representational Elaboration of Emotional Themes

Developmental Goals

• Can elaborate a number of ideas in both make-believe play and symbolic communication that go beyond basic needs (e.g., "want juice") and deal with more complex intentions, wishes, or feelings (e.g., themes of closeness or dependency, separation, exploration, assertiveness, anger, self-pride, or showing off).
• Creates pretend dramas with two or more ideas (e.g., dolls hug and then have a tea party). The ideas need not be related or logically connected to one another.
• Uses symbolic communication (e.g., words, pictures, motor patterns) to convey two or more ideas at a time in terms of complex intentions, wishes, or feelings. Ideas need not be logically connected to one another.

36 Months: Emotional Thinking

Developmental Goals

• Can communicate ideas dealing with complex intentions, wishes, and feelings in pretend play or other types of symbolic communication that are logically tied to one another.
• Distinguishes what is real from unreal and switches back and forth between fantasy and reality with little difficulty.

Clinical Observations

• In pretend play, involves two or more ideas that are logically tied to one another but not necessarily realistic (e.g., "The car is visiting the moon" [and gets there] "by flying fast"). In addition, the child can build on an adult's pretend play idea (i.e., close a circle of communication). For example, the child is "cooking a soup" and the adult asks what is in it. The child says, "rocks and dirt" or "ants and spiders."
• Engages in symbolic communication that involves two or more ideas that are logically connected and grounded in reality: "No go to sleep. Want to watch television." "Why?" asks the adult. "Because not tired." Child can close symbolic circles of communication (e.g., child says, "Want to go outside." Adult asks, "What will you do?" Child replies, "Play.").

42–48 Months: Emotional Thinking

Developmental Goals

• Is capable of elaborate complex pretend play and symbolic communication dealing with complex intentions, wishes, or feelings.

Clinical Observations

• Engages in "how," "why," or "when" elaborations, which give depth to play and communication. (Child sets up castle with an evil queen who captured the princess. Why did she capture the princess? "Because the princess was more beautiful." When did she capture her? "Yesterday." How will the princess get out? "You ask too many questions.")
• Deals with causality in a reality-based dialogue. ("Why did you hit your brother?" "Because he took my toy." "Any other reason?" "He took my cookie.")
• Distinguishes reality and fantasy. ("That's only pretend"; "That's a dream. It's not real.")
• Uses concepts of time and space. (Caregiver: "Where should we look for the toy you can't find?" Child: "Let's look in my room. I was playing with it there." Caregiver: "When do you want the cookies?" Child: "Now." Caregiver: "Not now; maybe in 5 minutes." Child: "No. Want it now!" Caregiver: "You can have the cookie in 1, 2, or 5 minutes." Child: "OK. One minute.")

Bibliography

For Parents
Greenspan S, Greenspan N. *First Feelings: Milestones in the Development of Your Baby and Child.* New York: Penguin Books, 1985.

Greenspan S, Greenspan N. *The Essential Partnership: How Parents and Children Meet the Emotional Challenges of Infancy and Childhood.* New York: Penguin Books, 1989.

For Professionals
Greenspan S. Clinical assessment of emotional milestones in infancy and early childhood. *Pediatr Clin North Am* 38(6):1371–1385, 1991.

Specific Management Strategies

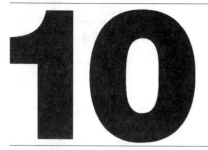

Managing Behavior Problems in an Office Practice

Barbara Howard

Behavioral and emotional problems comprise an estimated 25–50% of all pediatric problems raised by parents. Pediatric primary care clinicians are in an ideal position to deal with such concerns: they are well known to the family, generally respected, viewed as supportive by both parent and child, and already know much about the child and the family. Additionally, the office setting is seen as friendly, nonstigmatizing territory.

I. Identifying problems

A. Open-ended questions. The first requirement for addressing behavioral problems is their identification. This is not always easy since children rarely ask for help and the parents may not realize that the clinician has either the interest or the expertise to help. Open-ended questions, such as *"How are things going?"* allow the parent and child to express their own agenda for the visit. In other families, the clinician may need to ask specifically about "behavior at home, at school, or in day care."

B. Observations in the office. Observations of behavior in the office and waiting room can be revealing. Toys in the medical bag or examination room are an invaluable way to observe the child's behavior and development (as well as to enhance the enjoyment of the visit). These observations can then be used to start the discussion (e.g., *"I noticed that he is very active. How is that for you at home?"*). Such comments should be asked in a nonjudgmental way so that the parents' response can reveal if they view the behavior as problematic. The clinician's own feelings and intuitions about the child should be compared with parental and child reports and used to raise questions or to formulate clinical hypotheses about the child's behavior.

C. Screening questionnaires. Questionnaires can be a valuable time saver and tool for identifying behavioral problems. This method is discussed in Chapter 6.

II. Managing behavioral problems

A. Addressing the problem. The first step to successful problem resolution occurs during the initial discussion. It is important for the clinician to summarize the parent's (or his or her own) concern to demonstrate that their worries have been heard. The problem should be discussed nonjudgmentally and reframed in a more positive light (e.g., *"You would like him to listen to instructions* [rather than 'to behave']"). The initial discussion should set the stage for treatment by clarifying the problem, setting a positive tone, and not blaming or insulting the child (who may be listening). The next step is to convey some hope and confidence that a solution is possible.

B. Special "problem visits." Once a problem has been identified, one or more visits of longer duration than usual are generally needed. To arrange an effective "problem visit," all of the vitally important people in the child's life should be invited to attend. Boyfriends, distant cousins, and babysitters, for example, may be crucial to the solution of the problem. If a key person refuses to attend, a personal telephone call by the clinician that seeks his or her opinion and stresses this person's importance to the child can change a recalcitrant attitude.

1. **Visit duration.** Frequently, a longer (e.g., 1 hour) problem visit can be scheduled at the beginning or the end of the workday, when no sick children are waiting to be seen and telephone calls can be postponed. (It is often advantageous to schedule the problem visit at the beginning of the day, when

energy is high.) However, 1 hour is often inadequate to allow the family to express the range of their concerns and to provide counseling. Often the most delicate or powerful issue is not raised until the last moments of the visit in a "parting shot." Such important statements at the end of the hour need to be acknowledged with appropriate empathy, recorded in the chart, and promised as first agenda items at the next visit (which may need to be scheduled sooner, depending on the information revealed).

Another problem occurs when families or key family members arrive late for an appointment. This may be an important statement of that person's ambivalence about the issues being discussed. The emotional difficulty can be acknowledged directly and with empathy, but the visit should be kept on schedule.

2. **Space considerations.** Many offices lack an examining room large enough to seat all the family members. A conference room or even the waiting room may better serve and can be private enough before or after regular office hours.

3. **Documentation of the visit.** Since details of the session are critical to understanding and managing the problem, the clinician should leave adequate time to document the salient aspects of the visit. Note taking is possible during the session for some clinicians, but should be interrupted when it interferes with the therapeutic alliance with the family and patient.

4. **Billing for the visit.** It is important that the extended problem visit be adequately billed (i.e., commensurate to the time spent in counseling). Patients should be informed of the fee *before* the first extended visit. Offering to accept payment over time may decrease the burden of the extra fee for some families. Third-party reimbursement may be available depending on the diagnosis, the clinician's experience and training, and state insurance regulations. Clinicians generally cannot refer their own patients to themselves and record the visit as a consultation. Experience suggests that most patients *are* willing to pay for counseling if they are able. Many of the barriers to adequate billing are in the mind of the clinician, who is insecure about whether she or he really has something valuable to offer.

C. **Expanding counseling skills.** Books, journals, lectures, videotapes of master therapists, workshops, courses, and fellowships in behavior and development, child psychiatry, or family therapy are available to help clinicians strengthen their behavioral counseling skills. The best method, however, is through experience. For example, working as co-therapists with a more experienced clinician in the session with the family is a very valuable format. Case discussions with another clinician or in a group provides support and insight into the family's and clinician's emotional reactions, as well as input into the content and process of the management. This process is called *supervision* and can be either direct (another professional attends the counseling session or observes through a one-way mirror) or indirect (the other professional reviews cases later from audiotape, videotape, verbatim process notes, standard notes, and recall, and makes suggestions to be incorporated into future patient visits). The Bureau of Maternal and Child Health has funded a number of Collaborative Office Rounds demonstration projects to provide similar case discussion for groups of 8–10 practicing pediatric clinicians.

D. **Communicating with schools.** Some behavioral problems are situationally specific and occur only in school. In such cases it is useful to obtain an objective description of the problem from the school. A behavioral questionnaire can be sent to the teacher or a written note requested from the teacher. Ideally, direct telephone contact between clinician and teacher is the most revealing. (It is easiest to reach teachers at 7:30 A.M. or noon.) Teachers are generally very grateful for the clinician's interest and can be extremely helpful in providing more information about the family and the child. A single clinical visit to a school to meet the child's teachers, principal, and guidance counselors can facilitate communication for years to come.

E. **Making effective referrals.** One of the most important (and underrated) skills of the primary care clinician lies in making effective referrals. It is estimated that 68% of mental health referrals made for children are unsuccessful because the family has been poorly prepared, the referral is ill timed, the family has negative perceptions of mental health professionals, or there is a poor fit between the specialist's therapeutic style and the family's or child's expectations.

1. **Help the family to identify their distress.** The first steps in making an effective referral are to ensure that each member of the family feels that his or her voice has been heard and to identify the distress that will motivate the family and child to accept counseling. It is always better for a clinician to refer the family for a problem that bothers *them*, even if it is not the one that appears primary to the clinician (e.g., a referral for the child's truancy rather than the father's alcoholism). The therapist taking on the case may need to do further work before the family is able to face the central issue.

2. **Discuss issues in a constructive way.** Behavioral and family issues should be discussed in nonjudgmental terms, citing strengths and using issues from the family's current (rather than past) situation to suggest further work. In the case of a separation from an abusive spouse, for example, one might say, *"It took so much courage to make this break that I can see that you really want what is best for your son. Now you can focus on the work needed to free yourself from the memories of the past unkindness of your own father and get on with your life."*

3. **Find the appropriate referral.** The next step in making an effective referral is to identify an appropriate consultant for the family. The clinician should inquire about the family's past experiences with counseling and demystify the process of counseling (e.g., by pointing out that therapy is just like the talking that has been going on in the exploratory sessions).

    It is helpful to have ready the names and telephone numbers of several therapists who are available and have interest and skills in the type of problem at hand. This should take some preparation in getting to know the counseling style of a cadre of therapists:
    • Ask them what kinds of cases they prefer.
    • Ask whether their style is directive or free form and whether they offer groups.
    • Determine their fees and accepted insurance.
    • Consider a face-to-face meeting with a therapist. It allows some basis for discussing the therapist with a family and will facilitate future communications between physician and therapist.

    The clinician should provide the family and patient with details about the therapists so that they can make an informed choice. The gender of the therapist is not usually central to the success of treatment, although some family members may have a strong preference, which should be respected. The relationship of the family with this professional is vital to the treatment, so they should be actively involved in the initial referral. Additionally, they should be told that they can always change counselors, should the need arise. This is important so that their problems do not go unresolved simply because of an initial mismatch.

4. **Follow up.** Finally, it is important for the family to know that the primary care clinician will stay involved and will continue to manage other problems as before. This reassures them that they are not being rejected, especially if they have revealed undesirable information about themselves. The clinician should be clear in defining exactly what problems will be handled by which professional, and stay in touch with the referral therapist in order to assist or back up the therapist's plans and to facilitate ongoing communication with the family.

F. **Alternative counseling strategies in the office**

1. **Groups for families.** Group sessions for a number of families concerning common behavioral problems (e.g., temper tantrums, toilet training, discipline issues, choosing a day care provider, teenage risk-taking behaviors) can be an effective way to address those issues and to provide parents with a support system of other parents in similar circumstances. Other groups can be focused for parents of children with a specific problem, such as attention deficit hyperactivity disorder, oppositional defiant disorder, mental retardation, or substance abuse. Local branches of national diagnosis specific

organizations may already offer these or will arrange them when sufficient interest is shown. One-time sessions may be arranged to deal with crises, such as a suicide, disaster, abuse in a local day care center, or death of a public figure. For families, the existence of others with similar problems can be a tremendous relief in itself.

These groups can be led by a primary care clinician in the practice or by an outside consultant, or co-led by both. They may be offered in the office or elsewhere, sponsored by the practice, or simply made known to patients in the practice. It is important to remember that the needs of the individual child or family are frequently not entirely met by these groups, so the leaders must carefully monitor the participants and ensure that supplemental support, guidance, or management is given when needed.

2. **Group checkups.** The advantages of offering health supervision visits in groups are becoming evident. By seeing four 6-month-old babies together over 1 hour, rather than each one for 15 minutes, the clinician can spend much more time providing teaching, anticipatory guidance, and discussion of behavioral issues. What such group checkups lose in terms of chaos and intimacy, they gain in the time that is spent discussing behavioral and other issues. Most studies confirm that such an option is attractive to many parents.

3. **Call hour.** Many offices have a designated call-in hour for health questions. While telephone consultations have obvious major disadvantages, when supervised carefully they can be part of a spectrum of office services for dealing with behavioral problems.

4. **Housing other professional disciplines within the practice.** Many practices are choosing to provide offices for specialists from other disciplines to deal with specific behavioral and emotional problems. In private practices, the specialist may receive the space free, share in the costs and income of the group, set lower fees for patients from the practice, be paid a salary by the group, or be a totally independent contractor renting space and billing independently. The practice benefits by having a known, trusted, and readily available person to whom to refer their patients. The entire practice can be strengthened by the comprehensive care that ends up being delivered within its walls.

Bibliography

Allmond BW, Buckman W, Gofman HF. *The Family Is the Patient.* St. Louis: Mosby, 1979.

Constantino JN. Parents, mental illness, and the primary health care of infants and young children, *Zero to Three* 13:1–10, 1993.

King M, Novick L, Citrenbaum C. *Irresistible Communication: Effective Communication for Health Professionals.* Philadelphia: Saunders, 1982.

Kramer CH. *Becoming a Family Therapist.* New York: Human Sciences Press, 1980.

Smith CK, Leversee JH. Basic interviewing skills. In Rosen GM, Geyman JP, Layton RH (eds), *Behavioral Science in Family Practice.* New York: Appleton-Century-Crofts, 1980.

Stein MT. Interviewing in a pediatric setting. In Dixon SD, Stein MT (eds), *Encounters with Children, Pediatric Behavior and Development* (2nd ed). St. Louis: Mosby Year Book, 1992.

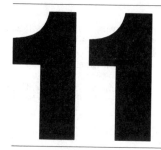

Behavioral Management: Theory and Practice

Edward R. Christophersen

Traditional behavioral management techniques can be very useful to the primary care clinician. This chapter describes the concepts and techniques that parents can routinely use in interacting with their children.

I. Techniques to teach or improve behaviors

A. Time-in and verbal praise

1. **Time-in** refers to the way parents interact with their children when they do not necessarily deserve praise but when their behavior is acceptable. Parents should be encouraged and educated to provide their children with frequent, brief, nonverbal, physical contact whenever their child is *not* engaging in a behavior the parents consider unacceptable or offensive. They do not have to wait for "good behavior."

2. **Verbal praise** is used only when a child has done something "good." The best time to use verbal praise is during natural breaks in an activity. For example, while a child is coloring, the parent should provide lots of brief, nonverbal, physical contact (time-in); simple physical contact, without any praise, is much less likely to distract a child. When the child has finished coloring or stops coloring to show it to a parent, verbal praise is appropriate.

3. **Advantages.** Time-in and verbal praise encourage children to continue to engage in acceptable behaviors. These techniques take no additional parent time and do not distract children.

B. Incidental learning.
Children learn behaviors by being around individuals who engage in those behaviors naturally. This is called *incidental learning*. For example, if both parents smoke cigarettes, their child is significantly more likely to become a smoker than if neither parent smokes. A surprising number and variety of children's behaviors appear to have been learned incidentally, including language, gestures, and even activity levels.

1. **Advantages and disadvantages.** Incidental learning can be achieved without any additional effort on the part of the parents. They need only be aware that such learning occurs naturally and be cognizant of incidental learning during the time they spend with their children. The negative side is that children also learn behaviors the parents never intended for them to learn (e.g., swearing).

C. Modeling

1. **Peer responses.** Two basic modeling techniques exist: live and videotape. Most modeling procedures work best if the model is approximately the same age as the target child. For example, a 6-year-old girl who has previously had her teeth cleaned by a dentist and who behaved appropriately during the procedure could be observed live or could be videotaped while being examined. A second child who observes the dental procedures being performed on this model can learn both what to expect of dental procedures and how to react to those procedures.

2. **Advantages and disadvantages.** Children are more likely to believe what they see a peer doing than what their parents tell them to do, particularly if the two messages are contradictory (e.g., one a verbal message that the child should relax, and the other the anxiety that a child feels in the dental

chair). However, modeling can teach maladaptive behaviors as well as adaptive behaviors. For example, if a child is observing a peer model in the dentist's office and the peer model becomes very upset, the target child will probably have a more difficult time when it is his turn for the procedure.

D. **Reinforcement.** No other topic in the behavioral literature has been more misunderstood than reinforcement. An item or activity can be said to have reinforcing properties for an individual child only if that child has previously worked in order to obtain access to that item or activity.

1. **Choosing rewards.** Under the right circumstances, reinforcement, by definition, will work with virtually any age group and under almost all circumstances. However, no item or activity can be accurately described as a reinforcer unless and until it has produced a change in behavior. For example, although candy is reinforcing for the vast majority of children, it cannot be referred to as a reinforcer until it has been demonstrated that the child will either work to obtain the candy or stop a behavior that prevents him or her from receiving it.

    Principles of reinforcement, or the manner in which the reinforcer is made accessible to a child, are extremely important:

    a. **Small rewards offered frequently are better than large rewards offered infrequently.** A physical hug offered several times during a household chore will usually be more effective than a big reward at the end of the chore. Small rewards during the chore and a reward at the end will also work nicely.

    b. **Repetition, with feedback, enhances a child's learning.** A child will learn more from performing the same task repeatedly, with help from his parent, than from performing it once. While parents will often expect their child to perform a task correctly the first time, the child will actually learn the task better if he has many opportunities to practice. For example, a child who helps one of his parents do the laundry several times each week for two years will probably be able to do the laundry for the rest of his life.

    c. **Children learn more quickly and retain the learning better if they are relaxed while they are learning.** While children can be very frustrating, the parent who becomes angry or impatient only exacerbates the situation. Similarly, an upset child does not learn as rapidly or as permanently as a calm child.

    d. **Warnings only make children worse.** While parents have a natural tendency to warn their children, it is far more effective to discipline the child for not performing the task and then give the child another opportunity to do it, rather than frequent warnings that the tasks must be done.

    e. **A behavior should be already learned before it can be reinforced.** If the child doesn't know how to perform the expected behavior, offering a reward, in lieu of teaching the child how to perform the behavior, is ineffective.

2. **Advantages and disadvantages.** Reinforcing items and activities frequently can become part of normal, everyday life without substantial planning on the parents' part. Reinforcing items and activities may sometimes be inadvertent. For example, when a parent picks up a child who has been crying in bed after bedtime, the parent may be reinforcing that child for crying.

    Additionally, the child's behavior may return to its prereinforcement level as soon as the reinforcers are no longer available. For example, in research on the use of reinforcers for automobile seatbelt use, many children stopped wearing their seatbelts as soon as the reinforcers were no longer available. Procedures that have been shown to be successful in maintaining desired behaviors after reinforcement ceases include gradually making the reinforcer available less often (e.g., on the average, every second behavior is reinforced, then every third behavior, then every fourth behavior). Once a behavior becomes *habitual,* the individual will engage in it whether it is reinforced or not.

E. **Conditioned reinforcers.** Many items and activities that have no intrinsic reinforcing properties can take on reinforcing properties. Money, for example, is not usually a reinforcer to a small child. When the child learns what he or she can purchase with money, it begins to take on reinforcing properties. As another example, to a distressed child in the middle of the night, even the sound of the bedroom door opening can take on reinforcing properties, as the child associates the sound of the door opening with being rescued by a parent.

1. **Advantages.** Conditioned reinforcers are usually more readily available than the actual reinforcer, and most children work just as hard for a conditioned reinforcer as they will for the actual one. Conditioned reinforcers, such as money, also have the advantage that they can be traded for a wide variety of items or activities as the child's tastes and preferences change.

F. **The token economy.** Conditioned reinforcers must use a consistent method of exchange. In the case of money, the exchange system is already in place, and the money becomes a "token" of what can be purchased. Entire "token economies" have been devised as treatment programs for children from age 3 years to adulthood. The term *token economy* refers to the organized manner in which tokens are gained and lost, as well as what can be purchased with them. The success or failure of a token economy depends almost entirely on how it is implemented and on how many reinforcing activities are realistically available to the individual who must earn, lose, and spend tokens.

Token economies are most effective when they are used as motivational systems to encourage children to engage in socially appropriate behaviors. Three different types of token economies are widely used with common behavioral problems.

1. The **simple exchange system** provides a means of keeping track of the child's appropriate and inappropriate behaviors. A list of behaviors can be taped to the door of the refrigerator. As the child completes assigned or volunteered tasks or chores, she or he marks these on the "positive side" of the exchange chart. Similarly, as the child engages in inappropriate behaviors, she or he marks these on the "negative side." When the child wants a special privilege or activity, there must be more positive marks than negative marks to "afford" the special privilege. The simple exchange system is appropriate for children ages 5–12 years.

2. Under **chip systems,** the child earns poker chips for positive behaviors. Each time chips are earned, the parent acknowledges the child's appropriate behavior while offering two chips. The child is then expected to take the chips from the parent's hand, look the parent in the eye, and say, "Thank you." In this way, the child not only receives the tokens for the appropriate behavior but also practices appropriate social behaviors. Similarly, when the child engages in a behavior that loses chips, he or she is expected to hand the chips to the parent politely but may receive one chip back for "taking the fine so nicely." The chip system is useful for ages 3–7 years.

3. The **point system** is similar to the chip system but can be much more sophisticated. Points can be used to motivate children and teenagers to practice the behaviors they are lacking, such as taking feedback well and sharing their feelings appropriately. Each time they engage in these types of behaviors, they earn points that can be used to purchase items and activities they want. The point system is useful for children ages 6–16 years. (Manuals that describe how to set up a chip system and a point system are available in Christophersen 1994.)

G. **Fading** refers to changing something gradually instead of abruptly changing it. For example, instead of taking away a toddler's bottle, a cup can be available with milk in it while the bottle is gradually diluted from 100% milk to 90% milk/ 10% water, then 80% milk/20% water, and so on, until the toddler is drinking pure water from the bottle and pure milk from the cup. Fading works better with younger children, who lack the cognitive skills for noticing the changes that are taking place. Other examples of fading include:
• Raising training wheels on a bicycle 1/8 in. every 2 weeks until they are about 3 in. off the ground and no longer necessary.

- Changing a child's bedtime 15 minutes each night at daylight savings time instead of abruptly changing it the entire hour in one night.
- Teaching a child how to swallow pills by starting out with very small cake sprinkles to wash down with a favorite beverage, then moving to slightly larger pieces of candy.

   1. Advantages and disadvantages. Fading often helps to avoid confrontations with a child. It can be used to accomplish something without incident that otherwise may have been difficult to accomplish. The disadvantage of fading is that parents have to spend more time than they would if their child could abruptly make the desired changes.

II. Procedures to decrease or discourage behaviors

   A. Time-in and time-out. Probably the most often recommended disciplinary technique is time-out. As initially used, time-out referred to "time-out from pleasant interaction." Over the past decade or so the term has been shortened to *time-out,* and, in doing so, the idea of removing a pleasant interaction has been ignored or forgotten. Time-in and time-out are effective from less than age 1 year to early adolescence.

   The following variables have the most impact on the effectiveness of time-out:
   - It must be presented immediately after an inappropriate behavior.
   - It must be presented *every* time the inappropriate behavior occurs.
   - The inappropriate behavior should occur frequently.
   - The time-out must remove or make unavailable an otherwise pleasant state of affairs (i.e., time-in).
   - The time-out should not be considered over until the child has quieted down.
   - All warnings of using time-out should be carried out.
   - The child should be completely ignored during the time-out, regardless of how outrageous the behavior might become. One study demonstrated that time-out becomes more effective when the time-in is "enriched" (more fun, more enjoyable) and becomes less effective when the time-in is "impoverished."

   1. Advantages. Time-in and time-out provide parents with an effective alternative to nagging, yelling, or spanking. Their consistent use also encourages children to develop self-quieting skills (a child's ability to calm herself or himself without the assistance of a parent). It encourages these skills because the parents are modeling the ability to cope with an unpleasant situation and because the child is learning how to cope with feelings when he or she does not like something the parents have done.

   B. Extinction is defined as the withdrawal of all attention after a child engages in undesirable behaviors. The most common example of extinction is letting a child cry at bedtime instead of paying attention to the whining, fussing, or screaming. When used properly, extinction involves completely ignoring a child's behaviors and protests.

   A major problem with using extinction is an initial sharp increase in the child's inappropriate behavior, called an *extinction burst.* For example, when a child is ignored during a temper tantrum or when whining at bedtime, these behaviors usually increase at first, perhaps discouraging the parents from continuing the extinction procedure. If the parents continue with the extinction procedure, however, the change in the child's behavior will usually be forthcoming.

   Although extinction procedures are often successful, parents may not be able to tolerate the technique. Several modifications have been made to make extinction techniques more acceptable to parents. For example, the day correction of bedtime problems technique involves teaching the parents to use extinction for whining and fussing *during the day.* The parents then gain confidence in their ability to use it properly, and the child learns that the parents will follow through with the use of extinction once they start it. The day correction technique is actually more effective than using extinction only at bedtime.

   1. Advantages and disadvantages. Extinction procedures have been effective with many different childhood problems. The time necessary to educate parents on the use of these procedures is reasonable, given the constraints of primary care practices. The main disadvantage is the extinction burst and the parents' inability to tolerate their child's initial distress at being ignored.

C. Planned ignoring. The parents gradually ignore their child's behavior more and more (as opposed to introducing complete extinction abruptly). Planned ignoring may result in less of an extinction burst, but it takes longer to work.

D. Spanking. With spanking, caregivers can vent their own frustration at the same time they are discouraging a child from engaging in the behavior that resulted in the spanking. Additionally, spanking will often produce an immediate decrease in the child's behavior.

    1. Advantages and disadvantages. Spanking teaches a child that hitting is acceptable. The child, after being spanked, is likely to avoid or try to escape from the caregiver who administered the spanking. Spanking can also result in other discipline methods losing their effectiveness. Thus, a child who is frequently spanked at home is less likely to be responsive to the use of extinction. Since time-in and time-out can produce virtually the same effects as spanking but without the side effects, spanking should not be one of the alternatives that professionals recommend for parents.

E. Job grounding, a form of grounding whereby the child has control over how long the grounding is in effect. When a child has broken a major rule (e.g., gone to a shopping center by bike without telling parents), he or she is grounded: the child loses all privileges (including television, telephone, having a friend over, playing with games, snacks and desserts). The grounding lasts until the child has completed one job properly. The jobs, which should be written on a 3- by 5-in. card, should be agreed upon by both parent and child during a quiet, peaceful period of time. The child, upon being grounded, is asked to pick from a stack of cards that are held face down by the parent. Once the job is chosen, the child is restricted from most activities until the job is completed. The parents are instructed to refrain from nagging, prodding, and reminding. As soon as the child has completed the job (most jobs should take only 5–10 minutes to complete and be tasks that the child has done many times before), he or she is "off grounding."

    Job grounding differs from traditional time-based grounding in that the child determines how long the grounding lasts and, under most circumstances, the child has the option of getting the job done without missing a valued social activity.

    1. Advantages and disadvantages. Job grounding is usually effective, it lets the child practice a job that he or she probably did not want to do in the first place, and it gives him or her the opportunity to avoid losing a valued activity. The disadvantage is that if the child has no planned activities, he or she may stall on completing the job until some external motivation is present.

F. Habit reversal. Habit reversal procedures were developed for use with habit disorders. Habit-reversal training requires a level of cognition not reached before age 4–5 years.

    1. Components of habit reversal:

        a. Keeping a **daily record** of the number of habit episodes.

        b. Making a **list of the annoyances** and inconveniences the habit is causing the child.

        c. Describing exactly **how and when the child performs the habit.**

        d. Teaching the child to **relax when nervous** by changing her posture and breathing slowly.

        e. Identifying the **situations, activities, and people that cause the habit to occur.**

        f. Teaching the child **mentally to rehearse and act out how to deal with the habit** in different situations.

        g. Arranging for the **child's friends to comment on her or his progress** and to remind her or him of habit episodes.

        h. Seeking out **situations the child has avoided** because of the habit.

        i. Having the child **practice the objectionable habit repeatedly** for a period of time each day (*massed practice*).

j. Teaching the child to **practice a behavior that cannot be done at the same time as the habit to be changed** (e.g., teaching the child to grip the bottom of the chair when he or she feels the urge to pull his or her hair) (*competing-response training*).

2. **Advantages and disadvantages.** Habit reversal training is effective and has no physical side effects. The overall reduction in habit disorders and tics is also far greater with this technique than with medication. The disadvantage is the time it takes to teach and monitor, as well as the time it takes to reduce the habit disorder (usually days).

G. **Positive practice,** the procedure of having a child practice an appropriate behavior after each inappropriate behavior. For example, when a previously toilet trained child wets his pants, he is required to practice "going to the bathroom" 10 times—5 times from the place where the accident was discovered and 5 times from such alternative sites as the front yard, the back yard, the kitchen, and the bedroom. When used correctly, with no nagging or unpleasant behavior on the caregiver's part, positive practice can produce dramatic results.

1. **Advantages and disadvantages.** Positive practice gives a child a lot of opportunities to practice appropriate behaviors. This technique is typically effective quickly. The disadvantages include the length of time necessary to implement the practice, as well as the fact that the practice should be done immediately after the inappropriate behavior, which is not always convenient.

III. **General remarks and conclusions.** Although the term behavior management frequently has been used to refer to coercive action taken in an effort to discourage a child from engaging in inappropriate behavior, many positive alternatives are now available. Generally, the emphasis should be on teaching children appropriate behaviors, rather than concentrating on reducing inappropriate behaviors.

The single most important consideration in implementing such behavior management strategies is taking a history that can help to identify precisely what strategy should be offered to the caregiver and how to offer that strategy. The primary care provider now has a variety of behavior management strategies available for dealing with situations encountered in the provision of care to normal children with minor behavior problems.

Bibliography

For Parents

Christophersen ER. *Little People: Guidelines for Commonsense Child Rearing* (3rd ed). Kansas City: Westport Publishing Group, 1988.

Christophersen ER. *Beyond Discipline: Parenting That Lasts a Lifetime.* Kansas City: Westport Publishing Group, 1990.

Schmitt BD. *Your Child's Health* (2nd ed). New York: Bantam Books, 1991.

For Professionals

Azrin NH, Nunn RG. *Habit Control in a Day.* New York: Simon & Schuster, 1977.

Christophersen ER. *Pediatric Compliance: A Guide for the Primary Care Physician.* New York: Plenum, 1994.

Schmitt BD (ed). Pediatric Advisor. Inglewood CO: Clinical Reference Systems. *Computer software.*

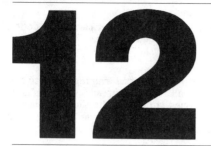

Coping with Stressful Transitions

W. Thomas Boyce

The primary care clinician is often the principal source of assistance for a family or a child during periods of stressful transitions. As such, he or she is especially well placed to offer advice, construct effective interventions, and provide encouragement and empathic care during critical moments in a family's life course. It is precisely during such moments that patients and families may find themselves unusually receptive to the words, reflections, and concerns of a caring professional. What may seem at first an insurmountable difficulty can become, under the guidance of the primary care provider, an occasion for growth and renewal. Stressful transitions may become turning points in a child's life and, through an alchemy of crisis, the pain of a seemingly catastrophic event can be memorably transformed into a moment at which life was indelibly changed for the better.

I. **Types of childhood transitions.** A childhood transition is a period of swift, challenging change that may alter a child's experiences of self, life circumstances, or future possibilities and expectations. Childhood is a period of rapid and dramatic developmental change and is filled with transitional events, ranging from the birth of a sibling or starting school to the death of a beloved grandparent or a parental divorce. Such transitions can be regarded as normative or nonnormative, biological or psychosocial, and 'on-time or off-time' events.

A. **Normative and nonnormative transitions.** Normative events (e.g., entering kindergarten) are those experienced by most children under ordinary conditions growing up in the Western world. Nonnormative transitions (e.g., the death of a parent) are those that represent unexpected deviations from the normal, anticipated sequence of life events. Events deemed as nonnormative within a given society may be regarded as normative in other social or cultural circumstances. Divorce, for example, has become so prevalent in North American society that it could arguably be viewed as a nearly normative stressor for many children. Normative transitional events may be planned, as in a family's move to a new home, or unplanned, as in the changes in a family's economic condition that typically follow the loss of a parent's job.

B. **Biological and psychosocial transitions.** Transitions in childhood can attend both biological and psychosocial changes. The onset of puberty is an example of a transition with biological origins, but it is also a transition with social and psychological consequences. The endocrine processes in early adolescence that set into motion a cascade of intricately interconnected changes ultimately transform the individual's reproductive capacity, self-identity, relationships with peers, and social role within the context of the family and community. On the other hand, religious rites of passage (such as a bar mitzvah or confirmation) are transitions that constitute points of psychosocial demarcation in the young person's emergence into the adult world.

C. **On-time and off-time transitions.** On-time or off-time transitions depend on the timing of the event in relationship to personal and societal expectations. Pregnancy, for example, is a fundamentally different event in the life of a married 23-year-old woman than it is in the life of a 13 year old. While the onset of puberty in a 14-year-old boy may be an occasion for celebration or relief, the same event may be bewildering and distressing to an 8-year-old boy. The meaning and adaptive significance of a transition depends in part on whether its timing conforms to cultural and biological norms regarding its location within life-course development.

II. Factors defining stressful transitions

A. Manifestations of stress. Not all transitions in childhood *are* stressful but many are accompanied by the behaviors and expressions of emotion that signal a child's efforts to overcome and adapt to stress. Transitions are capable of invoking a child's neuroendocrine stress response systems. Starting preschool or kindergarten, for example, has been shown to activate the hypothalamic-pituitary-adrenocortical axis, resulting in measurable elevations in the cortisol levels found in both blood and saliva and alterations in immune and cardiovascular function. Stressful transitions therefore appear capable of changing not only the child's behavior and emotional experience but may also set in motion physiologic processes that may be plausibly linked to the development of disease.

B. Aspects of stressful transitions

1. **Adaptation to new situations.** Transitions are, by definition, processes that expose the child to novelty and challenge. A move to a new home, for example, is an event that brings with it the challenges of new neighborhoods and communities, new friends, new schools, and new patterns of living. Although the novelties inherent in such transitions can be invigorating and growth promoting, they often require the simultaneous processes of reorientation, reintegration, and reexploration of the surrounding physical and social landscapes. Each of these processes can result in the experiences and feelings of emotional stress.

2. **Exacerbation of existing problems.** Transitions can create stress by exacerbating or inflaming previously existing problems. A young girl who is struggling with the new academic demands of middle school may find herself overwhelmed by such demands at the time of menarche and its associated biological changes. A 4 year old who is experiencing difficulty self-regulating his aggressive impulses in preschool may feel (and be) out of control following the birth of a sibling. Points of transition carry with them a tendency to uncover, accentuate, or bring into focus struggles in the psychological life of the child.

3. **Coping with changed relationships.** A family systems perspective on child development teaches that major changes in the life of any family member can be expected to alter systematically each of the relationships that comprise the family unit. With events such as divorce, these changes in relationships are glaringly self-evident. Even more subtle transitions, such as a grandparent's coming to live with the family, will be reliably accompanied by shifts and disequilibria in the various relationships among siblings and parents.

4. **Beginnings and endings.** Transitions may be experienced as stressful by virtue of their capacity either to open up or to close down the opportunities available to the child or family. When a child begins kindergarten, a landmark is passed in the relationship of child and parents. This child has begun a journey that will end almost certainly in eventual parting from the family that conceived, loved, and raised him or her. While school may open new visions of possibilities and promise, school also signals—for both the child and parents—the end of something: the final, nonnegotiable conclusion of life as a "little girl or boy."

III. Management. While some changes and transitions may be eagerly anticipated, others will be painful, saddening, or even frightening. At such times, a clinician can be of great assistance to the family by offering professional advice, suggesting practical interventions for the family to pursue, and providing small packages of wisdom about the transition and its likely effects.

A. Parents should be taught or reminded of the powerful effects created by their simple **presence and encouragement in their children's lives.** Within the typically hurried pace of a contemporary family's existence, it is easy to forget that one of the greatest and most lasting expressions of a parent's love—beyond the gifts of protection, security, and provision for physical needs—is the gift of time. The cultural myth of "quality time"—so much a part of the late-twentieth-century's parenting lexicon—should be debunked. Parents should be encouraged to be near and available to their children for as much time as possible, particularly during periods of significant transition. The economic requirements of modern life put undeniable constraints on the amount of time many parents can spend with their children. Nonetheless, even single, working parents can be encouraged to put aside the 30–40 minutes it takes to talk to their children about the day or play a family game. Parents often underestimate the efficacy of simple encouragement, but there is no question that the support and love of a parent can do more than almost anything else to sustain children through times of difficulty and change. In both words and behavior, parents should be encouraged to convey to their children the message: "This is a difficult time for you and for our family. But I know that better times are ahead, and I know that you, and we, can move through it together."

B. It may be helpful for parents to make special efforts to uphold and adhere to **family rituals and routines** during times of transition. For children at all developmental stages, clinging to the enduring, predictable aspects of day-to-day life may be especially helpful during periods of overwhelming change. Parents may know this already, having observed the tenacity and persistence with which children follow routine. Events as mundane as eating dinner together each night, reading together as a family, or taking a daily walk may take on special significance for children during times of upheaval in their family's life.

C. Families may find that it is helpful to children, when possible, to **reduce the rate of environmental changes.** Stress research suggests that it is usually not the isolated stressor that is deleterious to children's health and well-being but rather the cumulative effects of multiple stressors over a relatively brief period of time. A proliferation of such stressors is likely to occur, for example, during a divorce, when the painful loss of a parent's presence is attended by a wide variety of other changes, such as the selling of the family home, residential moves to new communities and schools, the loss of peer relationships, and the alterations in routine that accompany change in a parent's employment status. When possible, parents should consider slowing the rapidity with which such changes occur, allowing children to spread their adaptive efforts over a longer span of time.

D. **Fantasy and play** are natural, effective means of coping for young children in difficult transitions. Most children instinctively use imaginative play to process and work through the emotionally conflictive aspects of a transitional event. Parents may support these adaptive efforts by allowing children sufficient time for play, by engaging them in imaginative games and conversations about the event, by encouraging the use of art and drawing, and, most important, by not stifling or discouraging their playing through troubling or difficult aspects of their experiences. It has been noted, for example, that among children living in war-torn areas of the world, those children able to "play war" are more likely to show adaptive strengths and sustain positive developmental outcomes.

E. Clinicians and parents should share with children the **personal coping strategies** that have helped them to lighten the difficulties they have encountered during major life transitions. Adaptive hints—such as approaching transitions a single day at a time or dividing the task into smaller steps of graded intensity—may provide substantial benefits to children who have attained sufficient cognitive development to understand such concepts. Among latency-age and older children, parents can teach the importance of pacing oneself by allowing adequate time during periods of stress for sleep, relaxation, and play. With adolescents and young adults, parents and clinicians can encourage the displacement of emotional distress onto physical activities, such as vigorous exercise and competitive athletics.

F. Parents should be encouraged to provide for their children, as a preventive measure for later stressful experiences, opportunities for the **development of competence and mastery.** Parents often fail to place meaningful responsibilities in the hands of children, thereby disallowing the discovery of their own competencies and talents. Even preschool children can be given meaningful household tasks that support the collective life of the family. Responsibilities of increasing difficulty and significance can be progressively shared as children grow. Taken together over the span of years, these opportunities for the production of meaningful work can support the development of a child's sense of mastery and personal confidence in facing the vicissitudes of life. Parents may also need, at times, to foster the development of mastery by gently urging children into situations that tax or stretch their abilities. An extremely shy or inhibited child, for example, may need to be quietly but persistently encouraged to join a soccer team in order to discover her or his innate athletic abilities. Through such experiences of bearing responsibility and engaging in controlled risk taking, children become increasingly aware of their internal strengths and their adaptive capabilities.

Bibliography

Boyce WT. Life events and crises. In Green M, Haggerty RJ (eds), *Ambulatory Pediatrics* (4th ed), Philadelphia: Saunders, 1990.

Haggerty RJ, Garmezy N, Rutter M, Sherrod LR. *Stress, Risk, and Resilience in Children and Adolescents: Processes, Mechanisms, and Intervention.* Cambridge: Cambridge University Press, 1993.

Rutter M. Pathways from childhood to adult life. *J Child Psychol Psychiatry* 30(1):23–51, 1989.

Shonkoff JP, Jarman FC, Kohlenberg TM. Family transitions, crises, and adaptations. *Cur Probl Pediatr* 17(9):507–553, 1987.

13

Self-Regulation Therapy

Karen Olness

Training in self-regulation is useful for health professionals and for the children and adolescents they serve. Ongoing studies are comparing the cost-effectiveness and societal impact of self-regulation training methods with other treatments. For example, training in self-hypnosis prevents migraine episodes in children, and this may reduce the enormous morbidity associated with adult migraine. Early training in self-regulation may extinguish negative conditioned physiologic responses, such as tachycardia, and thereby avoid more complex adult problems. Perhaps most important, such training provides a sense of coping ability and mastery in children. The average child learns quickly, and initial training requires only a few office visits.

I. Definitions

A. Cyberphysiology is the process of governing or controlling one's own physiologic responses.

B. Biofeedback is a strategy of cyberphysiology that provides visual or auditory evidence of physiologic changes. A bathroom scale and a blood pressure monitor, for example, are biofeedback devices. Machines designed to provide feedback of autonomic responses (e.g., galvanic skin resistance, peripheral temperature, heart rate, and electromyographic responses) have been used therapeutically.

C. Hypnotherapy is a strategy of cyberphysiology that refers to focusing attention on specific mental images for therapeutic purposes. It often, but not always, involves relaxation. Children, for example, may be physically active when practicing self-hypnosis. All hypnosis is, in fact, self-hypnosis. When those who teach self-hypnosis choose methods consistent with a patient's interests, learning styles, and imagery preferences, it is likely that any motivated person can learn self-hypnosis.

II. Self-regulation in pediatrics

A. Applications. The child health professional may recommend training in a cyberphysiologic strategy as primary or adjunct treatment for a number of problems (Table 13-1). Numerous clinical reports and prospective controlled studies have documented the efficacy of self-regulation in general categories of pain management, chronic illness, habits, and individual performance. In general, training in self-hypnosis is a suitable adjunct to reducing pain, anxiety, nausea, vomiting, and other symptoms associated with chronic disease.

B. Principles of self-regulation treatment

1. Assess the **presenting problem** to rule out biologic causes that may require other types of treatment.

2. Assess the interest of the child and his or her **willingness to practice self-regulation techniques.** If the problem is primarily of concern to the parent and not the child, the child may not wish to invest the requisite time.

3. Determine the **child's interests, likes, dislikes, fears, and learning patterns** in order to choose an approach that is likely to be appealing and practical. For example, a 10-year-old boy who likes computer games may be highly motivated by relaxation training associated with computer feedback of his peripheral temperature and galvanic skin resistance.

4. Because self-regulation is the job of the child, not the parents, **teach the**

Table 13-1. Applications of self-regulation in pediatrics

Pain management
  Acute (procedures in office or emergency room)
  Chronic (sickle cell disease, hemophilia, recurrent headaches, etc.)
Habit problems
  Thumbsucking
  Trichotillomania
  Simple tics
  Enuresis
  Habit cough
Reduction of anxiety in chronic conditions
  Malignancies
  Hemophilia
  Sickle cell disease
  Lupus erythematosus
  Tourette syndrome
  Diabetes
Improved performance
  Sports
  Drama
  Music
  Tests
Control of conditions involving autonomic dysregulation
  Raynaud's phenomenon
  Reflex sympathetic dystrophy
  Dyshydrosis
  Conditioned hyperventilation
  Conditioned dysphagia
Other
  Insomnia
  Warts
  Conditioned hives
  Eating problems

---

child without the presence of parents, although they may be present during the initial part of the interview. It is important to say, in the presence of both child and parent, "Your mother is not allowed to remind you to practice. On the way home you can discuss a way to remind yourself to practice, for example, a sign on your bedroom door."

5. Be certain the child **understands something about the mechanism of the problem.** This can be achieved by simple drawings and concrete language (e.g., diagramming the urinary tract or a pain pathway).

6. Emphasize your **role as a coach or a teacher.** You are not forcing the child to practice; you only coach him or her to do so. The child decides if and when he or she will do it.

7. Communicate in a way that increases the **child's sense of coping and mastery.** For example, say to a child who is in an isolation room after a bone marrow aspiration, "You've done very well in your biofeedback practice. You can decide whether to practice in the morning or afternoon and, when you're ready, you can show your mom how you do it."

8. Help the child **predict how life would be different if she or he no longer had the problem.** What would be different? What is the desired outcome? A child with no picture of the benefits may not be ready for the self-regulation intervention.

9. Plan, with the child, some **system to record progress,** such as a calendar or sticker chart. It is important to record not only symptoms and their severity but also the frequency of practice.

C. Self-regulation training

1. **Imagery.** Self-regulation involves directing a child's imagination to focus attention, at which time the child can give herself or himself instructions to regulate or control a sensation, physiologic function, or action. The teacher or coach suggests imaginary involvement that is appealing and asks the child to focus on this until she or he is ready to accept suggestions related to the problem. The child can indicate readiness by lifting a "yes" finger, nodding, or saying, "I'm ready." For example, a child can imagine riding a bicycle to a favorite place and take all the time she or he needs to arrive there. Most children enjoy being offered such control and, after a few minutes, signal their arrival at the special place.

2. **Control.** Giving a child some control in a training session is not only therapeutically sound but also aids in determining if she or he is interested in resolving a habit or performance problem. If the child does not reach the special place on the imaginary bicycle, for example, this may be evidence that she or he is not motivated to change or has not understood what is being taught (or perhaps does not like bike riding). The use of "canned" instructions removes the child's ability to choose and is therefore contraindicated.

3. **Therapeutic suggestions** should be consistent with the child's wishes and previous explanations. The health professional and child should have agreed on the purpose of the visit and should be very clear about what the child wishes to achieve. Suggestions to a child to awaken herself or himself to get out of bed and go to the bathroom will seem strange to the child if they have not been previously discussed. Suggestions should be concrete and refer to language used in earlier explanations and drawings—for example, "When you're ready, you can tell your bladder to send a message to your brain to wake you up when the bladder is full. Tell your brain to wake you up completely and send a message to your legs to get out of bed and walk to the toilet."

4. **Access to the child health professional.** Because parents should not be reinforcers, the child must be able to ask the teacher about the practice, when necessary. Ordinarily a follow-up review visit should take place within 10 days.

5. **Early training for children with chronic diseases.** It is much more efficient and effective to train very young children with chronic diseases such as hemophilia or sickle cell diseases in self-regulation. Children who have developed conditioned anxiety, nausea, and other symptoms associated with procedures can also benefit from self-regulation training, but in general, much more training time is required.

D. **Anticipatory guidance.** Clinicians may choose to include teaching self-regulation in their anticipatory guidance. For example, preschoolers may be encouraged to tell stories during physical examinations. They can be asked, "Where would you like to be?" If the child responds, "At the playground" or "Playing on the swings," the clinician says, "Good. Pretend you're there right now. Tell me about it." This type of interaction can be repeated and becomes useful if painful procedures are required at some later time. For younger children who must undergo procedures, nurses, clinic assistants, and parents can be instructed in holding techniques that give a child a sense of control (e.g., sitting upright on a nurse's lap). A supply of pop-up books, headphones, tapes of appropriate music or stories, or bubbles are excellent distractors that mitigate the distress of procedures.

Regardless of whether the child health professional decides to study this area in formal workshops, he or she can practice using language in a way that is encouraging and inspires confidence. For example, during a visit for a minor injury, the clinician may say, "When you go home, what's the first thing you will do?" or "Your blood looks strong and healthy." These simple messages reiterate that a positive outcome is expected and engender, hopefully, a self-fulfilling prophecy.

III. **Training for the professional.** The most practical training is a beginning pediatric hypnotherapy course sponsored by the Society of Behavioral Pediatrics or the Society

Table 13-2. Organizations providing training in hypnotherapy

American Society of Clinical Hypnosis
2200 East Devon Avenue, Suite 291
Des Plaines IL 60018
(708)297-3317

Association for Applied Psychophysiology and Biofeedback
10200 West 44th Avenue, #304
Wheat Ridge CO 80033

Society for Behavioral Pediatrics
241 East Gravers Lane
Philadelphia PA 19118
(215)248-9168

Society for Clinical and Experimental Hypnosis
6728 Old McLean Village Drive
McLean VA 22101
(703)556-9222

University of Minnesota Department of Continuing Medical Education
UMHC Box 203
Room 3-110, Owre Hall
University of Minnesota Medical School
Minneapolis MN 55455
(612) 626-7600

Note: When writing to these societies for information, include a self-addressed stamped envelope.

for Clinical and Experimental Hypnosis. These 3-day workshops are organized for those who work with children and adolescents.

The American Society of Clinical Hypnosis provides 3-day workshops in basic hypnosis on a monthly basis in cities around the United States. These focus primarily on problems of adults. Several universities, such as the University of Minnesota, provide annual 3-day workshops in basic or advanced hypnotherapy (Table 13-2).

The Association for Applied Psychophysiology and Biofeedback provides some basic training in biofeedback instrumentation. In general, unless one is anticipating doing research in this area, it is not necessary to become familiar with complex biofeedback systems. Simple devices such as bio-bands, bio-dots, Radio Shack thermistors, or Calmpute products provide sufficient feedback for most children and are inexpensive.

Bibliography

For Parents

No Fears, No Tears Canadian Cancer Society, 955 West Broadway, Vancouver BC. V5Z 3X8, Canada.
Videotape for parents of children with cancer.

Mind Body Medicine Consumer Reports, Coleman D, Gurin J (eds). Yonkers, NY: Consumer Reports Books, 1993.

For Professionals

Olness K, Gardner GG. *Hypnosis and Hypnotherapy for Children* (2nd ed) Philadelphia: Saunders, 1988.

Hilgard H, Hilgard E. *Hypnosis in the Relief of Pain*. Los Altos CA: William Kaufmann, 1983.

Kohen DP, Olness K. Hypnotherapy with children. In Rhue J, Lynn S, Kirsch I (eds), *Handbook of Clinical Hypnosis*. Washington DC: American Psychological Association, 1993.

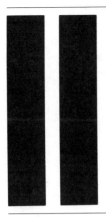

Specific Child Problems

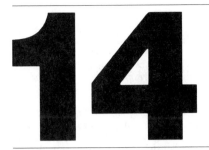

Anorexia Nervosa and Bulimia

Alain Joffe

I. **Description of the problem.** There is no simple definition for the eating disorders termed anorexia nervosa and bulimia nervosa. In fact, a young woman may suffer from both disorders simultaneously or develop one after having first manifested symptoms of the other. More useful than a definition is a description of the behaviors and feelings that are so intimately associated with each disorder that they have come to define the illness itself:

- With **anorexia nervosa,** the young woman has such an overwhelming fear of fatness and an unrelenting drive to be thin that she restricts food intake even as her weight continues to fall further below ideal body weight (usually at least 15% below). In this regard, *anorexia* is a misnomer; until the advanced stages of the illness, these patients experience hunger but deny it.
- Patients with **bulimia nervosa** also manifest a persistent concern with body shape and weight but, in addition, recurrently experience a loss of control and binge eat. They subsequently attempt to prevent the anticipated weight gain through a variety of means, such as vomiting, exercise, or laxative use.

A. **Epidemiology**
- It is estimated that up to 1% of white females may have anorexia nervosa, especially with certain risk factors, such as high socioeconomic status or groups for whom thinness is essential for success (such as ballet dancers and models). The age of onset is bimodal, with peaks at 13–14 and 17–18 years of age.
- The prevalence of bulimia is not known. Estimates are that as many as 3% of college-age females meet strict psychiatric diagnostic criteria for this disorder. The age of onset is slightly older than that for anorexia.
- Males account for less than 10% of individuals with eating disorders.
- Anorexia and bulimia are most prevalent among Caucasian women, although the disorders are being seen increasingly among diverse racial and ethnic groups.

B. **Genetics**
1. The concordance rate among monozygotic twins is 55% (versus 7% for dizygotic pairs) for anorexia, suggesting a genetic basis for this disorder. First-degree relatives of probands are eight times more likely to develop anorexia than suitable controls.

2. The concordance rate for monozygotic twins with bulimia (22.9%) is higher than that for dizygotic pairs (8.7%).

3. Some studies suggest an increased risk for affective disorders in the first-degree relatives of patients with eating disorders compared to the general population.

C. **Etiology**
1. **Environmental.** Our society places a premium on being thin, especially for women. Thinness is often equated, implicitly or explicitly, with success, attractiveness, and self-control. Not surprisingly, women who must be thin to be successful have the highest rates of eating disorders.

2. **Organic.** During female puberty, there is a widening of the hips and increased deposition of adipose tissue. These normal changes run counter to social messages to be thin, leading to a preoccupation with weight and a dissatisfaction with one's emerging body shape.

Patients with anorexia nervosa, bulimia nervosa, or both have been shown to have a large number of metabolic, hormonal, and neurotransmitter abnormalities. However, many (perhaps most) of the abnormalities noted can result from starvation or from the binging-purging behaviors associated with eating disorders, thereby precluding a straightforward cause-and-effect relationship from being established.

3. **Developmental.** Anorexia can be viewed as a defense against the increasing demands of maturity. Because these young women have a sense of personal ineffectiveness (despite academic achievement), difficulty in separating from their families, and obsessive personalities, the focus on control of appetite and food refusal provides a measure of success, a sense of identity, and a feeling of control.

Enmeshment is characteristic of the families of patients with eating disorders. In the case of anorexia nervosa, families are often described as overprotective and rigid, with an inability to express emotion and resolve conflicts. Bulimic patients tend to have family relationships that are chaotic and characterized by hostility.

4. **Transactional.** Our cultural emphasis on thinness provides the backdrop against which the intrapersonal and intrafamilial factors can operate in an individual who is biologically vulnerable. Once weight loss or abnormal eating behaviors or both are established and secondary physiologic changes develop that sustain the abnormal behaviors, the young woman becomes locked into a stereotypic pattern that is all but impossible to break.

II. Making the diagnosis

A. **Signs and symptoms.** Young women rarely disclose their eating disorder to their primary care clinician. Just as anorexics deny hunger as they pursue the ideal body shape, so too will they ignore or cover up various manifestations of their illness. For example, they may wear bulky clothing in an attempt to hide their weight loss. Similarly, patients with bulimia will be quite secretive about their binging (which occurs alone) and about their use of laxatives or diuretics to minimize weight gain. Hence, the clinician must maintain a high index of suspicion and gently but firmly pursue the diagnosis when symptoms suggest or are consistent with an eating disorder.

The signs and symptoms associated with eating disorders are highlighted in Table 14-1. The adolescent who has both anorexia and bulimia will manifest signs and symptoms of both. Girls who develop anorexia early in puberty will present with failure to gain the weight normally expected with physical maturation or with the delayed onset of secondary sexual characteristics and primary amenorrhea.

B. **Differential diagnosis.** In developing a differential diagnosis, clinicians should remember that patients with illnesses whose signs and symptoms are similar to anorexia and bulimia generally indicate discomfort with these manifestations and do not have a persistent and overriding concern with body shape and weight. While they may initially be pleased with an unexpected weight loss, they become alarmed as their weight continues to fall. A list of diseases that can mimic these disorders is presented in Table 14-2. A careful physical examination and a few screening tests (such as an erythrocyte sedimentation rate and thyroxine level) will generally exclude these diagnoses.

C. **History: Key clinical questions.** Clinicians should focus their questions in the following areas:
- weight and dietary history
- patient concerns about being fat
- perceptions of body image
- methods used to lose weight or prevent weight gain
- exercise patterns
- symptoms of concomitant affective disorder
- details of binging and purging episodes
- use of drugs and alcohol

Table 14-1. Signs and symptoms of eating disorders

	Anorexia Nervosa	Bulimia Nervosa
General	Hyperactivity or lethargy Irritability Sleep problems Dizziness, confusion Syncope Hypothermia	Puffy face
Skin	Subcutaneous fat loss Dry, brittle hair or loss of hair Lanugo hair Yellow skin	Ulcerations, scars, or calluses on back of hand (over knuckles)
Oral		Dental caries Enamel erosion or discoloration of teeth (posterior surface) Parotid gland hypertrophy
Cardiovascular	Hypotension Bradycardia	Arrhythmias
Gastrointestinal	Constipation Decreased bowel sounds	Epigastric tenderness Abdominal distension Ileus
Neuromuscular	Muscle weakness/wasting Decreased deep tendon reflexes	Muscle weakness/wasting (with chronic use of ipecac) Decreased deep tendon reflexes
Extremities	Cold, mottled hands and feet	Edema of feet (and perhaps hands)
Genitourinary	Thin, pale, dry, atrophic vaginal mucosa	
Musculoskeletal	Osteopenia/fractures	

Note: Patients with both disorders may have signs or symptoms of both.

Table 14-2. Differential diagnosis of eating disorders

CNS	Hypothalamic disorders (e.g., brain tumor)
Endocrine	Addison's disease Diabetes mellitus Hyperthyroidism
Gastrointestinal	Inflammatory bowel disease Achalasia Malabsorption syndromes
Immunologic	Systemic lupus erythematosus
Gynecologic	Pregnancy
Psychiatric	Depression Thought disorders
Miscellaneous	Any undetected malignancy Drug abuse (e.g., amphetamines, alcohol)

1. *How do you feel about your current weight?* Begins to elicit information about fear of fatness and distortion of body image (e.g., feeling fat or wanting to lose "just a few more pounds," even when the teenager appears emaciated).

2. *What is the most and least you have ever weighed, and how old were you at each of those times?* Establishes baseline measurements. Updating of growth charts will also be helpful.

3. *When you look at yourself in the mirror, which parts of your body look best or worst? Why?* Addresses the issue of body shape. Patients usually identify thighs, hips, and buttocks as being too fat.

4. *Tell me what you ate for breakfast, lunch, dinner, and snacks yesterday. Was this a typical day for you?* Establishes caloric intake and food preferences and may indicate distorted thoughts about food. Information must be obtained in great detail (e.g., what was on the sandwich, how much of it was eaten).

5. *Tell me about your exercise routine. Have you increased the amount of exercise you do lately?* Patients with eating disorders exercise intensely as a way to increase caloric expenditure; those with bulimia will do so to compensate for binge eating.

6. *How often do you weigh yourself and at what times?* Addresses concerns about being fat, as well as distorted thinking about weight and compulsive behaviors.

7. *How would you generally describe your mood—happy, sad, down, something else? How did you feel last year?* Depression is commonly associated with eating disorders, either as a primary or secondary phenomenon.

8. *Which of the following have you used to control your weight: laxatives, water pills (diuretics), enemas, ipecac, diet pills?* These represent commonly used weight loss methods. Any positive answers should be followed up with questions about current use and frequency of use.

For patients with bulimia (alone or in combination with anorexia), the following should also be included:

9. *How often do you binge? Tell me what you eat when you binge.* A true binge includes consumption of large quantities of food—often several thousand or more calories. Conversely, some young women mistakenly interpret eating a few cookies or an ice cream sundae as a "binge."

10. *How do you feel before and after you binge? Are there situations or feelings that trigger binge episodes?* Binge eating typically is associated with feelings of lack of control, self-deprecation, and guilt. Binges are often triggered by a specific set of feelings or situations.

11. *How often do you vomit after a binge episode? What do you do to make yourself vomit?* These questions elicit details of the binge-purge cycle. Use of emetics such as ipecac can lead to life-threatening complications.

D. **Behavioral observations.** While eliciting the history, it is important to note the patient's general affect and willingness to answer questions directly. Patients with eating disorders often minimize their symptoms, typically showing little concern for a degree of weight loss that others would find alarming. The interviewer should also note the quality of any interactions between patient and family, such as who answers questions and how family members regard each other.

E. **Physical examination.** Key aspects of the physical examination are noted in Table 14-1. Patients with a relatively greater degree of weight loss display more of these features. Conversely, patients with bulimia alone may display few physical findings and be of normal weight or even slightly heavy. Patients must be undressed completely (except for a gown and underpants) in order to assess their physical condition accurately.

F. **Tests.** Women with severe anorexia nervosa or bulimia will have many abnormal laboratory tests, but it is not essential to identify all of them. Table 14-3 sets out

Table 14-3. Laboratory values in eating disorders

Hematologic	Anemia (mild)
	Leukopenia
	Thrombocytopenia
Endocrine	Follicle-stimulating hormone/luteinizing hormone: low/low normal
	Thyroxine/thyroid-stimulating hormone: low/low normal
GI	SGOT/SGPT normal or elevated
	Salivary amylase increased
Renal	Hematuria, pyuria, proteinuria
	BUN normal or elevated
	Urine pH > 7
	Urine specific gravity normal or elevated
Metabolic	Metabolic alkalosis
	Decreased NA^+, K^+, Cl^-
	Ca^{++} normal or low
	Mg^{++}, $PO_4^=$ normal or low
	Increased $CO_2^=$
ECG	Low voltage
	Bradycardia
	Depressed T waves

the most commonly noted abnormalities, which can help to confirm or eliminate the diagnosis or identify potentially life-threatening conditions.

III. Management

A. Primary goals. Some restoration of weight is the primary goal in the treatment of patients with severe anorexia nervosa. Until this goal is achieved, disordered cognition and/or depression due to malnutrition may inhibit the success of other therapies. Other goals for patients with eating disorders include:
- education about nutrition and appropriate eating patterns
- improvement in personal and social functioning
- improvement in family functioning
- correction of medical complications
- treatment of concomitant conditions (e.g., depression, drug and alcohol abuse)

B. Treatment. Management of a young woman with an eating disorder depends on a number of factors: the stage of the illness at which the patient is diagnosed; whether the patient has anorexia, bulimia, or the two together; the clinician's assessment of the family dynamics and the level of support likely to be offered by her family; the presence of a concomitant affective disorder and/or substance abuse problem; and the skill of the clinician in working with these patients. In general, younger patients with supportive families who have had relatively brief symptoms of an eating disorder without significant comorbidity can be effectively managed by the primary care clinician on an outpatient basis.

The optimal outpatient treatment of most patients occurs with a multidisciplinary treatment team, consisting of a pediatric clinician, a nutritionist, a mental health worker, and a nurse. More complicated patients or those with a long-standing eating disorder will likely require an initial inpatient treatment program. Immediate hospitalization is necessary if any of the conditions in Table 14-4 is present.

The primary care clinician is ideally suited to serve as the coordinator of the treatment process. Often he or she has a long-standing relationship with the patient and her family and can best explain to them the nature and severity of the illness. The clinician can also assume the role of monitoring weight gain and the potential medical complications of the illness (such as amenorrhea or hypokalemia).

1. **Weight gain.** Patients should be weighed weekly dressed in a gown and underpants only. They should urinate before being weighed. Emphasis on a slow but steady weight gain (1–2 lb/week) is critical since patients with

Table 14-4. Indications for hospitalizing an anorexic or bulimic patient

Weight more than 30% below normal weight

Continued weight loss despite treatment

Rapid weight loss (over 3 months)

Cardiovascular compromise
  Cardiac arrhythmias
  Postural hypotension (so-called grayouts) or systolic blood pressure less than
    70 mm Hg
  Bradycardia (slower than 40–50 bpm)

Hypothermia (less than 36°C)

Psychiatric conditions
  Suicidal ideation or intent
  Out-of-control behavior
  Unsupportive family (family crisis)

Electrolyte disturbances (e.g., K^+ less than 2.5 mEq/liter)

Significant dehydration

Other stresses in a compromised host (e.g., infection)

Need to confirm diagnosis in the face of an unusual or uncertain presentation

From Joffe A. Too little, too much: Eating disorders in adolescents.
Contemp Pediatr 7:129, 1990. Copyright © 1990 Medical Economics Company Inc. Montvale,
NJ. Reprinted by permission.

significant malnutrition will not benefit from any additional therapy, and too rapid weight gain may increase anxiety about becoming fat, leading to purging behaviors. The target weight should be the fiftieth percentile for the patient's height and pubertal development. Restoration of menses is a reliable indicator that an appropriate weight threshold has been achieved. Generally, patients tolerate an initial caloric intake of 1200–1500 kcal/day, with increments of roughly 500 kcal/week until the patient gains at least 1 lb/week. It will be necessary for the clinician or nutritionist to be very specific about what kinds of foods the young woman will need to eat in order to reach her daily caloric requirements. Many young women with eating disorders will have developed a long list of "forbidden" foods and will need considerable support in changing their diet.

2. **Restrictions on activities and privileges,** perhaps in a written format, will likely be necessary, both as a means to ensure the safety of an underweight patient and to provide an incentive to gain weight.

3. **Body image.** Much of the ongoing treatment will revolve around addressing the young woman's concerns about her body shape and fear of fatness. The clinician can review with her what happens to a young woman's body as she matures (e.g., the hips widen) and that these changes do not indicate that the patient is becoming fat. Many young women find it helpful to know that their peers are struggling with the same issues and that our society creates unreasonable expectations for them in terms of defining characteristics for physical attractiveness and success.

4. **Nutrition.** In conjunction with the nutritionist, the role of proper nutrition as critical to appropriate physiologic functioning should be stressed. Since many patients with eating disorders are concerned with athletics, it may be helpful to indicate that optimal performance requires adequate intake of essential nutrients. Many adolescents (and their parents) have inaccurate information about the caloric content of various foods and the appropriate diet for a maturing adolescent. It is important to stress, for example, that a low calcium diet, coupled with a hypoestrogenic state, can lead to osteopenia, which may not be reversible with weight gain. Many of the symptoms the patient experiences and finds distressful are due to physiologic alterations secondary to weight loss; clarifying this relationship will lend credence to the team's insistence on weight gain.

5. **Purging products.** Teenagers may not be aware that regular use of diuretics, laxatives and weight loss pills can induce, at most, a weight loss of only 1–2 lb but can induce a variety of life-threatening complications. The clinician should routinely ask if patients have used or are using any of these products or to what extent they are purging. (Monitoring of a fractionated serum amylase for the salivary component can be useful in determining whether someone has indeed been vomiting.)

6. **Family dynamics and problems** that contribute to the eating disorder must also be assessed. Treatment goals and expectations among team members and the family must be clear so that the patient, family members, and members of the treatment team are not pitted one against another. The primary care clinician can play a critical role in coordinating these efforts and ensuring that everyone is in agreement with treatment plans.

Bibliography

For Parents

Pamphlets
Eating Disorders. Available from the American College Health Association, P.O. Box 28937, Baltimore, MD 21240-8937, FAX for orders: (301) 843-0159.

Organizations
American Anorexia/Bulimia Association, 418 East 76th Street, New York, NY 10021, (212) 734-1114.

Anorexia Nervosa and Related Eating Disorders (ANRED), P.O. Box 5102, Eugene, OR 97405, (503) 344-1144.

Bulimia and Anorexia Self-Help, 6125 Clayton Avenue, Suite 215, St. Louis, MO 63139, (314) 567-4080 or (800) 762-3334 (crisis hot line).

National Anorexic Aid Society, 5796 Karl Road, Columbus, OH 43229 (614) 436-1112.

National Association of Anorexia Nervosa and Associated Disorders, P.O. Box 7, Highland Park, IL 60035, (312) 831-3438.

For Professionals
Andersen AE. *Practical Comprehensive Treatment of Anorexia Nervosa and Bulimia.* Baltimore: Johns Hopkins University Press, 1985.

Comerci GD, Williams RL. Eating disorders in the young. Part 1: Anorexia nervosa and bulimia. *Curr Prob Pediatr* 15:7–57, 1985.

Coupey SM. Anorexia nervosa in Friedman SB, Fisher M, Schonberg SK (eds). *Comprehensive Adolescent Health Care.* St. Louis: Quality Medical Publishing, 1992.

Johnson C. Initial consultation for patients with bulimia and anorexia nervosa. In Garner DM, Garfinkel PE (eds). *Handbook of Treatment for Anorexia Nervosa and Bulimia.* New York: Guilford Press, 1985.

Yates A. Current perspectives on the eating disorders: Part I. History, psychological and biologic aspects. *J Am Acad Child Adolesc Psychiatry* 28:813–829, 1989.

Yates A. Current perspectives on the eating disorders: Part II: Treatment, outcome and research directions. *J Am Acad Child Adolesc Psychiatry* 29:1–9, 1990.

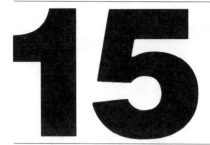

Articulation Disorders

Rebecca McCauley

I. **Description of the problem.** Articulation, or phonologic, disorders consist of a delay or difference in speech sound acquisition, resulting in speech that is difficult to understand or sounds immature. Many children with these disorders are at risk for social-emotional and learning difficulties because of their poor speech. When severe, these disorders are called "developmental dyspraxia of speech."

A. **Epidemiology.** Phonologic disorders have a prevalence of 5% in the school-aged population and 10% in younger children. Risk is increased for boys and children with mental retardation. Whereas almost all children (99.5%) will outgrow this disorder by adolescence, its academic and social-emotional consequences nonetheless make identification and treatment an important goal.

B. **Familial transmission/genetics.** A familial basis for severe forms of phonologic disorder has recently been suggested. Family histories of children with phonologic disorder are often positive for other speech and language disorders and dyslexia.

C. **Etiology/contributing factors**

1. **Organic.** Early and chronic periods of otitis media are an important risk factor, present in about one-third of children with phonologic disorders. There is little evidence that an abnormally short lingual frenulum affects articulation and ambiguous evidence for the role of infantile swallow (tongue thrust) in the disorder.

2. **Developmental.** Diagnosis before age 3 is difficult because young children are highly variable in their speech sound productions. However, infrequent vocalizations or feeding or swallowing problems may indicate oromotor problems that can predispose the child to phonologic disorders.

3. **Transactional.** Subtle neurologic differences are thought to underlie phonologic disorders and may be exacerbated by the fluctuating conductive hearing loss of otitis media or by other unknown factors.

II. **Making the diagnosis**

A. **Signs and symptoms.** See Table 15-1.

B. **Differential diagnosis.** Conditions resulting in delayed phonologic development include oral anomalies (e.g., submucous cleft palate), hearing impairment, apraxia or dysarthria, and mental retardation. Co-occurrence with language disorders is quite common (60%).

C. **History: Key clinical questions**

1. *How well do you and others understand your child's speech compared to the speech of other children his or her age?* Reduced intelligibility compared to peers is a strong indicator of a phonologic disorder.

2. *Has your child's speech changed much during the past 6 months?* For children up to age 5 years, any response suggesting little change over time is a cause for concern.

3. *How do you and others respond to your child's poor speech? How does your child respond to any negative reactions?* Teasing, frequent corrections, or requests to repeat can make the child frustrated or shy and withdrawn.

Table 15-1. Signs and symptoms of phonologic disorders

Any age	Speech is more difficult to understand than that of peers
	Teasing by others about speech (e.g., about a lisp)
	Shyness about speaking or excessive frustration when not understood
2 years or older	Intelligibility less than 50%
	Consistent errors in the use of the sounds /p,b,m,n,h,w/ or any vowel sounds
	Error patterns
	Consonants at the beginning of words are omitted (e.g., "ow" for "cow")
	A sound is overused (e.g., /p/ is used when /f,t,k/ is expected)
	/k/ or /g/ is used when /t/ or /d/ is expected (e.g., "ko" for "toe")
3 years or older	Intelligibility less than 75%
3½ years or older	Consistent errors in the use of the sounds /f,v,k,g/ or /j/ (e.g., "wu" for "you")
	Consistent errors that assume the following patterns:
	Consonants at the ends of words are omitted
	/t/ or /d/ is used when /k/ or /g/ is expected
4 years or older	Intelligibility less than 100%
5½ years or older	Errors on two or more speech sounds that are obvious enough to call attention to the child's speech

4. ***Does your child have a history of problems with chewing or swallowing?*** This question addresses the possibility of dysarthria or apraxia as part of differential diagnosis.

5. ***Do you ever think your child has day-to-day fluctuations or problems in hearing?*** This question addresses the differential diagnosis for chronic hearing impairment, as well as the issue of fluctuating hearing loss related to otitis media.

D. **Physical examination.** The physical examination can help rule out significant oral anomalies and frank neurologic abnormalities, and provide information about the child's middle ear status.

E. **Tests.** A certified speech-language pathologist can perform testing necessary for confirmation of phonologic disorder.

III. Management

A. **Primary goals.** The primary care clinician's principal goals in phonologic disorders are appropriate referral and management of middle ear status.

B. **Criteria for referral.** Refer to a speech-language pathologist if the child's speech demonstrates any of the signs or symptoms in Table 15-1. Speech-language pathologists in public school systems assess and treat children of all ages with communication disorders. Until recently, treatment before age 4 years was considered ineffective, but newly developed techniques may produce good results in younger children.

IV. Clinical pearls and pitfalls

- Tantrums or indications of extreme frustration from a child over age 3 years because of the parent's inability to understand the child's speech suggest a significant problem in speech development.
- To avoid judging the child in terms of their own speech dialect, clinicians should ask parents to gauge how well the child is understood compared to peers.
- Delays in referral not only can deprive the child of early treatment but can also result in increased parent-child conflict.

Bibliography

For Parents

Prather EM. Help your child learn to speak clearly. In Schrader M (ed), *Parent Articles*. Tucson, AZ: Communication Skill Builders, 1988.

Prather EM. Reasons for delayed speech development. In Schrader M (ed), *Parent Articles*. Tucson, AZ: Communication Skill Builders, 1988.

Williams N. Developmental apraxia. In Schrader M (ed), *Parent Articles*. Tucson, AZ: Communication Skill Builders, 1988.

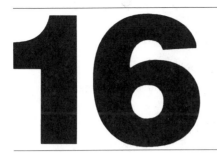

Autism

N. Paul Rosman

I. **Description of the problem.** Autism is a behavioral syndrome of neurologic dysfunction, characterized by impaired reciprocal social interactions, impaired verbal and nonverbal communication, impoverished imaginative activity, and a markedly restricted repertoire of activities and interests.

  A. **Epidemiology.** The prevalence of autism is 5–15 cases/10,000. It is three to four times more frequent in boys. There is no predilection for any racial, ethnic, or socioeconomic group.

  B. **Familial transmission/genetics.** The recurrence risk for autism in families with one affected child is 3–5%. Because many families with an autistic child choose not to have more children, the recurrence risk may be as high as 8½%. Most twin studies of autism have shown high concordance in monozygotic twins (35–95%) and a lower but substantial concordance in dizygotic ones (0–25%). Several studies have found first-degree relatives of autistic children to have an increased frequency of autistic spectrum disorders (e.g., speech-language disorders, learning disabilities, cognitive deficits, and psychiatric disorders).

  C. **Etiology/contributing factors.** Although the etiology of autism is unknown in most cases, an underlying brain disease can occasionally be identified. Examples include congenital infections (rubella, cytomegalovirus, and toxoplasmosis); developmental brain abnormalities (microcephaly or hydrocephalus, with or without accompanying cerebral dysgenesis); metabolic diseases (phenylketonuria and mucopolysaccharidoses); postnatally acquired destructive disorders (herpes simplex encephalitis, bacterial meningitis, and lead encephalopathy); neoplasm (temporal lobe tumor); and genetic disorders (tuberous sclerosis and fragile X syndrome).

  Because the majority of children with such disorders are not autistic, the *location* of the neuropathology, rather than its nature or severity, probably determines the development of autistic behaviors. Cases of idiopathic autism studied neuroradiologically and neuropathologically have shown two primary areas of brain abnormality: the limbic system and the cerebellum. It is unlikely that autism ever has a purely psychologic etiology.

II. **Making the diagnosis**

  A. **Diagnostic features.** It has been suggested that the disorder begins during infancy or childhood with clinical features that include:

    1. **Impaired reciprocal social interaction** (*at least two*)

      a. Lack of awareness of feelings of others

      b. Failure to seek comfort when distressed

      c. Absent or impaired imitation

      d. Absent or abnormal social play

      e. Impaired ability to make peer friendships

    2. **Impaired communication and imaginative activities** (*at least one*)

      a. Absent communication

      b. Abnormal nonverbal communication

      c. Absent imaginative activity

    d. Abnormal speech production

    e. Abnormal speech content

    f. Inability to initiate or sustain conversation

  3. Restricted repertoire of activities and interests (*at least one*)

    a. Stereotyped body movements

    b. Preoccupation with objects

    c. Distress with environmental change

    d. Insistence on following routines

    e. Restricted range of interests

B. Clinical features

  1. Age of onset. Autism has its clinical onset in the first year in about 25% of cases, in the second year in about 50%, and after 2 years in about 25%. Usually a disturbance of communication, both expressive and receptive, first brings the autistic child to attention.

  2. Language impairment. The child's language is nonexistent or immature. It is characterized by echolalia, pronoun reversals, unintelligible jargon, and abnormal melody. Speech content is abnormal, often with verbatim repetition of overlearned, irrelevant, pat sentences (e.g., television commercial jingles). The child typically has difficulty initiating and sustaining a conversation. In contrast with the linguistic deficiencies, the nonverbal abilities in the autistic child are often excellent.

  3. Affect and sociability. Affect varies in the autistic child. Some are withdrawn, others emotionally labile, others overtly anxious. Most seem unaware of the feelings of others. They avoid eye contact and have a profound inability to form friendships with peers or to engage in reciprocal play. Sociability is always deficient, ranging from a complete lack of interest in others to inappropriate intrusiveness with repetitive questioning. Children with autism may develop rote social skills, displaying them as part of a learned routine, rather than spontaneously. Some autistic children do express affection, although it may be indiscriminate.

  4. Play. The play of the autistic child lacks imagination and is often characterized by purposeless and repetitive manipulation of toys. Stereotypic behaviors, such as body rocking, toe walking, and hand flapping, are frequent. Some autistic children show tactile hypersensitivity, while others enjoy physical contact. Many autistic children respond poorly to sounds, while others show auditory hypersensitivity. Some autistic children demonstrate a love of music and an excellent sense of rhythm.

  5. Activity. Autistic children's activity levels are often increased, and their attention span is frequently short, except for things they find fascinating (such as rotating fans, running water, or moving lights). Insistence on following routines and distress when confronted with change are typical. Sleep disorders are common, with trouble falling asleep and nighttime awakenings.

  6. Changes over time. Although some symptoms of autism may diminish as the child grows older, there often are periods of worsening (such as during adolescence). At this time, the autistic child may show heightened overactivity, aggression, and destructive and self-injurious behaviors.

  7. Seizures. Seizures, either generalized or partial (often partial complex), occur in about 15–35% of autistic children. Infancy (often with infantile spasms) and adolescence or early adulthood are the two peaks of greatest frequency. The risk of seizures is highest in autistic children with greatest cognitive delays. The risk is greater still (>40%) when there are also accompanying motor deficits.

  8. Cognitive function. Most children (75%) with autism are mentally retarded, with verbal IQs much lower than performance IQs. Occasionally, the autistic child will show superior "splinter" skills. In such "savants," exceptional talent may be seen in areas such as music, art, memory, calendar calculation, and solving puzzles.

C. Differential diagnosis. Diagnoses to be excluded include the following.

1. **Hearing impairment,** an important cause of delayed and disordered speech.

2. **Developmental language disorder,** in which sociability, activities, and interests are much less deviant than in autism.

3. **Rett's syndrome,** affecting girls only, in whom autistic withdrawal is accompanied by growth failure and loss of hand use.

4. **Disintegrative psychosis,** with a longer period of normal behavior before the onset of regression, often following an environmental stressor.

5. **Landau-Kleffner syndrome** or acquired epileptic aphasia, in which the language disorder is associated with seizure activity and the deviant sociability and interests of autism are lacking.

6. **Schizophrenia,** seen in older children or adults who lack the cognitive deficits and language disturbance of the autistic child.

7. **Undifferentiated mental retardation,** which, when severe, can be accompanied by many of the behavioral characteristics of autism.

D. History: Key clinical questions

1. *What is it that concerns you about your child?* The parent is usually the best judge about the possible presence of a developmental problem in the child.

2. *Do you feel that your child's development is delayed or different?* In autism, there is always developmental delay (especially in speech), as well as developmental deviancy (especially in sociability, activities, and interests).

3. *Has your child lost previously acquired skills, or just failed to develop new ones on schedule?* The autistic child may lose previously acquired speech, especially if there is an accompanying seizure disorder. If many other skills have been lost in addition, a progressive neurologic disorder must be excluded.

4. *Has your child's speech always been delayed, or did it seem normal for a time?* Epileptic aphasia or hearing deficit can cause speech delay, loss of previously acquired speech, or both. In autism, receptive language is more affected than expressive speech.

5. *Are there times when your child simply does not respond to sounds?* Hearing loss and seizures particularly must be investigated.

6. *Are your child's social skills developing normally?* In autism, socialization is always abnormal, especially in playing with other children.

7. *Does your child's play seem to be normal for age?* In autistic children, patterns of play, particularly reciprocal play, are always abnormal.

8. *Does your child show unusual repetitive behaviors, strong likes or dislikes, or resistance to change?* Some repetitive play and insistence on sameness can be normal in a child. In autism these norms are greatly exceeded.

9. *Does your child seem to be improving? If so, what appears to be helping?* What works for one child may not for another, even with the same diagnosis. Treatment plans must always be individualized.

10. *How are you, your spouse, and other members of your family managing?* Autism is a family problem. All members need support.

E. Physical examination. The physical and neurologic examination of the autistic child is of limited value unless there is an identifiable underlying disease. In such circumstances, one may see a cataract (as in congenital rubella), hirsutism (as in Cornelia de Lange syndrome), a fair complexion (as in phenylketonuria), coarsened facies (as in Hurler's syndrome or hypothyroidism), outstanding ears and a long face (as in fragile X syndrome), hypopigmented skin macules (as in tuberous sclerosis), or café-au-lait spots (as in neurofibromatosis). The most common motor abnormality in autism is hypotonia; ataxia is second. There is also a high frequency of left-handedness or ambidexterity.

F. Tests and additional evaluations.

    1. Tests. When the cause of the autism, either from history or examination, is obscure, investigations should be limited. They should include:

        a. A hearing evaluation, including brainstem auditory evoked responses, which are abnormal in about one-third of autistic children.

        b. An electroencephalogram, abnormal in about half of autistic children.

        c. Magnetic resonance imaging of the brain, abnormal in about one-fifth of autistic children.

        d. In selected cases, other laboratory studies are indicated, such as **thyroid function tests; blood lead level; chromosome analysis** (including fragile X), **blood** and **urine amino acids; TORCH** (toxoplasmosis, other, rubella, cytomegalovirus, herpes simplex) **titers;** and **blood serotonin level** (elevated in one-third of autistic children).

    2. Evaluations. All autistic children should have a detailed evaluation by a developmental pediatrician, child neurologist, child psychologist or child psychiatrist, and a speech-language pathologist. Evaluation by an occupational or physical therapist will often prove useful as well.

III. Management

A. Educational/behavioral management. The cornerstones of treatment of the autistic child are special education (with a major focus on enhancement of communication skills) and behavioral management. Classroom structure is important and should include as much one-on-one instruction as possible. Routines should be followed in a regular, predictable fashion. The educational strategies employed should be carried over into the home, with the parents involved as "co-therapists." The child's oral communication often requires supplementation (with gestural language or sign, communication books or boards, computers, and voice-simulation devices). In concert with communication, socialization skills must be fostered. It is important that the child's instruction include teaching of basic life skills, and showing the child how to broaden these skills for use in a variety of settings.

    Behavioral management is an essential component of the treatment plan for every autistic child. Whenever possible, positive reinforcements should be used. It is crucial that such management be carried through in all of the autistic child's environments: home, school, workshop, or other. For periods of increased behavioral upset, physical exercise is often useful. When needed, medication can be employed in a time-limited manner to help make the autistic child more accessible to behavioral interventions. Classic psychotherapy is not useful in management of the autistic child's behavior.

B. Medications. Autistic children who develop seizures should be given anticonvulsants. With partial or generalized seizures, carbamazepine or valproic acid is usually the medication of first choice. Attentional difficulties may benefit from drug treatment. Psychostimulants (such as methylphenidate, dextroamphetamine, or pemoline) can be tried, though these medications are often less effective in autistic children than in nonautistic children with attentional difficulties. Neuroleptics (such as haloperidol or chlorpromazine) can also be useful on a short-term basis for severe behavioral upset. In general, however, psychopharmacology has proved disappointing in the management of autistic children.

C. Support for families. Support for the families of autistic children can include respite care, support groups for parents, sibling groups, and family counseling.

IV. Prognosis. A major determinant of prognosis in childhood autism is the presence or absence of an underlying disorder of the brain and its accessibility to treatment. In general, the previously healthy child with idiopathic autism (in whom autistic withdrawal occurred after a period of normal development) has a better outlook than the child with autism caused by an identifiable disease of brain. In the latter circumstance, the prognosis improves if the brain disease (e.g., herpes simplex encephalitis) or its accompanying symptoms (e.g., seizures) are treatable.

Speech is another important predictor of outcome. In most (but not all) autistic children, speech and language improve with age. In the child who has developed no useful speech by age 5 years, however, the prognosis is almost always poor.

Many autistic children can eventually be integrated into the community: 5–10% will become independent adults (some of whom will seem normal, although vestiges of earlier autistic characteristics often remain), and 25% will show notable developmental progress, achieving considerable vocational and residential independence. Even those who are of good intelligence, however, tend to be underemployed because of their concrete thinking and deviant social skills. The remaining two-thirds of autistic children will continue to be substantially impaired and require a high level of ongoing care. Placement in group homes or custodial institutions is frequently necessary. Not surprisingly, autistic persons with lower IQs have poorer outcomes than those who are brighter.

Bibliography

For Parents

Organization

Autism Society of America, 8601 Georgia Avenue, Suite 503, Silver Spring, MD 20910; (301) 565-0433; fax (301) 565-0834
Provides a wealth of written materials, including newsletters, book lists, meeting schedules, and research updates.

Publication

Powers MD (ed). *Children with Autism: A Parents' Guide*. Rockville MD: Woodbine House, 1989.

For Professionals

Denckla MB, James LS (eds). An update on autism: A developmental disorder. *Pediatrics* (suppl) 87:751–796, 1991.

Edwards DR, Bristol MM. Autism: Early identification and management in family practice. *Am Fam Physician* 44:1755–1764, 1991.

Rapin I. Autism: A syndrome of neurological dysfunction. In Fukuyama Y, Suzuki Y, Kamoshita S, Casaer P (eds), *Fetal and Perinatal Neurology*. Basel: Karger, 1992.

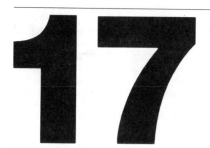

Biting

Barbara Howard

I. Description of the problem

A. Epidemiology
- Almost all children bite at some time during the first 3 years. For example, 50% of toddlers in child care are bitten three times every year. Bites constitute 6% of injuries to males and 3% to females in day care.
- As with most other aggressive behaviors, boys are more likely to bite than girls.
- Biting is more severe or persistent in children with family dysfunction, where physical punishment is used, or when there is chronic stress.
- Acceptability or modeling of violence predisposes to aggressive behaviors, such as biting.

B. Contributing factors

1. **Environmental.** Children are more likely to bite others when they are in social situations beyond their coping abilities. Biting in these situations is usually intended to obtain objects, to gain attention, or to express frustration. It is also a powerful way of acquiring attention from adults. For example, some parents remove the child from the day care setting for the day after a biting incident. Such *secondary gain* from the environment may prolong the biting phase.

2. **Developmental.** Biting emerges at predictable developmental stages.

    a. The first peak, at the **time of tooth eruption,** is rarely reported as a problem since caregivers interpret it as normal experimentation. Interestingly, breast-fed infants generally learn very quickly not to bite the breast, probably because of their mother's shriek, her affective distress, and the prompt removal of the infant.

    b. The next peak in biting occurs around **8–12** months when infants bite as an expression of excitement. A negative, firm response by caregivers generally leads to rapid extinction.

    c. The **second year of life** is normally a time when skills develop unevenly and there is a strong desire to act autonomously. Fledgling or delayed abilities in expressive language and fine motor skills serve to delay gratification and set the child up for frequent outbursts, especially in social situations. Under these circumstances, biting may be used to dominate, to acquire an object, or to express anger or frustration. Additionally, children undergoing stressful separation experiences (such as at day care) may derive satisfaction from causing distress to others by biting. This phase of biting typically disappears quickly.

    d. Biting in children **over age 3 years** should occur only in extreme circumstances (e.g., if they are losing a fight or perceive their survival to be threatened).

II. Recognizing the issue

A. History: Key clinical questions

1. *When did the biting start? What are acute stress events? Was the biting coincidental with new developmental milestones?*

Table 17-1. Techniques to diminish biting in toddlers

Directed to the child
  Provide close supervision.
  Ensure attention to positive behaviors.
  Redirect when anger or frustration appears.
  Verbalize feelings for the child.
  Assess all skill areas and habilitate deficiencies.
  If a bite occurs, shout and place child in time-out.
  Be sure the child receives no interaction in time-out.
  Offer teething ring or cloth to bite.
  If most bites are toward a certain peer, separate the children.
  If biting persists, remove to home or smaller day care.
Directed to the caregivers
  Set consistent limits, especially on aggressive acts.
  Avoid physical punishment or exposure to violence.
  Express negative emotions verbally and stay in control.
  Do not bite back. This models the undesirable behavior, elicits fear and anger in
    the child, and makes the adult feel so guilty that his or her effectiveness in
    limit setting is diminished.
  Ensure that the child is not the least competent in his or her group.
  Ensure that all caregivers are properly responsive and not using physical punish-
    ment.
Directed to the parents if the child is about to be removed from day care
  Seek professional help promptly.
  Meet with day care staff.
  Determine exactly how incidents are being handled.
  Establish a consistent plan for managing incidents (which does not include taking
    the child home, if possible).
  Consider a shorter day in the day care if the child tires.
  Negotiate a time-limited trial of intervention, documenting incidents to determine
    improvement.
  If necessary, move the child to home or a smaller, closely supervised, structured
    setting or one with younger or less aggressive children, or staff who are more
    open to dealing with biting.

2. *In what situations does it occur?* Look for situations in which frustration is common and the child has poor coping skills.

3. *How have you handled it so far?* Determine the previous measures used to address the problem and whether there is any secondary gain for the child to continue to bite.

4. *What other concerns do you have about your child's behavior or development?* Other signs of aggressive behavior or specific developmental delays may point to a more pathological process.

5. *How is anger expressed in your home?* Children may model other family members' behaviors around expression of anger and violence.

6. *Have you had any concerns about how your child is cared for?* Abuse, neglect, violence, or poor-quality care may contribute to the problem.

III. Management

A. Information for the family.
Adults view biting as a very primitive behavior that elicits strong emotional reactions, especially in day care settings. Families need to understand that biting is usually a normal developmental phase and does not predict later aggression.

B. Treatment (Table 17-1)

1. **Determination of cause.** Before formulating a treatment plan, the clinician must determine the reason for the child's biting. Developmental assessment will dictate the need for management of specific delays. Children who are

frustrated by their relative weaknesses in skills compared with peers, for example, often do better when placed with younger children or in a less demanding setting. Other children push themselves to perform beyond their abilities. Such children may need support by arranging same-age peer play, placement in smaller groups, and avoidance of difficult tasks.

2. **Negative reinforcement and redirection.** The chronic biter will need to be observed closely so that appropriate social interactions can be praised and biting encounters interrupted quickly with a shout that declares the seriousness of the offense. The child should then be put in time-out, with a short explanation such as, "I know you are angry, but people are not for biting." Sympathizing with the victim is helpful and may also serve to avoid secondary gain for the biter. Later, the incident can be reviewed with the child and alternatives discussed for negotiating conflict and for expressing feelings. A teething ring can be offered or attached to the clothing, allowing the child expression of the feelings through an acceptable alternative outlet.

3. **Parental attitudes toward aggression.** Parental attitudes toward aggression need to be discussed. Since corporal punishment is a contributor to persistent biting, it should be eliminated. Parents often need coaching to develop appropriate expression of negative affect. Counseling regarding reasonable limits for the child's behavior and nonphysical ways to attain them are the centerpiece of treatment.

4. **Day care setting.** When biting occurs in a day care setting, a crisis often ensues. Having the parents of the victim meet the equally distraught parents of the biter (or even a meeting of the entire center) can help defuse these situations. The nature of the supervision and activities should be evaluated. Preschool children need an active curriculum focused on small-group play with responsive adults who are positive in their interactions and able to redirect untoward behaviors. There also should be enough toys to discourage disputes. Larger toys for shared play are associated with fewer struggles between others. A child in group care who persists in biting often will do better at home or in a family day care setting.

Bibliography

Block RW, Rash FC. *Handbook of Behavioral Pediatrics*. Chicago: Year Book, 1981.

Solomons HC, Elardo R. Biting in day care centers: Incidence, prevention and intervention. *J Ped Health Care* 5:191–196, 1991.

18

Blindness

Albert P. Scheiner

I. **Description of the problem. Legal blindness** is defined as visual acuity in the better eye with a correction of not more than 20/200 or a defect in the visual field so that the widest diameter of vision subtends an angle of 20 degrees. **Residual vision** is defined as insufficient vision to read print of any size. **Partial vision** is defined as vision that interferes with learning but still allows the child to read print. The term **visual impairment** encompasses less severe visual defects and may include such problems as photophobia, color blindness, severe myopia and hyperopia, and unilateral amblyopia.

A. **Epidemiology.** 0.7–3.0 per 10,000 children are considered to be legally blind.

B. **Etiology**

1. **Congenital causes.** Approximately 85% of blindness is congenital in origin. Table 18-1 describes the standard classification of causes and locations of severe congenital visual impairment.

2. **Acquired causes.** Acquired ocular visual impairment constitutes approximately 15% of U.S. children who are blind. Injury is the most common cause, followed by retinoblastoma. Acquired infectious diseases continue to be a major problem in developing countries, with trachoma, onchocerciasis, and vitamin A deficiency as the most common etiologic agents.

3. **Associated disabilities.** Of all children who are blind, 50% have associated disabilities, including mental retardation, cerebral palsy, and epilepsy.

II. **Making the diagnosis**

A. **Neonatal period.** The visual acuity of the newborn has been estimated at somewhere between 20/50 and 20/200. The evaluation of neonatal visual capacity should include:

1. **Careful observation** of the shape and size of the eye and the position of the pupil.

2. The **response of the pupil** to light and the presence of a red reflex in the absence of any opacification.

3. The **ability of a term infant to track** a human face or a patterned black and white object visually for 30–60 degrees horizontally.

B. **Infancy and early childhood.** Initially, eyes may move independently, but a conjugate gaze should be achieved by 6–12 weeks. The presence of strabismus is easily identified by an asymmetrical reflection of light from each pupil. Eyes that do not see well tend to deviate or drift, and this may be the first indication of poor vision. Pupillary responses and a view of an unblemished red reflex with the ability of the infant or child to track are reasonable assurances of adequate vision.

Infants and children who are visually impaired can often be identified by:
• their visual behaviors (Table 18-2)
• abnormal head positions or an effort to view objects at close range.
• parental concern about the infant's inability to fix and follow visually.

C. **Acuity testing.** By age 3 years, many children can cooperate with visual screening. The Allen Card and Multiple E have proved to be the most specific and sensitive measures of visual acuity in preschool children. Any questions con-

Table 18-1. Site and frequent lesions in congenital blindness

Site	Lesion	Approximate percentage
Retina	Retrolental fibroplasia	22.0
	Macular degeneration	2.0
	Retinitis pigmentosa	0.5
Optic Nerve	Optic nerve atrophy and other	20.0
Lens	Cataracts	20.0
Eyeball in general	Albinism	6.0
	Myopia	3.0
Uveal tract	General disorders	5.0
Cornea, sclera		1.0
Vitreous		0.5
Other	Nystagmus	8.0

Table 18-2. Visually related developmental milestones

Term neonate	Alertness to visual stimulus presented 8–12 in. from eyes
1 mo	Follows 60 degrees horizontally, 30 degrees vertically, blinks at approaching object
2 mo	Follows person at 6 ft away, smiles in response to face, raises head 30 degrees from prone
3 mo	Track through 180-degree arc, regards own hand, begins visual motor coordination
4–5 mo	Social smile, reaches for cube 12 in. away, notices raisin 12 in. away
7–8 mo	Picks up raisin by raking
8–9 mo	Pokes at holes in pegboard, neat pincer grasp, crawling
12–14 mo	Stacks blocks, places peg in round hole, stands and walks

cerning vision should be referred to an ophthalmologist, who can provide a comprehensive evaluation.

D. The **differential diagnosis** of the infant who demonstrates a reduced visual response from birth includes:

1. **Severe visual impairment** due to significant ocular problems.

2. **Persistent neurodevelopmental abnormalities** such as mental retardation or cerebral palsy.

3. The presence of **perinatal problems,** such as sequelae of hypoxic-ischemic encephalopathy.

4. **Visual impairment of unknown cause.**

E. **Developmental assessment of blind children**

1. **Cognitive development.** It is difficult to assess the developmental status of the blind infant or child. Sightedness not only plays a role in the ability to perform fine motor tasks, but it also contributes to the development of such concepts as object permanence. Children who are blind and who do not have associated neurological abnormalities achieve developmental milestones at a slower pace but should not be considered delayed.

    The slower developmental milestones are the result of the increased difficulty in apprehending relationships between objects in space. For example, the infant is unable to witness the disappearance of food as it falls to the floor. As a result, object permanence develops with difficulty, occurring only after the infant accidentally touches a toy that has been moved or finds a displaced cookie through taste and smell.

2. **Motor development.** The blind infant achieves motor milestones later than the sighted infant:

   a. **Head raising to 90 degrees in a prone position** is a visually motivated activity and may not be established until 10–12 months.

   b. **Coming to a sitting position** is delayed because of the infant's inability to assess the environment in terms of his or her body's position in space. Although the blind infant can usually sit at the normal 6–8 months, coming to a sitting position and returning to prone is delayed.

   c. **Pulling to stand** and **walking** are similarly delayed due to difficulty in spatial orientation. The child may not crawl at all. Some infants may not walk independently until 2 years.

   d. Many **fine motor activities** are delayed, especially the superior pincer grasp, which may not occur in the presence of a more efficient method of exploring the environment (i.e., a raking movement).

   e. The mouthing of objects along with the tactile exploration, shaking, and banging are **indispensable compensations** for the absence of visual exploration.

3. **Language development.** Language is not delayed except for words and concepts that have visually mediated meanings (such as *big* and *small*).

4. **Emotional development.** The separation/individuation process may be impaired because of the infant's inability to track parents' movements visually. The infant may then be unwilling to separate physically from the tactile security of the parent.

III. **Management**

A. **Primary goals.** The responsibility of the primary care clinician is to interpret and facilitate the infant's behavior and development, to facilitate the family's adaptation to and understanding of the blind child, to coordinate the diagnostic evaluation, and to refer for needed services, such as early intervention programs.

B. **Emotional support**

   1. **Normal grieving.** The typical emotional response of a family is to grieve the loss of the expected sighted child. It is the clinician's task to support parents through the stages of normal grieving and to allow them to express their sadness and anger. While most grief reactions lead to an adaptive accommodation to the child's blindness, some parents do not transcend their grief and become chronically depressed and emotionally unavailable to the infant. This is a devastating experience for any child, and especially so for the blind child. Identification of parental depression and appropriate counseling and referral may be necessary.

C. **Developmental interventions.** Guidelines for developmental interventions with blind children are listed in Table 18-3.

   1. **Infant.** Mobility and orientation should be the early ingredients of any program. Touching, labeling, smelling, and exploring toys and objects encourage the infant to learn about her surroundings and prepare her for preschool education.

   2. **Preschoolers.** Preschoolers without associated significant handicaps can attend a regular, well-structured program with extensive consultation from a teacher of the visually handicapped. The curriculum must be rich in sensory experiences, including objects that can be manipulated and audio programs that will expand the child's knowledge of the world.

   3. **School age.** An individualized curriculum is essential. The school-aged child without significant associated handicapping conditions should participate in regular community-based classroom activities that will prepare him or her for higher education, as well as for independent living.

      Braille continues to be the mainstay of nonvisual communication. The use

Table 18-3. Methods of facilitating the development of the infant who is blind

Developmental skill	Activity
Affective	Supplemental carrying, touching, hugging, comforting
Fine and gross motor (awareness of body image)	Putting bells on extremities; encourage reaching on sound cues; exposing to textured surfaces; placing objects in the infant's hand
Language	Labeling objects, activities; consistently responding to utterances
Cognitive	Searching for objects with sound, smell; touching and labeling objects
Feeding	Providing early exposure to textured foods and self-feeding
Personal and social behavior	Facilitating self-quieting behavior; encouraging self-help skills

of records and tapes presents significant adjuncts to reading. Such instruments as the opticon, which converts the printed word into a form that can be felt with the finger, hold a great deal of promise.

4. Orientation and mobility skills (peripatology)

  a. Orientation requires that a child know his or her present position and space, the destination, and the route he or she will travel.

  b. Mobility refers to the technique for safely and efficiently traveling to a predetermined destination. These skills can later be enhanced with the use of a guide dog or electronic travel aids.

Bibliography

For Parents
American Foundation for the Blind, 15 West 16th Street, New York NY 10011.
A source of a wide variety of information for professionals and parents involved with children who are blind.

American Printing House for the Blind, P.O. Box 6085, Louisville KY 40206.
Assessment and curriculum techniques for children who are blind.

Recording for the Blind, Inc., 215 East 58th Street, New York NY 10022.
Texts and tapes of books for secondary and college students who are blind.

Your state commission for the blind.

Scott EP, Jan JE, Freeman RD. *Can't Your Child See?* Baltimore: Baltimore University Park Press, 1977.

For Professionals
Fraiberg S. *Insights from the Blind.* New York: Basic Books, 1977.
The best description of the developmental characteristics of infants and young children who are visually impaired.

Jan JE, Freeman RD, Scott EP. *Visual Impairment in Children and Adolescents.* New York: Grune and Stratton, 1977.
An excellent, easily readable review of the cause and management of children with visual impairment.

Robinson GC, Jan JE. Acquired ocular visual impairment in children 1960–1989. *AJDC* 147:325–328, 1993.
Epidemiology of blindness in Vancouver BC.

Robinson GC, Jan JE, Kinnis C. Congenital ocular blindness in children 1945–1984. *AJDC* 141:1321–1324, 1987.
Epidemiology of blindness in Vancouver BC.

Scheiner AP, Moomaw M. Care of the visually handicapped child. *Pediatr Rev* 4:74–81, 1982.
Brief overview of the care of the child who is visually handicapped.

Warren DH. *Blindness and Early Childhood Development* (2nd ed). New York: American Foundation for the Blind, 1984.
A comprehensive review of the developmental evaluation of infants and children. An excellent reference that is especially useful for professionals working with children who are blind.

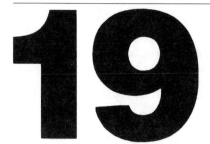

Breath Holding

Barry Zuckerman

I. Description of the problem. Breath-holding spells involve the involuntary cessation of breathing in response to a painful, noxious, or frustrating stimulus. If prolonged, they can lead to loss of consciousness and/or seizures. There are no reported long-term adverse outcomes associated with breath holding.

A. Epidemiology
- The peak frequency is between 1–3 years, although they may begin in the newborn period.
- Breath-holding spells after age 6 years are unusual and warrant further investigation.
- They occur equally in males and females.
- There is a positive family history in approximately 25% of cases.

B. Types

1. Cyanotic spells. The most common type is a cyanotic spell, which is precipitated by anger or frustration. A short burst of crying, usually less than 30 seconds, leads to an involuntary holding of the breath in expiration, resulting in cyanosis that can lead to a loss of consciousness and occasionally a seizure (Table 19-1).

2. Pallid spells. The second type is precipitated by fright or minor trauma (e.g., occipital trauma due to a fall). Following the precipitating event, there is an absence of crying or a single cry, followed by pallor and limpness. This sequence of events is thought to be due to a hyperresponsive vagal response that results in bradycardia (and often asystole), causing pallor and loss of consciousness. Some of these children go on to faint when they are injured or frightened as adults.

II. Making the diagnosis. The key to diagnosis is to differentiate breath-holding spells from seizures (Table 19-2). The presence of a precipitating factor followed by crying and cyanosis before the loss of consciousness and/or seizure is specific to a breath-holding spell. An electroencephalogram is rarely necessary unless a clear precipitating event is not apparent.

III. Management

A. Information for parents.
Breath-holding spells need to be explained and demystified for parents. The clinician should explain, in simple, concrete terms, the sequence of events leading to the loss of consciousness and seizure. The benign nature of these events should be emphasized because parental concerns about epilepsy, brain damage, or death are common.

B. Management strategies

1. For cyanotic spells, an **intense stimulus** (e.g., a cold cloth on the face) may terminate the breath holding if applied within the first 15 seconds of apnea. Although the window of opportunity for this intervention is brief, many parents find it comforting to have *something* to try, rather than just feeling helpless.

2. If the event progresses for either type of breath-holding spells, the **child should be placed on the floor to prevent falling.**

Table 19-1. Progression of breath-holding spells

Cyanotic spell
    Precipitating event (anger or frustration associated with temper tantrums)
    Period of crying (frequently less than 20 secs)
    Holding of breath in expiration
    Cyanosis
    Progressive loss of consciousness
    Occasional twitching, opisthotonos, or clonic movements
Pallid form
    Precipitating event (minor trauma, especially occipital trauma or fright)
    Absence of crying or single cry
    Bradycardia and often asystole
    Simultaneous loss of consciousness and breath holding
    Pallor
    Occasionally generalized seizure or twitching

Table 19-2. Distinguishing breath-holding spells from seizures

	Severe breath-holding spells	Epilepsy
Precipitating factor	Always present	Usually not present
Crying	Present before convulsion	Not usually present
Cyanosis	Occurs before loss of consciousness	When it occurs, it is usually during prolonged seizure
Electroencephalogram	Almost always normal	Usually abnormal but may be normal

    3. When the child awakes (usually immediately after the seizure or loss of consciousness) **parents should not fuss over the child** so that inadvertent secondary gain does not occur.

C. Prevention. Prevention involves avoiding unnecessary struggles and setting firm, consistent limits to increase the child's ability to cope with frustration.

Bibliography

Lombroso CT, Lerman P. Breathholding spells (cyanotic and pallid infantile syncope). *Pediatrics* 39:563–581, 1967.

Gordon N. Breath-holding spells. *Dev Med Child Neurol* 29:805–814, 1987.

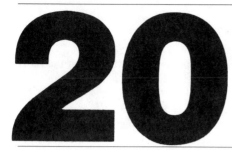

Cerebral Palsy

Frederick B. Palmer and
Alexander H. Hoon

I. **Description of the problem.** Cerebral palsy (CP) is a disorder of movement and posture caused by a static defect or lesion of the immature brain. Rather than a specific diagnosis, it encompasses a spectrum of neurodevelopmental syndromes characterized by persistent motor delay, abnormal neuromotor examination, and often an extensive range of nonmotor-associated deficits in cognitive, neurobehavioral, neurosensory, orthopedic, and other areas. These associated deficits reflect the fact that motor areas of the brain are rarely affected in isolation. Although the brain lesion is, by definition, nonprogressive, its motor and nonmotor manifestations can be expected to change with the child's development.

A. **Epidemiology**
  - About 2/1000 live births (half-born at term, half-born preterm).
  - Evidence over the past decade of an increase in CP birth prevalence in very low birth weight babies (with a decrease in mortality in this group).

B. **Classification.** Clinical classification is based on the nature of the movement disorder, muscle tone, and topography. Classification by type is essential to management and anticipation of associated deficits (Table 20-1) and future needs.

  1. **Spastic CP** (65% of children with CP). Most children with CP are "spastic," with an upper motor neuron syndrome consisting of persistently increased muscle tone with clasp-knife character, increased deep tendon reflexes, pathologic reflexes, and spastic weakness. Spastic CP is further subclassified based on topography:

     a. **Hemiplegia** (30% of children with CP): Primary unilateral involvement, often with the arm more involved than the leg.

     b. **Quadriplegia** (5% of children with CP): Four-limb involvement with legs often more involved than arms but with substantial arm involvement.

     c. **Diplegia** (30% of children with CP): Four-limb involvement with legs much more involved than the arms (which may show only minimal impairment and no functional handicap). Diplegia should be distinguished from "paraplegia," which implies entirely normal arms and suggests a spinal cord lesion, not CP.

  2. **Dyskinetic CP** (19% of children with CP). The other major physiologic category is designated "dyskinetic" due to the prominent involuntary movements, fluctuating muscle tone, or both. **Choreoathetosis** is the most common subtype. Most children with dyskinetic CP have relatively symmetric four-limb involvement and require no further topographic designation.

  3. **Ataxic CP** (10% of children with CP). This type of CP has a relatively good motor prognosis.

C. **Etiology/Contributing factors.** Despite 150 years of research, specific etiologic factors responsible for the motor impairment remain unknown in most children with CP, especially in children born at term. Large studies have shown that birth injury is the cause in only 8–12% of cases. Prenatal defects or insults are the most common etiologies. In premature children, both prenatal and perinatal factors are felt to play a role in what is most commonly a spastic diplegia or

Table 20-1. Selected nonorthopedic associated deficits in cerebral palsy

Cognition
Mental retardation (present in 30–77%)
   The most important factor influencing habilitation
   Hemiplegia and diplegia associated with higher cognition
   Easy-to-underestimate cognition in choreoathetosis
   Epilepsy associated with lower cognition
Language disorder, learning disability (present in about 40%)
   Heterogeneous group with deficits due to oromotor dysfunction, dysphasia, hearing loss
   Often "superimposed" on mental retardation
   Very high risk for learning disability in child with CP and "normal" IQ

Neurobehavior (present in up to 50%)
Entire spectrum of neurobehavioral disorders (attention deficit hyperactivity disorder to
   autism) seen
No symptom typical
Behavior dysfunction often primarily a neurologic symptom

Sensation
Visual disorders (present in 50–90%)
   Most common ones amenable to treatment
   May have a bearing on education (acuity, field deficits)
   Hemianopsia in 25% of hemiplegia (easily missed as gaze may compensate to side of
      field cut)
   Refractive errors seen in 50% overall, 67% in diplegia; amblyopia develops in 14%
Hearing disorders (present in 10%)
   Easily missed
   Higher prevalence (45–60%) in postkernicteric choreoathetosis and other etiologies
      (toxoplasmosis, other, rubella, cytomegalovirus, herpes simplex)
Somatosensation (present in up to 50% of hemiplegia)
   Deficits in stereognosis most common
   May be the limiting factor in arm/hand functioning in hemiplegia
   Repeated clinical examination essential to recognition
   Associated with linear undergrowth but not muscular atrophy

Seizures (present in 30–40%)
Often associated with spasticity and lower cognition

Growth failure
Undernutrition a frequent problem
Empiric nutritional goal of 10% weight for height
Multifactorial in origin: increased caloric needs, oromotor dysfunction, gastroesophageal
   reflux, chronic infection, "neurogenic," syndromic
Limb length asymmetry associated with hemisensory abnormalities

Other health problems
Genitourinary complaints common; pathogenesis unclear
Drooling a major cosmetic problem: may be exacerbated by antispasticity drugs;
   treatment with anticholinergics, surgery, and biofeedback disappointing

quadriplegia. Postneonatal etiologies (e.g., traumatic brain injury, meningitis)
account for about 10% of CP.

II. Making the diagnosis

   A. Symptoms. CP usually presents with significant motor delay, although the delay
   may not be recognized in the first months of life. Other common presenting
   concerns include poor head control, hypertonia (especially during activities such
   as bathing or diapering), generalized hypotonia, early preferential hand use,
   absent weight bearing, and feeding problems.
      The nonprogressive nature of "the lesion" is essential to the diagnosis. If
   etiology is not clear or if the clinical picture is not static, then evaluation for a

progressive process (metabolic, structural, neurodegenerative, etc.) should be undertaken. This may require assistance from a subspecialist.

B. Neurologic signs

1. Sole reliance on the neuromotor examination in diagnosing CP can lead to both under- and overdiagnosis. Instead, the clinician should initially focus on the **presence or absence of motor delay.** If there is no delay, CP is unlikely even if the neuromotor examination is abnormal (although children with such "minor neuromotor dysfunction" may have other neurodevelopmental disabilities, such as mental retardation or learning disability). An exception to this "no delay, no CP" rule is seen in hemiplegia, in which the prominent upper extremity handicap causes substantial neuromotor asymmetry rather than gross motor delay.

2. On neuromotor examination, **muscle tone** may vary from excessive hypotonia to hypertonia (spastic, dyskinetic, or mixed in character). Hypotonia may be manifest as head lag on pull to sit, slip through at the shoulders, or an exaggerated curve in ventral suspension. Hypotonia with significant weakness is uncommon in CP and suggests a neuromuscular disorder. Early hypotonia may persist, normalize, or evolve into hypertonia.

3. Spastic hypertonia—**persistent clasp-knife catch or hitch**—is part of the upper motor neuron syndrome and is brought out by rapid movement of the limb by the examiner.

4. The **hypertonus** seen in dyskinetic forms (lead pipe rigidity) is variable in nature and can usually be "shaken out" by the examiner with rapid movements of the limb. Involuntary movements, such as choreoathetosis, dystonia, and tremor, are often associated. Facial and oromotor involvement are often prominent.

5. All children are born with a constellation of primitive (e.g., Moro) and "pathologic" (e.g., Babinski) **reflexes,** probably mediated at the brainstem level. In normal infants, brain maturation leads to the disappearance of these reflexes and the emergence of postural and equilibrium reactions that precede the attainment of motor skills. In infants with CP, primitive reflexes are often increased in intensity and delayed in disappearance. Recognition of these phenomena may aid in diagnosis, especially in the first 6–12 months of life when motor delay is less apparent.

6. The examination should include a careful assessment of **oromotor and ocular function** and a search for **orthopedic abnormalities,** including joint contractures. The general physical examination should focus on dysmorphic features, neurocutaneous signs, retinal abnormalities, organomegaly, and other findings that could suggest a specific etiology. Ophthalmologic and genetic consultations may be helpful.

C. Tests. Table 20-2 lists the indications for various tests for CP. A neuroimaging study is an important part of the evaluation. Although it may not directly affect management, it can provide a structural correlate of the motor impairment and insight into the timing of the insult. Often parents find this information quite useful as they try to come to terms with their child's impairment.

In children with *atypical* clinical findings, especially choreoathetosis, metabolic disorders should be suspected. Plasma amino acids, urinary organic acids analyses, and selective use of other tests can be important. A karyotype may be revealing in children with apparent prenatal onset of CP and dysmorphic features.

III. Management

A. Primary Goals

1. To allow the child with CP to **function as effectively and normally as possible** in the home, school, and community.

2. To provide a foundation for the child to **function independently as an adult,** within the constraints imposed by the neurologic and other impairments.

Table 20-2. Suggested indications for diagnostic or screening tests in children with motor disorders

---

Magnetic resonance imaging of the brain
  Cerebral palsy or motor asymmetry
  Abnormal head size or shape
  Craniofacial malformation
  Loss or plateau of developmental skills
  Multiple somatic anomalies
  Neurocutaneous findings
  Seizures
  IQ<50
Cytogenetic studies
  Microcephaly
  Multiple (even minor) somatic anomalies
  Family history of mental retardation
  Family history of repeated fetal loss
  IQ<50
  Skin pigmentary anomalies (mosaicism)
  Suspected contiguous gene syndromes (e.g., Prader-Willi, Angelman, Smith-Magenis)
Metabolic studies
  Dyskinetic CP (choreoathetosis, dystonia, ataxia)
  Episodic vomiting or lethargy
  Poor growth
  Seizures
  Unusual body odors
  Somatic evidence of storage
  Loss or plateau of developmental skills
  Sensory loss (especially retinal abnormality)
  Acquired cutaneous disorders

Adapted from Palmer FB, Caute AJ. Mental retardation. *Pediatr Rev* (in press).

3. To **assist the parents** in accepting and assuming their role as advocates for their child's needs.

4. To **coordinate the recommendations of the many medical providers** into an integrated health care plan. Table 20-3 outlines common clinical indications and goals for referral to *nonmedical* professionals. These guidelines and comments reflect personal experience rather than rigid rules and should be interpreted in the context of available resources.

B. **General principles of treatment**

1. **The severity of disorder should help determine the aggressiveness of treatment.** For example, an infant with a motor quotient below 0.5 generally requires complete evaluation by a physical or occupational therapist, or both, and ongoing intervention. Children with milder delays (motor quotient 0.5–0.7) may only need a one-time consultation and suggestions for home management.

2. Although most **traditional interventions** are not of clearly proved efficacy (like many traditional medical therapies), they can be useful if used with clear indications and goals in mind.

3. **Parents** should be included in any therapy and should incorporate techniques into their everyday activities with the child.

4. **Therapists and intervention programs** should be kept informed about the child and, in turn, should keep the clinician informed of their activities.

5. Clinicians should be familiar with available **local intervention programs,** their services, and details of eligibility, access, and payment.

Table 20-3. Suggestions for use of nonmedical specialties

Service	Common useful indications	Comments
Special nutrition services	Weight for height less than 5% or declining Suspected insufficient caloric intake due to poor swallow, gastroesophageal reflux	Nutritional problems require extensive medical workups Significant gastroesophageal reflux common in severe CP Gavage or gastrostomy feeding may be needed to meet caloric requirements Ideal body weight is tenth percentile for height
Occupational therapy	Fine motor delay (DQ < 0.50)[a] Presence or risk of contractures in the upper extremities Overdependence on others for activities of daily living for child's cognitive level Oromotor dysfunction, excess drooling, poor oral intake, excessive feeding time Equipment needs	
Physical Therapy	Gross motor delay (MoQ < 0.50)[b] Difficult or inefficient ambulation in the absence of prominent delay Abnormalities of tone or reflexes interfering with function or management Presence or risk of contractures in the lower extremities Adaptive equipment needs	Videotaping motor function, or formal gait analysis, may be helpful in assessment Helpful to have physical therapist present for orthopedic evaluations One-time consultations for children with MoQ 0.50–0.70 may be useful
Audiology	All patients with CP due to high prevalence of hearing loss Recommend and apply amplification, if indicated	Office-based hearing screening is unreliable and insensitive Brainstem auditory evoked responses (BAERs) nonspecific measures of hearing loss in high-risk premature infants in the newborn period; more specific results using BAERs, behavioral audiometry, and acoustic impedance audiometry are obtained after 6 months of age Early treatment of hearing loss can significantly improve outcome
Speech and language	Global language delay Isolated expressive language delay Dysarthria May assist occupational therapy with feeding concerns	Receptive language may be surprisingly better than expressive language Language may be underestimated in choreoathetoid patient with oromotor involvement Repeat evaluations necessary Isolated articulation lessons usually not rewarding

Table 20-3 (continued)

Service	Common useful indications	Comments
Psychometric testing	All children with CP due to high prevalence of cognitive disorder Reevaluate in patients with suspected plateau, degeneration, or difficulty in school	Academic achievement testing may be handled by school Parent and teacher input needed in assessing discrepancies between IQ and achievement Special testing methods for children with severe motor or sensory impairment
Special education (private or school based)	Upon entering first grade or when change in placement is suggested To develop an individualized education plan (IEP)	Classroom teacher input is invaluable Evaluation in conjunction with psychometric testing advised May not be necessary to have a special education evaluation if IQ < 55
Behavioral psychology	Parental or teacher difficulty in managing behavioral problems When caretakers use excessive physical punishment	Behavior techniques may be enhanced by medication (e.g., methylphenidate) Teachers and other caretakers should be involved in program Planned management should be adaptable to home, school, and community
Social work	Often useful at initial diagnosis When difficulties in parent adaptation are noted Suspected child abuse When services are not easily accessed	To aid the clinician in attending to the many details involved in supervising care by the intricate network of agencies Respite care services may enhance the long-term outlook for family-provided care Evaluation in suspected child abuse is essential

Source: Adapted from Rosenblatt AI, Palmer FB. Cerebral palsy. In RT Johnson (ed), *Current Therapy in Neurological Diseases* (3rd ed). Philadelphia: Decker, 1991.
[a]Developmental quotient (DQ) = Fine motor age (milestone-based) divided by chronologic age.
[b]Motor quotient (MOQ) = gross motor age (milestone-based) divided by chronologic age.

    6. Assistance in identifying needs and appropriate intervention options is often available through **neurodevelopmental disability programs in tertiary centers.**

  C. Criteria for referral.

    1. An **orthopedic evaluation** is needed of any child with limitation in range of motion of any joint(s). Orthopedic surgery may be indicated when function is impaired, care is limited, or pain is caused by deformity, contracture, or muscle imbalance. Goals of surgery should be clearly understood by families. The common parental expectation for unreasonable functional gains should be anticipated. Orthopedic and neurodevelopmental pediatric consultants should work closely with physical and occupational therapists in nonsurgical interventions. They can assist in prescribing appropriate adaptive equipment and bracing. Such equipment includes seating and positioning devices and transportation implements.

    2. Neurosurgical interventions in CP have a long history. Stereotactic ablation surgery and implanted stimulators have been unrewarding and are seldom indicated. Selective lumbar dorsal rhizotomy may offer help in lower extremity spasticity, especially spastic diplegia. However, long-term functional outcome data are not yet available, and the procedure remains controversial.

3. If **pharmacological adjuncts** are to be used, specific treatment goals are essential and should include functional improvement, not just reduction in tone. It is generally best to have the child's physical or occupational therapist assist in objective measurement of agreed-on outcomes to avoid basing dosage decisions solely on "he's better [or worse] today" reports from family or treatment programs.

Medication is sometimes effective in reducing hypertonus in spastic and mixed forms of CP. However, striking functional improvement is rarely seen. Diazepam, and occasionally other benzodiazepines, are most commonly used. Baclofen, a gamma-aminobutyric acid agonist, is used less frequently (usually in older children). Baclofen has been given by intrathecal pump with questionable functional effects. Further research is necessary if any reported benefits are to be confirmed. Medications to control involuntary movements are sometimes useful as an effective adjunct in severe dyskinetic CP. Dopamine agonists and anticholinergics have been employed in treating dystonia and rigidity.

Bibliography

For Parents

Associations

American Academy for Cerebral Palsy and Developmental Medicine, 1910 Byrd Avenue, Suite 118, P.O. Box 11086, Richmond VA 23230; (804) 282-0036.

Council for Disability Rights, 343 South Dearborn #1503, Chicago IL 60604; (312) 922-1093.

National Handicapped Sports and Recreation Association, 1145 19th Street, NW, Suite 717, Washington DC 20036; (202) 393-7505.

National Information Center for Handicapped Children and Youth, 1555 Wilson Boulevard, Suite 700, Rosslyn VA 22209; (703) 893-6061.

United Cerebral Palsy Associations, 66 East 34th Street, New York NY 10016; (212) 481-6300.

Publications

A Reader's Guide: For Parents of Children with Physical or Emotional Disabilities. Publication [HSA] 77-5290. Washington DC: US Government Printing Office.

Batshaw ML, Perret YM. *Children with Handicaps: A Medical Primer* (2nd ed). Baltimore: Paul H Brookes, 1986.

Exceptional Parent.
Magazine for parents of handicapped children. 1170 Commonwealth Avenue, Brighton MA 02134; (617) 730-5800.

Finnie NR. *Handling the Young Cerebral Palsied Child at Home* (rev ed). New York: EP Dutton, 1975.

Fraser BA, Hensinger RN. *Managing Physical Handicaps: A Practical Guide for Parents, Care Providers, and Educators.* Baltimore: Paul H Brookes, 1983.

Pueschel SM, Bernier JC, Weidenman LE (eds). *The Special Child: A Source Book for Parents of Children with Developmental Disabilities.* Baltimore: Paul H Brookes, 1988.

For Professionals

Bleck EE. *Orthopaedic Management in Cerebral Palsy.* Clinics in Developmental Medicine, Nos. 99/100. London: MacKeith Press, in association with Blackwell Scientific Publications and Lippincott, 1987.

Capute AJ, Accardo PJ (eds). *Developmental Disabilities in Infancy and Childhood.* Baltimore: Paul H Brookes, 1991.

Rosenblatt AI, Palmer FB. Cerebral palsy. In RT Johnson (ed), *Current Therapy in Neurological Diseases* (3rd ed). Philadelphia: Decker, 1991.

Rubin IL, Crocker AC (eds). *Developmental Disabilities: Delivery of Medical Care for Children and Adults.* Philadelphia: Lea & Febiger, 1989.

Ellen C. Perrin

I. Description of the problem. A chronic health condition is defined as one that
- lasts, or is expected to last, for 3 months or longer, and
- affects the child's usual age-appropriate activities, or
- results in extensive hospitalization, home health services, or utilization of medical care in excess of that generally considered appropriate for a child of the same age.

Children with chronic health conditions are of increasing interest and importance to primary care clinicians because of (1) their increasing prevalence; (2) the growing recognition that these children and their families are at higher than usual risk for family stress, social isolation, and difficulties with social and psychological adjustment; and (3) the additional challenges they present for comprehensive pediatric care and coordination.

The true prevalence of chronic health conditions in childhood is unknown because the inclusiveness of definitions of "chronic health conditions" has been extremely varied. Their prevalence is increasing with advances in perinatal care and medical and surgical technology. In addition, improved systems available to collect data and more effective delivery of health services have increased the identification of children with chronic health conditions.

Up to 30% of all children have been reported to have at least one of the large range of chronic health problems that affect children, of which asthma is the most common. Approximately 3.5 million, or 5½%, of U.S. children have a chronic health condition that limits their usual activities to some degree.

II. Salient issues. There are considerable commonalities in the experiences of children who have a chronic health condition and the experiences of their families (Table 21-1). In addition to those issues they share, important characteristics of children themselves, of parents and families, and of the specific conditions have considerable effects on the experience of having a chronic condition (Table 21-2).

A. Characteristics of children. The age at which a child develops a chronic health condition, and the child's age at any particular time, independently contribute to the child's experience of the condition and the particular issues associated with its management (Table 21-3). For example, congenital conditions generally are associated with greater resiliency than conditions whose onset is during early adolescence.

Children's ability to manage their condition is related not only to their age but also to their understanding of the illness. Children with chronic health conditions are no more sophisticated than their healthy peers in their conceptual sophistication about the processes of illness causation and treatment. Healthy children and their peers with a chronic condition gain conceptual understanding of the processes of bodily functioning and of the prevention, causation, and treatment of illness along a predictable sequence of developmental stages parallel to those described in other domains by Piaget and others (Table 21-4).

It is important to assess the level of the child's cognitive sophistication about illness prior to instituting specific health education efforts, providing information about the condition, or determining appropriate expectations for the child's participation in the care and management of the condition. The child's intelligence, temperamental style, locus-of-control beliefs, self-concept, gender, and ethnic background all contribute to his or her resiliency in adapting to the extra stresses of a chronic health condition.

Table 21-1. Issues common in the presence of chronic health conditions

---

For children

  Limitations in usual childhood activities because of the condition itself and
    medical care requirements

  Need for medications, other treatments

  Experience with doctors, nurses, other providers

  Pain and discomfort

  Experience with hospitalization

  Feeling different from peers

  Loneliness

  Worry about the future

  Dependency, loss of control

For families

  Extra burden of care

  Financial drain

  Interactions with complex medical system

  Multiple doctors, nurses, other professionals

  Restricted social networks

  Difficulties with child care, short and long term

  Special requirements of school

  Necessity to inflict pain and discomfort

  Interference with needs of other family members and of family system

  Worries about long-term care, insurance

  Uncertainty in daily life planning

  Loneliness

  Guilt

  Anger

B. **Characteristics of conditions.** Certain kinds of health conditions present children with greater risks for difficult adjustment than do others. Unpredictable conditions and those that involve CNS or cognitive dysfunction appear to present special challenges to children and families.

   The adjustment of children, of their siblings, and of their parents cannot be predicted simply from the severity of the condition. Some children with only moderate disease experience a greater impact on their lives and challenges to their psychological and social adjustment than do children who are more severely affected. The confusing experience of marginality, in which a child is neither clearly sick (and in need of special services and attention), nor clearly well, may result when a health condition is not obvious to peers and important adults and does not interfere noticeably with normal activity but still requires a special diet, medication, and medical care.

C. **Characteristics of families.** Parents, siblings, and extended family interactions play a very major part in children's successful adjustment. Parental reactions to a diagnosis of a chronic health condition and their adaptation to its long-term implications affect the coping resources of the child and his or her siblings. The risk of parental discord and divorce is somewhat greater for families that include a child with a chronic health condition, reflecting the additional stresses presented by the parenting and care of these children. Siblings also are at risk to feel less important than the child on whom so much worry and attention is directed.

   The development of children's positive views of themselves is supported by their family's perception of their health condition as an incidental difficulty requiring shared problem solving, rather than as an intrusion on the family's functioning. The family's ability to attend to each member's needs for nurturance and attention, to express and deal with conflict, to support the independence of all members, and to provide both structure and flexibility are critical to children's successful adaptation.

III. **Management.** Maintaining optimal growth and development in the presence of a chronic health condition is a challenge to families, to primary care clinicians, and to the children themselves. While there is a somewhat greater risk of psychological,

Table 21-2. Factors affecting children's experience of a chronic health condition

Characteristics of the child
  Age of onset
  Personality/temperament
  Intelligence
  Self-concept
  Gender
  Ethnic background
  Developmental level
  Understanding of illness
  Locus-of-control beliefs
Characteristics of the illness
  Age of onset
  Stable or unpredictable
  Prognosis
  Interference with mobility
  Interference with normal activities
  Visibility
  Academic effects
  Medications and other treatments
  Intensity of care requirements
  Discomfort
  Nervous system involvement
Characteristics of the family
  Marital status
  Number and ages of children
  Parents' education
  Parents' occupations
  Financial situation
  Strength of parents' relationship
  Parents' self-esteem
  Extended family support
  Social support network
  Ethnic background

social, and educational difficulties for children with chronic health conditions, most of them and most of their families adapt successfully to the extra challenges they confront.

Primary care clinicians have the opportunity—and therefore also the responsibility—to be available to families over a long period of time. They are often the first professional person consulted about issues of concern to children and their parents. Thus, they are in a unique position to **support families and to help them to coordinate their child's care**. In addition to ensuring that these children receive all usual preventive and acute illness care and health supervision, the primary care clinician should serve as an effective interface among subspecialty and surgical teams, early intervention and family support programs, schools, third-party payers, nursing services, and a large variety of other care providers.

Primary care clinicians also should provide regular **monitoring** of the child's development, the emotional and social adaptation of children, parents, and siblings, and referral for appropriate mental health services when indicated. Such comprehensive attention to overall health care supervision for children with ongoing health conditions has been made easier with new coding guidelines that allow supplemental third-party reimbursement for extended office visits, case conferences, and sometimes lengthy telephone-assisted care.

Primary care clinicians need to know the **resources available** in their own community. They should have, or be able to develop, effective contacts with local school systems, the resources of the department of public health, home nursing and respite care services, and sources of specialty medical and surgical care. In addition, they can provide community-specific information regarding supportive networks of children with health conditions and of their parents and their siblings.

Table 21-3. Challenging tasks for children with chronic health problems

	Primary task	Challenges
Infants and toddlers	Development of trust and security	Parental grief Altered eating/feeding experiences Restriction of movement Hospitalizations Painful procedures Chronic discomfort
Preschoolers	Development of autonomy	Medication requirements Dietary restrictions Mobility restrictions Need for adult supervision Repeated separations Impaired limit setting Limitations on peer interactions
School-aged children	Development of sense of mastery	Differences from peers Dependence on medical care Restrictions on independence Requirements for adult monitoring Medication and dietary requirements Activity restrictions School absence
Adolescents	Development of personal identity separate from family	Altered body image Decreased growth Visible deformity Requirements of medical supervision Medication and dietary requirements Vocational limitations Challenges to sexuality Enforced dependency

The clinician also has a responsibility to **assure appropriate education** of children and their families about the health condition and its management. In addition, they should help parents to plan for an appropriate school program, with attention to the integration of the child's medical and educational needs. Excessive school absences that result from the course of a condition itself and from requirements for its care can be made less disruptive by home tutoring services for long-term and for predictable short-term absences. Effective communication among the school system, the pediatrician, and the family can make overall health care management and transitions between school and home care efficient and effective.

Bibliography

For Parents
Association for the Care of Children's Health (ACCH), 36-5 Wisconsin Avenue, Washington DC 20016; (202) 244-1801.

Federation for Children with Special Health Needs, 95 Berkeley Street, Boston MA 02116; (617) 482-2915.

Sibling Information Network, 991 Main Street, East Hartford CT 06108; (203) 282-7050.

For Professionals
Hobbs N, Perrin JM, Ireys HT. *Chronically Ill Children and Their Families.* San Francisco: Jossey-Bass, 1985.

Table 21-4. Typical progression in children's understanding of illness concepts

Cognitive level	Approximate age	Understanding of illness	Typical responses to "How do children get sick?"	Typical responses to "How do children keep from getting sick?"	Typical responses to "How can children get better?"
1		No response; do not know; inappropriate or off-task response			
2	4–6	Phenomenism: circular or phenomenistic response	"By catching something"; "sometimes you just do"; "from throwing up"	"Stay healthy"; "go to doctor for checkups"	"Go to the doctor"; "take medicines"
3	7–9	External agents: concrete, external causes cited; no explanation of how the agents interact with the body to result in, prevent, or cure illness	"If you go out in the rain without your boots"; "eating bad foods"; "from other people"	"Get shots"; "stay away from sick people"; "eat good foods"; "rest enough"	"Eat foods that are good for you"; "rest a lot"; "do what the doctor says"
4	10–13	Internalization: internalization and/or relativity in understanding of illness; once agent is internalized, illness follows invariably	"Germs get in and spread all over your body"; "when you breathe in sick people's germs"	"Take special vitamins that will keep your body strong"; "rest/food/exercise . . . give your body what it needs"	"Do different things for different illnesses"; "get more sleep than usual"; "take the right kind of medicine to give your body what it needs"
5	10–13	Interaction: interaction of host and agent described; some effect of agent on body	"Germs get in your system and start to eat/kill your cells"; "interference with normal body parts"	"If your body is strong from eating what you should, it will be able to resist the germs"; "exercising keeps the bones in place so they can work right"	"Resting allows your body not to waste its energy so it can fight the germs better"; "vitamins help the body to repair what's not working right"
6	>14	Mechanisms: processes of illness causation, prevention, or treatment described; includes notion of bodily response	"Germs take away food from the body and then the body has nothing to use for power"; "eat something that messes up your muscles so your heart doesn't work right"	"The right foods nourish the fighting cells so they are powerful enough to kill germs that get inside you"	"Good food/vitamins help your body to make more blood so the cells can fight off the germs"; "make your heart stronger so your body has better defenses"

Newacheck P, Taylor W. Prevalence and impact of childhood chronic conditions. *Am J Public Health* 82:364, 1992.

Perrin EC, Gerrity PS. Development of children with chronic illness. *Pediatr Clin North Am* 31:19, 1984.

Perrin EC, et al. Issues involved in the definition and classification of chronic health conditions. *Pediatrics* 91:787, 1993.

Wallander J, et al. Family resources as resistance factors for psychological maladjustment in chronically ill and handicapped children. *J Pediatr Psychol* 14:157, 1989.

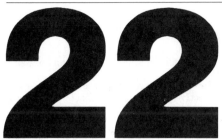

Colic

Steven Parker

I. **Description of the problem.** There is no reliably objective definition of colic. Wessel's criteria define colic as crying for more than 3 hours per day for 3 or more days per week. By these standards, however, half of all infants would be classified as colicky! Additionally, parental tolerance for infant crying is quite variable: some are stoic in the face of constant crying, while others come to the primary care clinician for the occasional whimper. The best definition of colic may be a purely clinical one: colic is *any recurrent inconsolable* crying in a *healthy and well-fed infant* that is experienced by the parents or caregivers as a problem.

A. **Epidemiology**
- Estimates range from 7–25%, depending on the criteria for diagnosis.
- No differences by gender, breast- versus bottle-fed, full term versus preterm, or birth order.
- ? Whites > nonwhites.
- ? Industrialized countries > nonindustrialized.
- ? More frequent the farther away from the equator.
- Increased incidence of physical abuse in colicky infants.

B. **Clinical features**
1. Colic typically begins at **41–42 weeks gestational age** (including preterm infants).
2. **Two patterns** of colic have been noted.
   a. **Paroxysmal fussing** typically occurs between 5–8 P.M. The infant is contented and easily soothed at other times of the day. These infants do not cry more frequently over 24 hours; rather, they sporadically cry for a longer period of time.
   b. **The hyperirritable infant** is one whose crying occurs at all hours of the day, often in response to ambiguous external or internal stimuli. They may also exhibit increased tone and other signs of hyperarousal.
3. Colic **stops as mysteriously as it starts,** by 3 months in 60% and by 4 months in more than 90% of infants.
4. There are no **predictable long-term outcomes** (behavioral, temperamental, or psychological) that emerge from a colicky infancy.

C. **Etiology.** Theories of causation abound (Table 22-1), but evidence for any one is scant. It appears likely that there is no single cause of colic and that it represents the final common pathway for a number of etiologic factors.

II. **Making the diagnosis**

A. **History: Key clinical questions**
1. *When does the crying occur? How long does it last?* The timing of the cry provides useful information. For example, if it occurs directly after a feeding, aerophagia or gastroesophageal reflux may be considered. If it occurs reliably 1 hour after feedings, a formula intolerance is possible. If the crying occurs only from 5–7 P.M. every day, it is difficult to posit an organic problem that would cause pain at only one time of the day.
2. *What do you do when your baby cries?* It is important to determine how the parents have tried (successfully and unsuccessfully) to console the infant.

Table 22-1. Theories of the etiology of colic

Gastrointestinal
    Cow's milk protein intolerance (an equal number of studies have found an association
        of cow's milk with colic as have not)
    Lactose intolerance (higher breath H_2 level in some colicky infants)
    Immature gastrointestinal system (ineffective peristalsis; incomplete digestion; gas)
    Faulty feeding techniques (e.g., under- or overfeeding, infrequent burping)
Hormones causing enterospasm
    Increased motilin levels (one study showed higher levels of motilin, but not vasoactive
        intestinal peptide or gastrin, in colicky infants)
    Increased circulating serotonin (hypothetical only but an attractive hypothesis because
        serotonin has a circadian rhythm in infancy, which could explain the curious timing
        of paroxysmal fussing)
    Progesterone deficiency (one study in 1963, never repeated)
Temperamental
    Difficult temperament (but there is poor correlation of colic and later temperament)
    Hypersensitivity (crying at end of day represents discharge after a long day of shutting
        out intrusive environmental stimuli)
Parental handling
    Most studies do not show a relationship between parental anxiety, psychopathology,
        and/or emotional difficulties and colic; at most, nonoptimal handling may exacerbate
        but not cause the symptoms.

In some cases, their techniques may have inadvertently worsened the situation (e.g., anxiously overstimulating a hypersensitive infant); in other cases, the technique may be inappropriate (e.g., giving half-strength formula).

3. *What does the cry sound like?* Most parents can distinguish a cry of pain from that of hunger. Additionally, the description of the cry provides insight into parental distress, empathy, or anger with the cry.

4. *Tell me how and what you feed your baby.* Underfeeding, overfeeding, air swallowing, and inadequate burping have all been implicated in colic.

5. *How does it make you feel when your baby cries?* History taking is an opportune time to begin the process of parental support. Opening up the subjects of parental guilt, helplessness, and anxiety sends the message that these topics merit discussion. Some parents are especially worried about their anger toward the screaming child, believing that such anger is the mark of a bad parent. Others seek pediatric attention because they are afraid of actually harming the infant during a crying spell.

6. *How has the colic affected your family?* Colic is a *family* issue. In some cases it may disturb the parents' relationship with each other, cause distress in a sibling, or serve as a forum for blaming the parents (e.g., by grandparents).

7. *What is your theory of why the baby cries?* In order to support the family, their hypotheses for the crying must be understood. Some may view it as a curse, others as a rebuke to their parenting skills, and others as a sign that something is terribly wrong with the baby.

B. **Physical examination.** A thorough physical examination serves to rule out medical problems that cause pain or discomfort, as well as to reassure the parents that the infant is physically well.
    Any problem that causes pain can lead to hyperirritability (but rarely to paroxysmal fussing):
    • Infections (otitis media, urinary tract, oral herpes).
    • Gastrointestinal (diarrhea, constipation, gastroesophageal reflux).
    • Genitourinary (posterior urethral valves).
    • CNS (intra- or extracranial hemorrhage, hydrocephalus).
    • Ophthalmologic (corneal abrasion, glaucoma).
    • Cardiac (supraventricular tachycardia).
    • Narcotic withdrawal syndrome (especially methadone).

• Fracture, hernia, anal fissures.
• Tourniquet (on toe or finger).

The diagnosis of colic is predicated on the infant being healthy and well fed. Only after a thorough history and physical examination do not reveal an obvious source of pain should the diagnosis of colic be considered.

III. Management

A. Shotgun approach. Because the cause of colic is rarely clear, a shotgun approach is often helpful. Table 22-2 lists suggestions for parents to help them deal with colic. The history and physical examination may point to one line of treatment as potentially more useful than another. As a general rule, **most treatments for colic work in 30% of infants, but none works for all infants.** It is best to try only one or two interventions at a time. This allows for the effective measure to be more easily identified. Additionally, since *nothing* may work very well, it is helpful to keep a few suggestions in reserve, at least until the process runs its course at 3–4 months.

B. Parental support. Colic is a benign, self-limited problem with no untoward sequelae. Its impact on the early parent-child relationship should be of primary concern. Long after the crying abates, the consequences of an impaired parent-infant relationship can do damage. Therefore, the primary role for the clinician in the management of colic is to support the family through a difficult period and ensure that no untoward interactions are set up.

   1. Inform the family. The mysterious but benign nature of colic should be reiterated. The family will need constant reassurance that nothing is physically wrong with the infant. This is best accomplished by frequent physical examinations to assure the family that nothing has been missed and an emphasis on the otherwise normal growth and development of the infant. The usual time course should be explained but not to downplay the family's current distress (e.g., "I know how distressing it is to care for an inconsolable infant. I've seen a lot of colicky babies, and fortunately it almost always disappears by 3–4 months. In the meantime, let's see what we can do to help things here and now").

   2. Lessen parental feelings of guilt. Most parents (especially inexperienced ones) feel that the crying occurs because of *something* that they are doing wrong. They require reassurance that this is not the case and that colic occurs with even the most attentive, loving, and experienced of caregivers.

   3. Empathize and depathologize parental feelings of resentment and anger. Many parents are mortified by the ambivalent and frankly negative feelings engendered by their crying infant. They should be reassured that *all* parents feel some resentment and anger toward their colicky infant, that it does not make them bad parents, and that these feelings are short-lived. In some cases, parental fear of harming the baby during an episode should be taken seriously, and a brief hospitalization may be indicated to provide respite.

   4. Provide close and consistent follow-up. Parents should call the clinician within 48 hours of the first visit to report on progress. If no progress is evident, a second visit can be scheduled within a week for further discussion and to reassure them that there is no organic problem. The parents need to be able to count on the clinician's availability during this difficult time.

   5. Remind the beleaguered parents that it is permissible to take breaks from the baby. If the baby cries inconsolably despite all reasonable interventions, it is permissible to put the baby down and let him or her cry for increasingly longer periods of time before attempting another consoling maneuver. Parents can be reassured that crying is healthy for the lungs, that (especially since the infant is crying anyway) it is not emotionally damaging for the infant to cry alone for a while at this age, and that such isolation teaches some infants how to self-console. Some parents find letting their infant cry unattended to be intolerable. They should be supported in handling the problem in the way that is most comfortable to them.

   Parents should also be encouraged to take breaks from the baby by letting a friend, family member, or babysitter attend to him or her for a few hours while the parents go out of the house for some unrestricted free time. They

Table 22-2. Suggestions for parents to help colic

	Strategy	Comments
Feeding/ nutritional	Change formula from cow's milk to soy based	Emphasize to parent that it is a clinical trial, that it might not work, and that changing formulas does not mean that there is anything physically wrong with the baby
	Change formula from soy based to predigested	Expensive but sometimes effective
	If breast-feeding, have mother stop cow's milk, caffeine, etc.	One study showed increased bovine IgG in the breast milk of mothers of colicky babies
		Ask the breast-feeding mother which foods seem to be associated with increased irritability
	Change nipple or bottle; feed in upright position with frequent burping	Try to decrease air swallowing (e.g., by using bottle with a plastic liner)
Alternate sensory stimulation	Supplemental daytime carrying	One study found little benefit of supplemental carrying for truly colicky infants
	Front carrier (e.g., Snugli)	Allows hand to be free while carrying
	Car seat on dishwasher or drier	Must be observed, because the seat can shift
	Ride in the car	Not advisable in the middle of the night if driver is sleepy
	Change of scenery	New sights can distract from the distress
	Pacifier	In Herman Meyer's words, "If for no other reason than to obstruct the opening from which the cacophonous sound emanates"
	Swing	Rarely allows more than 30 min of relief
	Belly massage	Use a lubricating lotion
	Swaddling	Especially good for babies who are hypersensitive to body movements or touch
	Heartbeat tape or white noise generator	Especially good for babies who are hypersensitive to noise
	Hot-water bottle on belly	Should not be too hot
	SleepTight (device that generates white noise and vibrates the bed)	Some pediatric practices have the device available to loan to patients. If it works, they can purchase one (telephone, (800)NO-COLIC). Two controlled studies, however, have shown disappointing benefits.
	Warm bath	
Medications	Herbal tea	A study of chamomile/verbena/ licorice/fennel/mint tea found improvement in 57% of colicky infants
	Simethicone	Probably harmless, dubiously helpful
	Antispasmodics	**Should not be used.** Despite some evidence of efficacy, there have been case reports of respiratory arrests associated with their use in infants.

should be reminded that the crying is not as emotionally wrenching for a nonparent to hear and that they can best serve their baby when they themselves are refreshed.

Bibliography

Barr RG et al. The crying of infants with colic: A controlled empirical description. *Pediatrics* 90:14–21, 1992.

Brazelton, TB. Crying in infancy. *Pediatrics* 29:579–588, 1962.

Geertsma MA, Hyams JS. Colic—A pain syndrome of infancy? *Pediatr Clin North Am* 36(4):905–919, 1989.

Wessel MA et al. Paroxysmal fussing in infancy, sometimes called "colic." *Pediatrics* 14:421–434, 1954.

Depression
Linda Forsythe and
Michael Jellinek

I. **Description of the problem.** Childhood major depressive disorder (MDD) is characterized by a significant emotional and behavioral change from baseline to a dysphoric or irritable mood with decreased functioning in the home, in school, and with peers.

A. **Epidemiology/incidence**

   1. **MDD in the general population**

      a. **Infants and preschoolers: 1%.** Seen as failure to thrive, as well as attachment, separation, and behavioral problems.

      b. **School-aged children: 2%.** Typically heralds a more protracted, recurrent, or severe course.

      c. **Adolescents: nearly 5%.** Presents most like the adult syndrome and may involve suicidality.

   2. **MDD in specialized populations.** As many as 7% of general pediatric inpatients and 28% of child psychiatry clinic patients.

   3. **Comorbid diagnoses in children with MDD.** 60–80% of children meeting criteria for MDD have additional or comorbid disorders, such as anxiety, attention deficit, substance abuse, and conduct problems, such as lying, stealing, vandalism, and truancy.

B. **Etiology/Contributing factors**

   1. **Genetic.** The biologic offspring of depressed adults are up to three times more likely to have MDD, which may present earlier and recur more frequently. Research suggests a polygenetic inheritance.

   2. **Environmental.** Distinguishing etiologic environmental factors from those that are coincidental to or a consequence of MDD is difficult. Children identify with, learn from, and share the mood of their parents and siblings. They are greatly affected by losses, especially parental death and divorce, and other stresses, including trauma and abuse. The boundary between extended bereavement and MDD is particularly unclear.

   3. **Organic.** A biochemical imbalance in norepinephrine may contribute to the fatigue of MDD; an imbalance in serotonin may cause the problems of irritability and anxiety. Many acute medical conditions (including toxic ingestions, metabolic disturbances, and CNS infections) and several chronic medical illnesses can lead to changes in appetite, weight loss, decreased energy, or irritable mood.

   4. **Developmental.** Intrapsychic depressive experiences become more differentiated and specific as emotional, language, cognitive, and social development proceed. Young children with MDD may simply experience a vague and overwhelming discomfort, while older children may come to use *stomachache* and *headache* as words for internal mood states. Such abstract terms as *depression* and age-appropriate synonyms like *blue, bored, empty, down,* and *bothered* are more likely to be used in adolescence.

   5. **Transactional.** The interaction of environmental contributions from school, home, and peers differs at different developmental stages and is influenced further by genetic and organic factors. Some school-aged children with MDD lose their ability to concentrate in school, causing performance and peer

Table 23-1. Criteria for child and adolescent major depressive episode

	Comments
Depressed mood or loss of interest or pleasure in activities at home, at school, or with peers for at least 2 wk or more than 50% of time	Including sad, blue, bored, empty, oppositional, irritable, angry, and rageful feelings

Coincident with depressed mood, changes in at least four of the following

Appetite or weight	In relation to expected weight gain; may present in infants and preschoolers as a feeding difficulty and in adolescents as anorexia or obesity
Sleep patterns	Including insomnia, hypersomnia, and frequent wakenings
Agitation	Including restlessness and aggressiveness; infants may be fussy and school-aged children hyperactive
Social withdrawal	In infants and preschoolers, problems of attachment and separation or loss of spontaneous play; in school-aged children, school reluctance, school phobia, or a sudden drop in school performance or after-school activities
Energy loss	Including listlessness, fatigue, and lethargy
Self-esteem	In school-aged children, feelings of stupidity, clowning around, or engaging in self-reproachful boasting; in adolescents, expressions of guilt, self-deprecation, helplessness, or hopelessness
Concentration	In infants and preschoolers, speech and motor delays or regression; with children or adolescents in school, sustained change in ability to attend in class, complete assignments out of class, concentrate, or make decisions
Dangerousness	In infants, head banging; in school-aged children, accident proneness; in adolescents, lying, stealing, and truancy
Somatic symptoms	In infants and preschoolers, failure to thrive and rumination; in school-aged children, enuresis, encopresis, and vague complaints; in adolescents, complaints of abdominal or head pain
Suicidal ideation	Recurrent thoughts of death and morbid preoccupation with illness, accidents, and/or death
Substance use	Including various drugs and alcohol

relationships to suffer. Other children are able to control their mood swings while at school, only to collapse into a depressed or irritable mood on safe arrival home. In adolescence, peer attachments assume major importance.

II. Making the diagnosis (Table 23-1)

A. Signs, symptoms, and behavioral observations

1. **Infant/toddler.** Both the persistently passive, unresponsive infant and the irritable, unsoothable, crying infant may suffer from the mood dysregulation associated with MDD. Their clinical presentations may evolve into a quiet, inhibited toddler with arrested social development or an overactive, impulsive, and irritable preschooler.

2. **School age.** In school-aged children with MDD, the expected pride associated with industry and enthusiasm may be overwhelmed by humiliation, defeat, irritability, and self-doubt. The child may become isolated, rejected, and accident prone. Temper tantrums or morbid preoccupations with bodily injury, illness, abandonment, or death might emerge. There may be pediatric office visits for multiple somatic complaints.

3. **Adolescence.** Teenagers with MDD experience hopelessness and have difficulty containing intense negative feelings. In the heat of a crushing rejection, they have both the passion and the means to act on self-destructive urges. They may direct negative actions inward against themselves by disregarding food, sleep, and hygiene. Some turn to alcohol and drugs for numbing symptomatic relief or engage in destructive behaviors. Instead of appearing sad and eliciting sympathy (as adults with MDD might), adolescents with MDD often seem angry and resentful.

B. **History: Key clinical questions**

1. *How is your child's mood? How does the child feel about himself or herself? For how many days, weeks, months, has this been the case?* Diagnosis of MDD requires at least a 2-week period of prominent mood-related symptoms.

2. *Has there been a recent change in your child's behavior, school performance, or peer relationships?* A cross-situational decrease in function or significant change in behaviors can be a key indicator of mood-related stress and disability.

3. *Does your child have a past history of feeling down, or has he or she ever seen a mental health professional in the past?* Studies suggest that a past depressive episode increases the risk of recurrence.

4. *Does anyone in the extended family have a history of depression, anxiety, attentional deficits, or alcohol or substance use?* Family psychiatric history is an important predictor of childhood risk.

5. *Is your child often intensely worried? profoundly anxious? impulsively inattentive? prone to lie and steal?* Identifying and clarifying comorbid diagnoses makes for more effective treatment.

6. *If depressed, has your child ever brought harm to himself or herself, even accidentally? Has the child ever talked of wanting or threatened to hurt himself or herself or others?* (And to the child: *Have you ever felt so bad that you wanted to hurt yourself?*) Self-destructive acts or threats must be taken seriously and should automatically lead to a careful suicide assessment and referral for psychiatric evaluation and follow-up. (See Chapter 64.)

C. **Physical examination.** Physical examination is useful to rule out medical illness as a cause of the symptoms.

D. **Tests.** Screening laboratory tests should be performed only when suggested by the history and physical examination.

III. **Management**

A. **Primary goals.** Most children with MDD can be safely managed as outpatients. In general, the comprehensive biopsychosocial approach to treatment of childhood MDD is beyond the expertise of the primary care clinician and should be referred to a mental health professional. The primary care clinician should monitor the treatment through the ongoing relationship with the family. Urgent psychiatric consultation is indicated whenever the child or adolescent is thought to be psychotic, acutely suicidal, acutely manic, abusing substances, or otherwise difficult to manage safely.

B. **Treatment strategies.** More than one treatment strategy is often indicated.

1. **Psychodynamic therapy** attempts to provide a safe and supportive environment for the child to explore, understand, and learn to express inner feelings and conflicts. It is often most effective for children and adolescents with low self-esteem. Play therapy is used in younger children who do not yet effectively use words to convey inner experiences and emotions.

2. **Cognitive therapy** reviews and challenges negative thoughts, actions, and feelings in a systematic and logical way. It is often used with particularly verbal adolescents.

3. **Behavioral therapy** uses reinforcement techniques to enhance positive experiences and minimize negative ones. It is often best for school-aged children in cooperation with one or both parents.

4. **Family therapy** views the family as a system unto itself and attempts to identify behavioral patterns and alliances that keep the family from developing or changing. It is often best for multiply stressed families and can be an important avenue for early detection of depression in other family members.

5. **Group therapy** views the child in a social and interactive context. It is often useful for developing social skills and social support.

6. **Parent guidance** helps parents to learn to deal with depression in their children or in themselves. Parents who feel personally overwhelmed or confused by the parental role often find this approach helpful.

7. **Environmental interventions** aim to support academic performance and raise a child's self-esteem through the use of role models and positive experiences that foster industry, responsibility, and pride. A carefully chosen summer or after-school activity, hobby, or encouragement of a friendship can be invaluable.

8. **Medications** focus on correcting biochemical imbalances. Although desipramine and imipramine are most often prescribed for childhood MDD, studies of efficacy are inconclusive. Lithium is gaining favor as a treatment for juvenile bipolar illness.

C. **Primary care follow-up.** The clinician may follow specific psychological symptoms over time, watch for side effects of medications, monitor patient compliance, and encourage appropriate child psychiatric follow-up.

Bibliography

For Parents

Facts for Families . . . The Depressed Child. Washington DC: American Academy of Child and Adolescent Psychiatry, 1991.

Let's Talk Facts About . . . Childhood Disorders, Depression, Manic-Depressive Disorder. Washington DC: American Psychiatric Association, 1992.

For Professionals

Kashani JH, Eppright TD. Mood disorders in adolescents. In JM Wiener (ed), *Textbook of Child and Adolescent Psychiatry.* Washington DC: American Psychiatric Press, 1991.

Sarles RM, Haerian M. Depression and suicide. In RA Dershewitz (ed), *Pediatric Ambulatory Care.* Philadelphia: Lippincott, 1993.

Shafii M, Shafii SL (eds). *Clinical Guide to Depression in Children and Adolescents.* Washington DC: American Psychiatric Press, 1992.

Weller E, Weller RA. Mood disorders in children. In JM Wiener (ed), *Textbook of Child and Adolescent Psychiatry.* Washington DC: American Psychiatric Press, 1991.

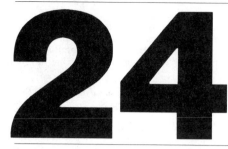

Disruptive Behavior: Lying, Stealing, and Aggression

Stuart Goldman

I. **Description of the problem.** The disruptive behavioral disorders (DBD) constitute a group of behavioral syndromes that are symptomatic of diverse underlying problems. They range from the irritable or oppositional child who is intermittently difficult to manage, to the child who breaks social rules (lying, cheating, etc.), to the child who breaks societal rules (truancy, stealing, assault, etc.). When a child, parent, or school raises questions about misbehaviors that compromise the child's functioning or are developmentally inappropriate, the disruptive disorders (Table 24-1) should be considered.

A. **Epidemiology**
   - Three to four times more common in boys than in girls.
   - Estimates of the milder forms of the disorders are unknown since some oppositional or dishonest behaviors are developmentally expectable.
   - Significant stealing is believed to affect approximately 5% of children.
   - Up to 9% of boys and 2% of girls have the most severe form of disruptive behaviors (conduct disorder).
   - Prevalence of oppositional defiant disorder is unknown but believed to be common.
   - Associated with familial psychosocial dysfunction and poverty.
   - No associations with ethnicity or race.

B. **Familial transmission/genetics.** There is a clear familial pattern of the DBD, due to both environmental and genetic components. The pattern of inheritance is unknown but believed to be complex.

C. **Etiology.** The vast majority of children have internal standards of conduct to which they aspire. Their antisocial behaviors can best be understood as an attempt to use the resources they have to solve the challenges they face (even if their "solutions" are maladaptive behaviors). Almost any factor that compromises their personal or social resources may have an etiologic role (Table 24-2). Any one of these factors may cause DBD, but multiple etiologies are the norm. Etiologic evaluation always involves evaluating the system from a dynamic, transactional perspective.

II. **Making the Diagnosis**

A. **Signs and symptoms.** Poorly controlled behaviors are the hallmark of these disorders. They may be primary or exist with comorbid diagnoses. Descriptively, they fall into three categories:
   - **Reactive** misbehaviors (adjustment disorder, posttraumatic stress disorder [PTSD])
   - **Endogenous** misbehaviors, characterized by impulsivity, inattention, and overactivity (attention deficit hyperactivity disorder [ADHD])
   - **Volitional** misbehaviors which may be mild (breaking social rules, oppositional defiant disorder) or severe (breaking societal rules, conduct disorder).

   1. **Developmental norms.** Although DBD is classified as pathologic, many of the described behaviors are developmentally predictable. For example, before age 6 years, children do not invariably follow rules (including those prohibiting cheating, stealing, and lying). Most children know these behaviors are wrong, but their ability to contain themselves is limited. By age 8 or 9 years,

Table 24-1. The disruptive behavioral disorders

Diagnosis	Onset	Duration	Key characteristics
Conduct disorder	Gradual after age 5 yr	> 6 mo	Breaking societal rules, stealing, assaults, truancy, may be antecedent to antisocial personality disorder
Oppositional defiant disorder	Gradual after age 3 yr	> 6 mo	Breaks social rules, irritable, argumentative, angry
Attention deficit hyperactivity disorder	Often noticed at school, usually congenital	> 6 mo	Impulsive, inattentive, distractible but often regrets behavior; coexisting secondary self-esteem problems
Adjustment disorder with disturbance of conduct	Within 3 mo of precipitating event	< 6 mo	Clearly identifiable precipitant; may mimic any of the above disorders but is transitory
Posttraumatic stress disorder	Variable	> 1 mo	Symptom of reexperiencing the event, avoidance of associated stimuli, and increased arousal

Table 24-2. Predisposing factors to disruptive behavioral disorders

Etiologic origin	Examples	Mechanisms
Environmental	Coercive discipline, abuse, neglect, chaos Emotional poverty Television violence Parental antisocial behaviors	Inappropriate models Cognitive distortions or disturbances Poor attachment and relationships Decreased self-esteem Unmet needs Defective internalization of rules Lack of alternative opportunities
Organic	CNS insult or injury (including lead, infection, cerebral palsy) Cognitive compromise, decreased IQ, learning disorders, attention deficit hyperactivity disorder Temperamental factors Certain psychiatric disorders, depression, psychosis	Poor modulation of impulses Decreased problem-solving abilities Decreased self-esteem Increased frustration
Developmental	Cognitive compromise Learning disorders Developmental failure/ deviations	Poor self-modulation Lack of relationships Decreased self-esteem Increased frustration

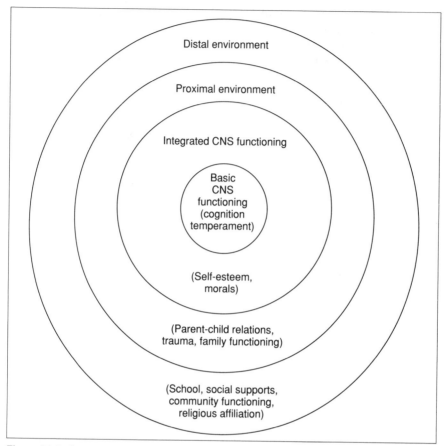

Figure 24-1. Concentric model for diagnostic assessment.

development has progressed enough so that clear and consistent encouragement by adults and peers to follow the rules generally results in the elimination of most of these behaviors.

Children who have not achieved the appropriate developmental mastery or are encouraged to misbehave will continue these behaviors. Other children carry out these behaviors sporadically in the context of personal, developmental, or environmental challenges. These children often need help in meeting the challenges of lowered self-esteem, resisting group pressures, or coping with a divorce.

B. **Differential diagnosis.** A concentric model (Fig. 24-1) allows one to assess the full range of the child's strengths and vulnerabilities. The clinician should inquire into all the potential etiologies of DBD starting with the child's cognitive, temperamental, and emotional development and moving outward. Diagnostic assessment then proceeds from the inner circle, as follows:

1. **Circle 1: Basic CNS functioning**

   a. **Strength:** No organic disorder, positive temperament, normal cognition.

   b. **Vulnerability:** Organic dysfunction.

   c. **Differential diagnosis:** ADHD, cognitive impairment, depression, psychosis, major developmental disorders, difficult temperament.

2. **Circle 2: Integrated CNS functioning**

   a. **Strength:** Strong sense of self, good self-esteem, well-integrated values, capacity for relationships.

   b. **Vulnerability:** Decreased self-esteem, depression, interpersonal deficits, character pathology, failure to internalize moral standards.

   c. **Differential diagnosis:** Oppositional defiant disorder, conduct disorder, depression, character pathology.

3. **Circle 3: Proximal environment** (parent-child relations, trauma, family functioning)

   a. **Strength:** Strong family function, supportive relationships.

   b. **Vulnerability:** Abuse, neglect, trauma, family dysfunction.

   c. **Differential diagnosis:** Adjustment disorder, PTSD, parent-child problems, primary parental diagnosis.

4. **Circle 4: Distal environment**

   a. **Strength:** Social supports through peers, school, church, outside agencies, community.

   b. **Vulnerability:** Conflicts with school, social isolation, community dysfunction.

C. **History: Key clinical questions.** These are geared to facilitate the multilevel assessment.

   1. *What happened just before the event?* Is there a readily identifiable precipitant? If so, consider an adjustment disorder or PTSD.

   2. *What were you thinking about or feeling when you . . . ?* Does the child appear to act volitionally? Premeditation, retaliation, and personal gain all suggest either conduct disorder or oppositional defiant disorder.

   3. *How did you feel afterward? What did you do?* True regret and remorse (not just to avoid punishment) indicate moral development and can be used to leverage change. True lack of remorse suggests conduct disorder.

   4. *What kinds of things make you angry? What do you do? What helps you to calm down?* How does the child modulate affect (anxiety, anger, sadness)? This question helps to explore for possible comorbid disorders.

   5. [To the parents:] *How do you (or the school) respond to these behaviors?* Is the message to stop unambiguous, or is there inadvertent encouragement? Are there clear consequences for misdeeds?

   6. *Is the behavior situation specific* (e.g., only in the home or school)? If so, focus on the interaction, rather than the child, as the primary source.

   7. *Are there escalating behaviors that put the child at risk* (e.g., firesetting, running away, violence, abuse)? If yes, the child may need protection and often needs psychiatric consultation.

   8. [To parent and child:]*What would you like help with?* and *How do you feel it could be accomplished?* This question establishes the family's initial position, which often serves as the foundation for negotiating a treatment plan.

D. **Behavioral observations.** The DBD are diagnosed primarily through history taking. Observational data can, however, be very helpful in making a differential or codiagnosis. The level of activity and impulsivity, affect, cognitive functioning, and disorders of thinking should be noted. Patterns of family interaction should also be observed.

E. **Tests.** Testing may be helpful in specific circumstances to define the problem. Examples include psychological testing to assess cognitive function, a lead screen, or a behavioral questionnaire. Sending the family home with the task of completing a behavioral log (over 1–2 weeks) for the behaviors in question can be extremely useful. This should include antecedents to the behavior (what was going on), the behavior (what the child did and said), and the consequences (what happened after the event).

III. Management

A. Information for the family. Families are able to collaborate fully only when they understand a disorder. A detailed review of the child's strengths and vulnerabilities at each level helps to achieve some perspective and places the behaviors in context. The description of the child, for example, should be reframed from "bad" to "troubled." This subtle but important shift in perspective may allow parents to deal with the child in a more sympathetic and constructive way. These families need reassurance that the vast majority of children do not become behaviorally disordered adults.

B. Treatment. The concentric circle model of assessment allows clinicians to plan and intervene in a multidimensional way. Starting from the center:

1. **Treat any underlying basic disorder.**

2. **Build social skills and promote self-esteem** through successful behaviors and skills. This can be done through identifying and supporting what the child does well (e.g., sports for strong, aggressive children).

3. **Encourage personal responsibility and provide alternate problem solving skills.** Help the child identify his or her own role in the problem. What would the child do differently next time? Generate with the child a list of alternative behaviors to specific stressful situations.

4. **Find out what the parent and child do together that is fun, and prescribe it at an increased frequency.**

5. **Identify a single problem behavior.** Prescribe a 2-week log to include antecedents, behaviors, and consequences.

6. **Help families to develop interpersonal management skills** focusing on clarity and consistency. Reassure the parents that it will take at least 2 weeks of consistent parental intervention to see results.

7. **Mobilize community resources,** including school, church, and social service agencies. The clubs, activities, and programs that are available in the geographic area can be matched to the child's interests and activities. Structured social interventions promote prosocial behavior.

8. **Review parental supports.** Social isolation and lack of parenting network or extended family make parenting more difficult. Encourage the parents to join groups, activities (church, support groups, etc.) that will be resources for them.

C. Backup strategies when things are going poorly

1. **Reexamine the etiologic model** for a missed diagnosis. Underlying disorders may be hidden by more dramatic behaviors. Certain factors (abuse, familial dysfunction) are often occult.

2. **Reexamine the intervention.** What made it fail? Parental compliance may be problematic. Systemic conflict between the clinician and family or between multiple agencies often occurs.

D. Criteria for referral

1. **If the diagnosis is uncertain,** referral to the appropriate specialist for psychological testing or psychiatric evaluation may be indicated.

2. **If the child's behaviors are escalating out of control or self-endangering,** refer for psychiatric consultation, hospitalization, or legal intervention.

IV. Clinical pearls and pitfalls

- Disruptive behaviors are often a cry for help. What is missing in the child's life? What problems push this child to such damaging solutions?
- Parenting approaches or problems can be simply divided into too much intervention (overcontrolling, abuse, etc.) or too little intervention (neglect, no rules) or occasionally both. Restoring the balance is the task.

• Successful parental behavioral management relies on (1) defining a specific problem, (2) setting a reasonable goal (baseline frequency of behaviors minus one is the first step), (3) positive rewards without undue delay (immediate or at least daily), (4) consistency over time, and (5) knowing it may get worse before it gets better.

Bibliography

For Parents
Clark L. *SOS Help for Parents*. Bowling Green KY: Parents Press, 1985.

For Professionals
Greenberg MT, Speltz ML. Attachment and the ontogeny of conduct problems. In MT Greenberg, D Cicchetti, EM Cummings (eds), *Attachment in the Preschool Years: Theory, Research, and Intervention*. Chicago: University of Chicago Press, 1990.

Lewis DO. Conduct disorders. In M Lewis (ed), *Child and Adolescent Psychiatry*. Baltimore: Williams & Wilkins, 1991.

Wolff S. Nondelinquent disturbances of conduct. In M Rutter, L Herzok (eds), *Child and Adolescent Psychiatry*. Oxford: Blackwell, 1985.

Down Syndrome

Siegfried M. Pueschel

I. **Description of the problem.** The child with Down syndrome has recognizable physical characteristics and limited intellectual functioning due to the presence of an extra chromosome 21 or part thereof.

A. **Epidemiology**
   - Estimated incidence: 1 in 800–1200 live births. Each year approximately 3000–5000 children are born with this chromosome disorder.
   - Slight decrease of the incidence of live born children due to the utilization of prenatal diagnosis (including alpha fetoprotein testing, chorionic villus sampling, amniocentesis, and other procedures) and the subsequent termination of pregnancy.
   - Higher prevalence because of an increased life expectancy.

B. **Genetics.** There are three main types of chromosome abnormalities in Down syndrome.

   1. The vast majority (93–95%) of children with Down syndrome have **trisomy 21.**

   2. **Translocation** occurs in 4–6% of children with Down syndrome. Most translocations involve the attachment of the long arms of the supernumerary chromosome 21 to chromosome 14, 21, or 22. If translocation is identified in a child with Down syndrome, the parents' chromosomes need to be examined (about one-third of them may be a carrier of the translocation), with appropriate genetic counseling.

   3. **Mosaicism** occurs in approximately 1–3% of children with Down syndrome.

C. **Etiology.** Many etiologies of Down syndrome have been posited. Historically, syphilis and tuberculosis were implicated. Currently, radiation, viral infections, genetic predispositions, and autoimmunity are under discussion. Advanced maternal age may be associated with problems in production line, persistent nucleoli, hormonal imbalance, delayed fertilization, and relaxed selection. Recent reports from cytogenetic and epidemiologic studies favor the concept of multiple causality. However, most theories remain either unproved or tentative, and many questions remain regarding etiology.

II. **Making the diagnosis**

A. **Signs and symptoms.** There is a wide variability in the characteristics of children with Down syndrome (Table 25-1). Some individuals have only a few signs; others show most of the features.

B. **Differential diagnosis.** The main features of Down syndrome are frequently recognized by the clinician. However, occasionally children with other chromosome aberrations display a similar phenotype to Down syndrome. For example, newborns with 49, XXXXX syndrome may have similar facial features. Confirmation by chromosomal analysis is mandatory.

C. **Medical concerns.** Some of the medical concerns in children with Down syndrome may be life threatening and need to be corrected at once; others may become apparent only during the subsequent days and weeks.

Table 25-1. Percentage of positive phenotypic findings in a group of 114 young children with Down Syndrome

Sagittal suture separated	98
Oblique palpebral fissure	98
Wide space between first and second toes	96
False fontanel	95
Plantar crease between first and second toes	94
Increased neck tissue	87
Abnormally shaped palate	85
Hypoplastic nose	83
Brushfield spots	75
Mouth kept open	65
Protruding tongue	58
Epicanthal folds	57
Single palmar crease, left hand	55
Single palmar crease, right hand	52
Brachyclinodactyly, left hand	51
Brachyclinodactyly, right hand	50
Increased interpupillary distance	47
Short, stubby hands	38
Flattened occiput	35
Abnormal structure of ears	28
Abnormal implantation of ears	16
Other hand abnormalities	13
Other abnormal eye findings	11
Syndactyly	11

1. **Neonatal medical problems**

   a. **Congenital heart disease** is diagnosed in 40–45% of children with Down syndrome (atrioventricular canal most commonly, followed by ventricular septal defect, tetralogy of Fallot, patent ductus arteriosus and atrial septal defect). All newborns with Down syndrome should be examined by a pediatric cardiologist and undergo echocardiography.

   b. Approximately 10–12% of patients with Down syndrome have **anomalies of the gastrointestinal tract,** including tracheoesophageal fistula, esophageal atresia, pyloric stenosis, duodenal atresia, annular pancreas, aganglionic megacolon, and imperforate anus. Most of these anomalies require immediate surgical attention.

   c. **Congenital cataracts** are observed in approximately 3% of patients with Down syndrome. These cataracts must be extracted soon after birth.

2. **Medical problems during childhood**

   a. **Nutritional aspects.** During infancy, feeding problems and poor weight gain may be observed (especially in children with significant congenital heart disease). On the other hand, excessive weight gain often becomes a problem in many other children and adolescents. Parents need to be informed with regard to appropriate dietary practices, proper eating habits, avoidance of high-caloric food items, and regular physical exercise from early childhood on in order to avoid excessive weight gain.

   b. **Infectious disorders.** Children with Down syndrome, especially those with congenital heart disease and pulmonary artery hypertension, have a high prevalence of respiratory infections. Otitis media also has been noted to occur more frequently. Skin infections are often seen in adolescents with Down syndrome, mainly at the thighs, buttocks, and perigenital area.

c. Dental concerns. Problems with tooth eruption, tooth shape, and absence or fusion of teeth are sometimes seen. The most devastating dental problems are gingivitis and periodontal disease. It is important that persons with Down syndrome learn appropriate dental hygiene, follow good dietary habits, and be examined regularly by a dentist.

d. Visual impairment. Many children with Down syndrome have ocular disorders, including blepharitis, strabismus, nystagmus, hypoplasia of the iris, and refractive errors. It has been reported that up to 50% of these children are myopic, and another 20% are hyperopic. Children with Down syndrome should be examined by a pediatric ophthalmologist annually.

e. Audiologic dysfunction. Numerous reports from the literature indicate that 60–80% of children with Down syndrome have middle ear pathology, often resulting in hearing deficit. Most of these deficits are due to conductive hearing loss, but some children have neurosensory hearing impairment or a mixed hearing loss.

f. Seizure disorders. There is an increased frequency (6–10%) of seizure disorders in individuals with Down syndrome. Infantile spasms may be observed in the very young child with Down syndrome; grand mal seizures, as well as complex partial seizures, are more often noted during adolescence and adulthood.

g. Sleep apnea. There have been several reports of sleep apnea due to upper airway obstruction in children with Down syndrome. These children usually present with noisy breathing, snoring, and frequent apnea during sleep.

h. Thyroid dysfunction. Up to 20% of children with Down syndrome have some form of thyroid dysfunction (usually compensated or uncompensated hypothyroidism). Thyroid function studies should be carried out yearly.

i. Atlantoaxial instability. Atlantoaxial instability is due to increased ligamentous laxity at the upper cervical spine. Approximately 15% of children with Down syndrome have been found to have this disorder, although only 1–2% have symptomatic atlantoaxial instability requiring surgical intervention. Children with Down syndrome should have radiologic assessment of the cervical spine at age 2 1/2–3 years, before entering Special Olympics sport activities, and during adolescence. If asymptomatic atlantoaxial instability is present, it is recommended that the individual refrain from participating in sport activities that potentially could lead to injury of the neck and spinal cord compression.

j. Orthopedic problems. An increased prevalence of hip dislocation, patellar subluxation, and metatarsus valgus occurs in children with Down syndrome.

k. Dermatological concerns. Dermatological concerns are alopecia, folliculitis, and xerosis.

l. Hematological diseases. Immunologic and hematologic issues (e.g., increased prevalence of leukemia) have been observed in children with Down syndrome.

III. Management

A. Primary goals. The main objective of management is to provide optimal medical and surgical care to all persons with Down syndrome. No form of treatment should be withheld from any child with Down syndrome that would be given unhesitatingly to a child without this chromosomal disorder.

B. Information for families

1. Initial counseling. Although there is no completely satisfactory way of giving bad news to parents (see Chapter 5), the clinician's approach, tact, compassion, and truthfulness will have a vital influence on the parent's subsequent adjustment.

a. **Use proper terminology** and inform both parents together in a sensitive and honest way as soon as the diagnosis has been made.

b. **Time your remarks** to coincide with increasing parental adaptation.

c. **Schedule follow-up sessions** for review of basic considerations and communication of more details (chromosome analysis, developmental expectations, etc.).

d. **Spend extra time in talking about various concerns and issues** so the parents will be aware of the clinician's sincere interest in helping them and their child.

e. **Stress that most observable characteristics do not cause significant disability** in the child. For example, the slanting of the palpebral fissures or the presence of Brushfield spots does not interfere with the child's vision. On the other hand, other less obvious characteristics (such as congenital heart disease or duodenal atresia) are of a serious nature and require prompt medical attention.

2. **Treatment.** It is important to let parents know that, there is no cure for Down syndrome. In order to improve physical features and mental functioning, a multitude of "treatments" have been tried, including hormones, dimethylsulfoxide, glutamic acid, 5-hydroxytryptophan, Sicca cells, various vitamins, and minerals, as well as facial plastic surgery. These have all proved to be ineffective.

3. **Education.** Parents should be informed about early intervention programs, preschool nurseries, and special education strategies with integrated school programs that are available to children with Down syndrome. With appropriate education and positive learning experiences, many children with Down syndrome, although mild to moderately mentally retarded, will be able to function well in society. Most individuals will be able to hold a job, and many will be gainfully employed. There may be medical problems during adulthood, such as early onset of Alzheimer's disease in about 20–30% of individuals with Down syndrome. The average life expectancy is about 50 years.

Bibliography

For Parents

Organizations
National Down Syndrome Congress, 1800 Dempster, Park Ridge IL 60068; (708) 823-7550.

National Down Syndrome Society, 666 Broadway, New York NY 10012; (212) 460-9330.

Books
Pueschel SM. *A Parent's Guide to Down Syndrome: Toward a Brighter Future.* Baltimore: Brookes Publishing, 1991.

Tingey C. *Down Syndrome: A Resource Handbook.* Boston: College-Hill Press, 1988.

For Professionals
Cooley WC, Graham JM. Common syndromes and management issues for primary care physicians: Down syndrome—An update and review for the primary pediatrician. *Clin Pediatr* 30:233–253, 1991.

Pueschel SM et al. *New Perspectives on Down Syndrome.* Baltimore: Brookes Publishing, 1987.

Pueschel SM, Pueschel JK. *Biomedical Concerns in Persons with Down Syndrome.* Baltimore: Brookes Publishing, 1992.

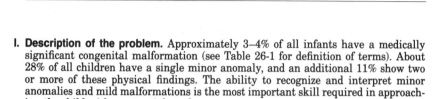

The Dysmorphic Child

John C. Carey

I. **Description of the problem.** Approximately 3–4% of all infants have a medically significant congenital malformation (see Table 26-1 for definition of terms). About 28% of all children have a single minor anomaly, and an additional 11% show two or more of these physical findings. The ability to recognize and interpret minor anomalies and mild malformations is the most important skill required in approaching the child with a potential syndrome.

The diagnosis of a dysmorphic syndrome is significant for the child, the family, and the health care professionals, for a number of reasons.

A. **Recurrence risk in genetic counseling.** The recognition of an established disorder of known etiology provides information on cause and heritable aspects of the condition, as well as potential prenatal options for future pregnancies.

B. **Relative prediction of prognosis.** Each disorder has its own particular natural history, risks for problems, and outcomes.

C. **Appropriate laboratory testing and screening.** Precise diagnosis eliminates the need for unnecessary tests; appropriate screening can be planned according to natural history.

D. **Treatment and management issues.** Knowledge of the natural history of a condition allows for the establishment of guidelines for routine care, including suggestions for educational interventions.

E. **Coping with the disorder.** In some families, the knowledge of a condition helps in dealing with the uncertainty of the situation.

II. **Making the diagnosis**

A. **Data collection.** The importance of a thorough history in the evaluation of a child with a potential syndrome cannot be overemphasized. Information on the gestational and birth history should include history of fetal movement, drugs and medications taken during pregnancy, alcohol consumption, intrauterine positioning, status of amniotic fluid, and maternal medical history. Documentation of a complete family history with a three-generation pedigree (including inquiry regarding consanguinity) is suggested.

B. **History**

1. Does the child in question have an **organized pattern of malformation** (i.e., a syndrome or sequence), or does the child exhibit a constellation of features that are consistent with the family and/or ethnic background (variant familial developmental pattern)?

a. If the child has a pattern, do the findings consist of multiple **primary** malformations of dysplasias (a syndrome), or do the findings represent **secondary** manifestations (deformations or disruptions) comprising a sequence?

b. If the child has a pattern, does it represent a **known syndrome** (or sequence,) or is it a **previously unidentified, provisionally unique pattern?**

2. What is the **date of the onset** of the physical abnormalities? Are they prenatal or postnatal? Some physical signs that are clues for syndromes are of postnatal onset and often provide signs for a metabolic disorder (e.g., the facial changes and joint contractures of the mucopolysaccharidoses).

Table 26-1. Definitions of commonly used terms

Term	Definition
Malformation	A primary morphologic defect of an organ or body part resulting from an intrinsically abnormal developmental process (e.g., cleft lip)
Deformation	An alteration of the form, shape, or position of a previously normally formed body part caused by mechanized forces (e.g., club foot due to oligohydramnios)
Sequence	Pattern of multiple anomalies derived from a single known anomaly; a primary defect with its secondary changes (e.g., Pierre Robin syndrome)
Syndrome	A recurring pattern of multiple defects due to a single etiology (e.g., Williams syndrome)
Dysmorphic	Structurally abnormal or malformed; more conventionally, used to refer to the presence of multiple minor anomalies or mild malformations, as in *dysmorphic* facial features

Source: Adapted from the recommendations of the International Working Group. Spranger J et al. Errors of morphogenesis: Concepts and terms. *J Pediatr* 100:160, 1982.

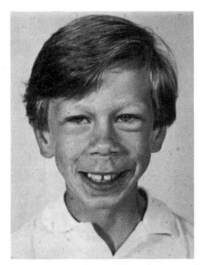

Figure 26-1. Child with Williams syndrome. Note the general facial gestalt, which is characteristic. Also, note that all of the features fall into the category of continuous features; none is a true malformation, minor or major. The mouth size measures above the 90%, but otherwise the features are not abnormal in the statistical or embyologic sense of the word.

C. **Physical examination of the craniofacies.** The practitioner needs to be observant and skilled in documenting physical variations and deciding what, in fact, is "normal" and what is not (Fig. 26-1). The evaluation of the face and hands is particularly important since most malformation syndromes have phenotypic variations in these areas. The common frustration of clinicians in approaching the potentially dysmorphic child probably helped lead to that pejorative, stigmatizing term, the "FLK" (funny looking kid), which should be eliminated from clinical practice.

   1. **The examination.** The clinician should examine the face as he or she would examine the heart or abdomen, looking at it in general and then examining each feature systematically (hair, forehead, eye slant, eyebrows, etc.) to

Table 26-2. Types of variations and malformations of the craniofacies

	Definition
Major malformations	Medically significant defects (e.g., cleft lip, microtia)
Mild malformations	Structural alterations that have no intrinsic medical significance (occur in < 4% of population, e.g., helical ear pit, cutis aplasia of the scalp)
Minor anomalies	
Continuous features with measurable alterations	Features that lend themselves to measurement and can be defined on standard curves (e.g., small ears) using the graphs in *Smith's Recognizable Patterns of Human Malformation*
Continuous features, not defined by measurements	Features that shade into normal variation and do not have a defined threshold (e.g., micrognathia, low nasal root, prominent nasal tip)

Table 26-3. Practical steps in the approach to the dysmorphic child

1. *Examine the child's family members.* Compare features to parents' or siblings'. When possible compare to photographs of family members at the same age as the index case.
2. *Consider ethnic background.* Certain features have different frequencies in different ethnic groups (e.g., eye measurements are different in African-Americans vs. persons of Hispanic descent vs. European Caucasians).
3. *Measure areas where standards exist* (e.g., ear size, palpebral fissure length). Do not trust the gestalt in deciding whether a feature is large or small; have plastic rulers available in the clinic setting.
4. *Look up the most distinctive and/or rarest defect for quick identification* (e.g., the white forelock suggesting Waardenburg syndrome).
5. *Become acquainted with the terminology and ways to describe the face and hands.*

determine what about this face makes it look different. Does one feature make the face look distinctive or unique, several features, or one area of the face? The gestalt should be noted (the whole is more than the sum of the parts). If the ears appear low set, the clinician should consider why they look that way. Are they small, posteriorly rotated, or overfolded, or does the low placement, in fact, represent an illusion?

2. **Classification.** Table 26-2 presents a classification of types of variations of the face. It is of note that most of the features of a child with Down syndrome fall into the minor anomaly category. This is the class of features that usually requires comparison to family members, especially parents and siblings, and also consideration of ethnic background. Photographing the patient is important for documentation. The pictures can be placed in the chart for future review.

3. **The approach.** Table 26-3 summarizes the practical steps that can be used in approaching the dysmorphic child.

The most useful and easily available reference source for looking up features and attempting to make a diagnosis is *Smith's Recognizable Patterns of Human Malformation* by Jones. In addition, a number of computer programs have been designed to help in the diagnostic process.

D. **Laboratory evaluation**

1. After initial evaluation of the child, if no secure diagnosis has been reached and it appears that the child has multiple anomalies, a **chromosome study** should be performed. There is a 5% yield of positive chromosome studies

among children with dysmorphic features and developmental delay. In most circumstances a routine G-banded karyotype is performed.

2. If there is suspicion that the child's features are suggestive of the fragile X syndrome (Chapter 33), then a **fragile X study** is warranted.

3. If one of the microdeletion syndromes is in question (e.g., Prader-Willi syndrome), then a **high-resolution study** or **FISH** (fluorescence in-situ hybridization) is indicated.

4. **TORCH (toxoplasmosis, other, rubella, cytomegalovirus, herpes simplex) titers** are usually not indicated in an infant who has multiple primary defects that are alterations in embryogenesis (e.g., cleft lip, polydactyly, or even minor anomalies).

5. **Amino acid studies** are not indicated in an infant with multiple primary malformations since none of the known aminoacidopathies is consistently associated with structural anomalies of prenatal onset. However, there are some inborn errors of metabolism that will have associated congenital or early-onset physical abnormalities that might raise the question of the child having a dysmorphic syndrome. Examples include the abnormal hair of an infant with Menkes syndrome and the dysmorphic features of the peroxisomal disorders. Imaging studies and referrals to subspecialists are indicated according to the presence of accompanying problems.

III. **Management**

A. **Specialty referral.** Consultation with a dysmorphologist or clinical geneticist skilled in syndrome recognition is indicated for any child who appears to be dysmorphic. Referral for consultation is also appropriate for any family with questions about the diagnosis, the natural history of the disorder, the recurrence risk, prenatal options, issues of reproductive decision making, and psychological support.

B. **Health maintenance and anticipatory guidance.** Once the diagnosis of a particular syndrome is made, the clinician can review the natural history of the disorder and help establish a plan for follow-up and screening.

C. **Psychological support.** The process of ruling out a syndrome can, in and of itself, be overwhelming and even stigmatizing for the family. Families often perceive the meticulous detail of the examination as a "picking apart" process. Discussion of the reasons for making a diagnosis is helpful, and acknowledging these potential feelings are important in the initiation of the referral process.

IV. **Clinical pearls and pitfalls**

• **The null hypothesis strategy.** The diagnosis of a syndrome should be approached in a hypothesis-generating manner. The clinician should state the null hypothesis— "This child does not have a dysmorphic syndrome"—and then review the evidence. This approach attempts to avoid overdiagnosis and puts the burden of proof on the person who makes the diagnosis. It also demands a certain amount of critical thinking about the use of the minor anomalies in the diagnostic thought process.

• **The eye doesn't see what the mind doesn't know.** This often-cited axiom underscores the importance of the knowledge of the disorder, as well as the need for astute observation. Recognition of the subtleties of physical variation, as well as clinical variability of a disorder, is crucial in the evaluation.

• Children with dysmorphic syndromes are not necessarily unusual or different in appearance. What is usually present is a **difference from their unaffected family members** rather than a clear-cut abnormality. In many syndromes, the features are consistent and show difference from the family background but are not very distinctive or striking.

• "You know my method. It is founded upon the observance of trifles." Sherlock Holmes, *The Boscombe Valley Mystery.*

Bibliography

For Parents

Alliance of Genetic Support Groups, 35 Wisconsin Circle, Suite 440, Chevy Chase MD 20815; (800) 336-GENE.
Offers an updated catalog of support groups for various disorders.

For Professionals

Aase JM. Dysmorphologic diagnosis for the pediatric practitioner. *Pediatr Clin North Am* 39 (1):135, 1992.

Cohen MM. *The Child with Multiple Birth Defects*. New York: Raven Press, 1982.

Hall BD. The state of the art of dysmorphology. *Am J Dis Child* 147:1184–1189, 1993.

Jones KL. *Smith's Recognizable Patterns of Human Malformations* (4th ed.) Philadelphia: Saunders, 1988.

Opitz JM. What the general pediatrician should know about developmental anomalies. *Pediatr Rev* 3:267, 1982.

POSSUM (Pictures of Standard Syndromes and Undiagnosed Malformations): An electronic reference.
Available through CP Export Pty. Ltd., 493 St. Kilda Road, Melbourne, Victoria, 3004, Australia. The program is found in many medical libraries and is often located in the office of a dysmorphologist or clinical geneticist. This is a very user-friendly system.

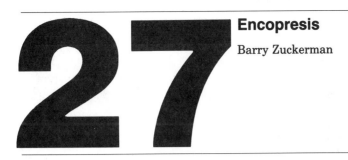

Encopresis
Barry Zuckerman

I. **Description of the problem.** Encopresis is defined as regular soiling of the underwear in children age 4 years and older with no organic disease. The soiling can range from staining the underwear to semiformed or formed stools. Encopresis can be *primary* (never toilet trained for stool) or *secondary* (previously trained).

A. **Epidemiology**
- Occurs in as many as 1.5% of school-aged children.
- Male preponderance.
- Unrelated to social class, birth order, or family size.

B. **Contributing factors.** The interaction of multiple biobehavioral factors contributes to stool retention and subsequent encopresis (Fig. 27–1).

1. **Constitutional predisposition.** Intestinal motility varies among individuals. Children with slower intestinal motility may be more vulnerable to stool retention.

2. **Temperament.** In response to the urge to have a bowel movement, distractible children on the way to the toilet may become engaged in another activity until the sensation to have a bowel movement abates.

3. **Toilet training/autonomy.** Forced toilet training may result in a child's withholding stool. Parents can control many aspects of young children's behavior, but children can always control their own body sphincters. Bowel and feeding issues are common manifestations of intense autonomy struggles.

4. **Pain.** A previously painful bowel movement (e.g., due to a rock-hard stool or rectal fissure) may make a child afraid to have a bowel movement, with subsequent voluntary stool withholding.

5. **Psychosocial stress.** Children going to a new school or camp may be uncomfortable if the bathroom does not allow for privacy. In response, children may have less frequent bowel movements, leading to stool retention over time.

6. **Medications.** Certain medications (e.g., narcotic-containing cough syrups, anticonvulsants) decrease intestinal motility.

7. **Pathophysiology.** Any one or some combination of the factors just noted can contribute to stool retention. As stool is retained, the simultaneous process of stretching the rectal wall and decreasing sensory feedback leads to less frequent bowel movements, which leads to further stool retention and larger stools. As water is reabsorbed, the stool becomes harder, and bowel movements may become painful. As this cycle progresses, the external and internal sphincters become compromised. Soft feces pass around the hard, immobile stool and leak out the anus. Sensitivity to rectal distension and control of rectal evacuation diminish in severe cases. The child soon loses the urge to have a bowel movement and habituates to the fecal odor.

II. **Making the diagnosis**

A. **Signs and symptoms**

1. **Staining of underwear.**

2. **Enuresis** coexists in approximately 25% of children due to decreasing bladder capacity and increased bladder irritability from pressure from the adjacent enlarged colon.

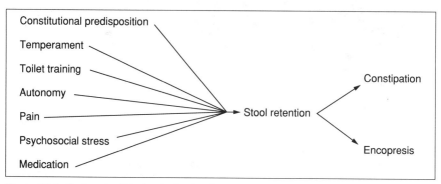

Figure 27-1. Factors leading to stool retention.

Table 27-1. Differentiating factors for encopresis and Hirschsprung's disease

	Encopresis	Hirschsprung's disease
Stool in ampulla	XXXX	X
Large-caliber stool	XX	
Avoidance of toilet	XXX	X
Onset of constipation in newborn period		XXX

Note: Number of Xs reflects relative frequency of occurrence.

3. **Recurrent abdominal pain,** especially in the early stages.

4. **Urinary** tract infections in females.

B. **Differential diagnosis.** In cases of stool retention, it is important to rule out organic pathology. Hirschsprung's disease is rare (1/25,000 children) and unlikely to lead to encopresis. Differentiating factors are listed in Table 27-1. Other diagnoses to consider include any condition that can cause constipation (e.g., hypothyroidism) and diseases that impair voluntary muscle control (e.g., cerebral palsy, amyotonia congenita, and spinal cord lesions). Finally, children who have experienced significant traumas (e.g., sexual abuse) may occasionally develop encopresis.

C. **History: Key clinical questions**

1. *When did this start? How often does the child stain the underwear?* The duration and pattern of staining provides important information. Eliciting this information in a sensitive and matter-of-fact way begins the therapeutic process of demystifying this embarrassing problem.

2. *Does your child have large caliber stools that may even clog up the toilet?* Large-caliber stools imply stool retention and functional megacolon.

3. [To the parent:] *Why do you think this happens? Is your child upset about it? What do you do about it?* Understanding the parents' hypotheses for the symptoms is revealing and can provide insight into their relationship with the child. Have the parents used punitive strategies or made degrading comments? Many parents think their child is "just lazy" and "doesn't seem to care" about the staining. However, just the opposite is often true. All children are ashamed because they know that "only babies have bowel movements in their pants." The shame is so great that they cannot even acknowledge it.

4. *How does your child get along with peers and parents? How does he or she do in school?* This question will provide information on the child's

strengths and weaknesses and whether the encopresis has affected social relationships.

5. [To the child:] *Do you want this problem to end? Are you willing to work hard to end it?* An affirmative response to these questions provides the clinician with the opportunity to empower the child to resolve the problem. The clinician must provide help and support but emphasize that the child alone must take responsibility to end this problem.

D. **Behavioral observations.** Observing the parents' interactions with the child will indicate whether their words and actions show sensitivity to or belittle the child (intentionally or not).

E. **Physical examination.** A complete physical examination is essential to rule out organic pathology, with special emphasis on the abdominal examination (looking for colonic masses) and the neurologic examination (looking for perineal reflexes and sensation). A rectal examination assesses the presence of fissures as well as stool in the ampulla. For most children, this examination can be deferred in order to support the child's taking control of his or her own body and to avoid undue emphasis on the rectum. A rectal examination can be performed at a later visit if the response to treatment is not satisfactory.

F. **Tests.** Abdominal x rays can confirm stool retention, but so too can the abdominal or rectal examinations or a history of large-caliber stool. Sometimes showing a child stool retention on x ray can be an important part of the intervention, but this should be used selectively. Manometric studies need be done only if Hirschsprung's disease is suspected and/or after management has failed.

III. **Management**

A. **Primary goals**

1. **To remove retained feces.**
2. **To retrain the child to defecate normally.**
3. **To help the child feel that he or she has mastered the problem.**

B. **Initial treatment strategies.** It is the clinician's job to form an alliance with the child, provide information about the mechanics of stool retention, support the child in taking control of his or her body, and provide a structured toileting program.

1. **Address the child's isolation and embarrassment.** Since children and parents are unlikely to know anyone else with encopresis, it is important for the clinician to tell them that he or she takes care of many other children with this problem. Additionally, acknowledging the child's embarrassment helps the parents to empathize with (and not castigate) the child.

2. **Take the child off the hook** by informing him or her that the staining is not his or her fault. A good analogy is a runny nose: as hard as people try to hold in mucus, they rarely succeed.

3. **Acknowledge the child's embarrassment.** The clinician explains that his or her goal is to teach the child control so that the youngster is no longer embarrassed by the symptoms.

4. **Demystify the process with developmentally appropriate explanations.** Drawings and diagrams can be used to explain in concrete terms the development of the stool retention that leads to soiling. Such demystification promotes compliance and engages the child to master a definable task. This may involve a description of how nutritious elements of food are absorbed and how the remaining "waste" is eliminated through the anus. The clinician explains how the buildup of stool stretches the tubelike colon, which then weakens the muscles of the bowel so they can no longer hold in the newly formed waste.

5. **Provide a structured toileting program.** The management strategy should emphasize the need for the child to eliminate the waste by "building up the muscles." This is done, like any other exercise, by having the child sit on the toilet after each meal and before bed for 5 minutes at a time and *strenuously* attempt a bowel movement. It is important to emphasize that this is not

passive sitting but rather an exercise for which the child has to strain hard (and even grunt "like a weightlifter") to build up his or her bowel muscles.

An exercise chart can be used with a circle for every time the child sits on the toilet and does the exercise. The goal is to sit on the toilet and exercise but not necessarily produce a bowel movement. If the child is successful in having a bowel movement, he or she will put an X in the circle. The parental role needs to be determined regarding how much they will remind their child to do the exercise. The child can be asked whether he or she wants parental reminders. If the parents become overinvolved and controlling, this plan will not work.

6. **Empower the child.** The child should send or bring each week's chart to the clinician and call the clinician once a week to report progress. It is important to emphasize that the child, not the parent, should call. This gives the child the clear message that he or she, not the parents, is in charge not only of his or her body but in working out this problem with the clinician. It is this appeal to the child's sense of mastery that engenders the motivation to succeed.

7. **Use bowel "clean-out" as a last resort.** An enema for initial evacuation of the colon can be impractical and stressful for the parent and child. Since the problem usually has been occurring for a long time, there is no need to conduct a rapid clean-out that may be psychologically stressful and give the child the message that other individuals control his or her body (e.g., sphincter). For many children, information and a behavioral approach with oral medications can be effective to clean out the colon. On the other hand, children with a significant megacolon will ultimately need enemas to facilitate clean-out. This should be the last, not the first, step.

C. Follow-up/back-up strategies

1. **Follow-up.** Children should be seen every 1 or 2 weeks to monitor progress and to provide support to the child. Charts should be brought in and sent by mail on alternate weeks. The charts should be reviewed with the child.

2. **Back-up step 1.** If after 2 weeks the child is not regularly having bowel movements in the toilet, the next steps are dietary manipulations and medication interventions. This includes eliminating milk, apples, bananas, and rice from the diet while simultaneously increasing dietary fiber and starting an oral laxative (e.g., Senokot).

3. **Back-up step 2.** If back-up step 1 is not successful in 3 weeks, a Dulcolax tablet should be prescribed before bedtime for 3–5 days.

4. **Back-up step 3**

   a. **Day 1:** Two hypophosphate enemas.

   b. **Day 2:** Dulcolax suppositories bid.

   c. Repeat both steps for two to four cycles until the impaction is cleared.

Bibliography

Nolan T, Oberklaid F. New concepts in the management of encopresis. *Pediatr Rev* 14:447–51, 1993.

Levine MD, Bakow H. Children with encopresis: A study of treatment outcome. Pediatrics 58:845–852, 1976.

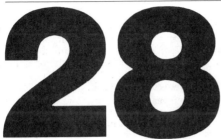

Enuresis

Leonard Rappaport

I. **Description of the problem.** Enuresis is defined as a lack of urinary continence beyond age 4 years for diurnal (daytime) enuresis, a lack of urinary continence beyond age 6 years for nocturnal (nighttime) enuresis, or the loss of continence after at least 3 months of dryness.

   A. **Epidemiology.** A universal definition remains elusive because the development of urinary continence varies by gender, cultural group, race, and country. Table 28-1 provides general guidelines for the attainment of urinary continence in the United States.

      1. **Subtypes.** Enuresis is divided into (1) **primary enuresis** (incontinence in a child who has never attained continence) and (2) **secondary enuresis** (when a child has attained continence for at least 3 months and begins to have episodes of incontinence). Enuresis is then further subdivided into **diurnal** (daytime) versus **nocturnal** (nighttime) enuresis. More than half of the children with diurnal enuresis also have nocturnal enuresis. Both secondary and diurnal enuresis are associated with a greater degree of organic pathology.

   B. **Familial transmission/Genetics.** There is a genetic predisposition to enuresis. If one parent had enuresis, 40% of his or her children will have enuresis. If both parents had enuresis, 70% of their children will have enuresis. Identical twins have the highest concordance rate.

   C. **Etiology.** In the vast majority of cases, the etiology of enuresis is unknown. There are, however, causes that should be considered.

      1. **Diseases/Structural abnormalities**

         a. **Increased urinary output.** Any process that increases urinary output can cause enuresis (e.g., diabetes mellitus, diabetes insipidus, sickle cell disease).

         b. **Increased bladder irritability.** The most common cause of secondary enuresis is increased bladder irritability, usually due to a urinary tract infection. Additionally, any mass impinging on the bladder (e.g., severe constipation) can increase bladder irritability.

         c. **Bladder capacity.** Bladder capacity is decreased in children with enuresis compared to their nonenuretic siblings. This reflects differences in functional, rather than absolute, bladder capacity, with contractions occurring earlier in filling.

         d. **Temperamental factors.** Diurnal enuresis is frequently complicated by a child's lack of attention to bodily signals. The child with a short attention span and/or a desire to persist in an activity will frequently ignore his or her need to urinate until it is too late.

         e. **Sleep and arousal factors.** Originally it was thought that enuresis was a non–rapid eye movement dysomnia (like sleepwalking and night terrors). Additionally, many parents believe that their enuretic child sleeps more soundly than their other children. This observation is probably due to selection bias (the child with enuresis is the *only* child the parents attempt to arouse from a deep sleep). Recent data suggest that enuresis occurs in *all* stages of sleep and that there is no difference in sleep patterns

Table 28-1. Prevalence of continence

Day	Night
50% by age 2½ years	66% by age 3 years
90% by age 4 years	75% by age 4 years
	90% by age 8 years
	98% by ages 12–14 years

between children with enuresis and their nonenuretic peers. Obstructive sleep apnea can be associated with nocturnal enuresis.

f. CNS factors. Recent research has focused on a lack of the usual nocturnal increase of antidiuretic hormone (ADH) secretion in children with nocturnal enuresis, leading to an increase in urinary output. These data remain relatively sparse and in need of replication, and they should be considered speculative. Enuresis is also more common in children with learning disabilities.

g. Psychopathology/stress. There are no data to support enuresis as a neurotic disorder. Similarly, although stress may exacerbate or contribute to enuresis, it is not a primary etiologic factor.

h. Abnormal sphincter control. Although abnormal urinary sphincter control is rare, insidious pathology (e.g., spinal cord abnormalities) can cause abnormal sphincter control. Some hypothesize that there is a group of children with decreased sphincter strength without obvious cause who may have a higher incidence of enuresis.

i. Structural abnormalities. Girls with ectopic ureters which empty into the vagina, for example, have constant wetting with no recognized episodes of incontinence.

j. Vaginal reflux. Overweight girls who sit with their legs together when urinating often reflux into the vagina. The urine will then leak out over the next several hours. This causes almost constant daytime wetting without nighttime episodes.

II. Making the diagnosis

A. History: Key clinical questions. A complete history should be obtained with a particular focus on a family history of enuresis, the child's pattern of wetting, and the previous interventions.

1. *Has the child ever been dry at night?* It is important to differentiate primary from secondary enuresis.

2. *Does the child have accidents during the day, as well as at night?* Treat the daytime enuresis first if it coexists with nocturnal incontinence.

3. *Was anyone else in the family late in achieving dryness at night or day?* A positive family history may make the family more (or less) sympathetic to the child's feelings. It may be helpful to elicit the parents' own experience with enuresis and how it affects their response to their child.

4. *What have you tried to fix the problem?* Evaluate the positive and negative interventions. Determine if they were appropriately implemented and their secondary effects (e.g., on the child's self-esteem).

5. [To the child:] ***How much of a problem is this to you?*** The child must be motivated to be cured if treatment is to be successful.

B. Physical examination. A full physical examination should be performed, with emphasis placed on the spine, neurologic, and genital examinations.

C. Tests. The laboratory evaluation should be very limited. A urinalysis should be obtained in all children (plus a urine culture in females). Further workup should be directed by findings in the history and physical examination. There is no

Table 28-2. Interventions for enuresis

Method	Initial success rate	Relapse rate
Nocturnal enuresis		
Alarms	70%	10%
Imipramine	50%	90%
Desmopressin acetate (DDAVP)	50%	90%
Bladder stretching	30%	?
Motivational	20%	?
Diurnal enuresis		
Urgency containment	75%	?
Alarms	?	?
Oxybutynin	?	?

indication for the use of imaging techniques or urodynamic studies unless suggested by the history or physical examination.

III. Management

A. Primary goals. The primary goals in the treatment of enuresis are to alleviate the problem and to limit its impact on the child's self-esteem and interpersonal relationships. Although a cure is possible for most children, a small percentage will have to learn to live with this problem. Initial interventions should be directed both at helping the child cope with the problem and working on a solution.

B. Information for the family. The family should be told how common enuresis is and made to understand that it is usually a developmental problem over which the child has little to no control. Punishments only lower the child's self-esteem without improving the symptoms. Finally, parents should understand that effective treatments are available and that most treatments require cooperation between them, the child, and the primary care clinician.

C. Treatment strategies.

1. **Nocturnal enuresis.** The spontaneous remission rate for nocturnal enuresis is 15% per year. Table 28-2 lists the cure and relapse rates for the common treatments.

   a. **Alarms** have become the preferred treatment for nocturnal enuresis over the past several years because of their high efficacy, low cost, ease of use, and almost negligible regression rate. However, the use of an alarm requires a considerable commitment from the parents (at least for the first month or two) when the child may not awaken to the alarm. The parents and child should be instructed in its use:
      • Use the alarm every night.
      • Parents should wake the child when the alarm rings and take the child to the bathroom (even if an accident has already occurred). After several weeks, the child will awaken independently when the alarm sounds.
      • Restart the alarm after the underwear is changed.
      • Use star or sticker chart for dry nights.
      Most children who respond to alarms do so within 4–6 months. (See the list of alarms at the end of the chapter.)

   b. **Medications**

      i. **Imipramine,** a tricyclic antidepressant, has been shown to be very successful in the treatment of nocturnal enuresis, although the mechanism for this improvement remains uncertain. There are two problems with imipramine in the treatment of enuresis: the high relapse rate when stopped and the very high toxic index if taken in overdosage.

      ii. **Desmopressin acetate (DDAVP)** is a synthetic analog of 8-arginine vasopressin and has been used in the treatment of enuresis for several years. There has been some literature to support its efficacy when taken intranasally at night. However, long-term data are sparse. Because of its high cost (approximately $100/month) and high relapse rate after stopping, DDAVP cannot be considered a first-line treatment for nocturnal enuresis. It can be useful in certain situations, such as a child going to overnight camp or a child who is discouraged by previous treatment failures.

   c. **Bladder stretching exercises** are a moderately successful form of treatment. In these exercises, children are asked to hold their urine for as long as they can, as frequently as they can. In several studies, the children who increased their functional bladder capacity the greatest amount with these exercises had the greatest improvement in their enuresis.

   d. **Motivational incentives** (e.g., star charts and other reward systems) generally provide a positive focus on a child's remaining dry at night. Their relatively low efficacy makes them a useful adjunct but not a primary treatment of nocturnal enuresis.

2. **Diurnal enuresis.** When a child has both nocturnal and diurnal enuresis, the daytime component should be addressed first.

   a. **Bladder stretching exercises.** Treatment for diurnal enuresis involves the use of bladder urgency containment exercises:
   • The child goes into the bathroom when he or she has to urinate.
   • Once there, he or she holds the urine for as long as possible.
   • When the child does urinate, he or she is asked to stop and start the urine flow frequently.
   The objective is to increase the muscle strength of the urethra, as well as to give the child confidence that he or she can control the urinary stream. In most children, the enuresis will resolve over several months.

   b. **Contingent and noncontingent alarms** are helpful for some children. Contingent alarms go off when the child starts to wet, but these can be socially embarrassing. Noncontingent alarms involve wearing a watch that beeps about every 2 hours to remind the child to urinate.

   c. **Medications** for diurnal enuresis are rarely indicated. Some believe that anticholinergic agents (e.g., oxybutynin chloride) have shown some efficacy, but there are no conclusive trials supporting their use.

D. **Improving self-esteem/family function.** Self-esteem is best preserved by a nonpunitive response to the enuresis. The child should understand that enuresis is common and that it is not a sign of emotional, psychological, or medical dysfunction. The child can be empowered to take responsibility for dryness at night following an accident via the "double bubble" technique:
   • Place a plastic sheet over the mattress, followed by the usual sheets and blankets.
   • Place another plastic sheet over those sheets, again followed by another set of sheets and blankets.
   • Keep a dry set of pajamas by the bedside.
   • During the day, rehearse with the child how to take the wet set of sheets off the bed, uncovering the dry second set, and how to change pajamas.
   This technique can defuse family tensions by allowing the child to handle his or her own needs at night and not awaken the parents.

E. **Criteria for referral.** The child should be referred to a urologist, when genitourinary pathology is suspected. Psychological counseling should be sought when the child's social function appears to have been impaired by the enuresis or when the family's response appears to be unduly punitive.

IV. **Clinical pearls and pitfalls**
   • *Always* do a full history and physical when beginning the treatment of a child with enuresis.
   • Parents may have not shared with the clinician all the information pertaining to enuresis unless they are asked directly. Parents need to be asked about previous interventions and, in particular, how these interventions were instituted. Frequently parents will have tried an intervention inappropriately.

- Success is contagious. A child who has had multiple failures in the treatment of enuresis might be helped by trying a medical therapy (e.g., DDAVP or imipramine) to achieve some success immediately. A more definitive but difficult therapy (e.g., an alarm) can follow after the child and family have the sense that success is possible.
- Involvement of the child is essential. No intervention will be successful without the motivation and commitment of the child.
- Always pay attention to the evolution of the child's self-esteem. Punitive techniques should be avoided at all costs.

Bibliography

For Parents
Mack A. *Dry All Night*. Boston: Little, Brown, 1989.

For Professionals
Foxman B, Valdez RB, Brook RH. Childhood enuresis: Prevalence, perceived impact, and prescribed treatments. *Pediatrics* 77:482, 1986.

Rappaport L. The treatment of enuresis: Where are we now? *Pediatrics* 92:464, 1993.

Rappaport L. Enuresis. In MD Levine, W Carey, A Crocker (eds), *Developmental-Behavioral Pediatrics*. Philadelphia: Saunders, 1992.

Schmitt BA. Nocturnal enuresis. In MA Green, RJ Haggerty (eds), *Ambulatory Pediatrics*. Philadelphia: Saunders, 1990.

Wille S. Comparison of desmopressin and enuresis alarms for nocturnal enuresis. *Arch Dis Child* 61:30, 1986.

Selected Enuresis Alarms

Nite Train'r Alarm, Koregon Enterprises, 9735 Southwest Sunshine Court, Beaverton OR 97005; (800) 544-4240.

Nytone Medical Products, 2424 South 900 West, Salt Lake City UT 84119; (801) 973-4090.

Wet Stop Alarm, Palco Laboratories, 8030 Soquel Avenue, Santa Cruz CA 95062; (800) 346-4488.

29

Failure to Thrive

Deborah Frank

I. **Description of the problem.** Failure to thrive (FTT) refers to children, usually under age 5 years, whose growth persistently and significantly deviates from the norms for their age and sex on the National Center for Health Statistics (NCHS) growth charts.

A. **Epidemiology**
  - Nutritional growth failure is seen in 8–12% of low-income children. However, the prevalence of FTT in the general population is unknown.

B. **Family transmission/genetics.** Familial short stature may be considered when the child's weight is appropriate to height and when linear growth velocity follows the normal curve on the growth chart. It is, however, perilous to assume that poor growth in children is secondary to familial predisposition for several reasons:
  - Parental height may be a poor guide of the child's growth potential if parents themselves were nutritionally deprived as children and therefore did not attain their optimal growth (as is often the case with immigrant and impoverished families).
  - The parents may have an eating disorder and be excessively concerned with obesity.
  - The child may share an organic problem with the parents (e.g., lactose intolerance).

C. **Etiology**

  1. **Organic versus nonorganic.** Traditionally, the etiology of FTT was considered either organic or nonorganic. However, this dichotomy is of limited use since children with so-called nonorganic FTT are suffering from malnutrition, a serious organic insult, while children with major organic diagnoses may, in part, have growth failure attributable to social and nutritional factors. Diagnostically and therapeutically, it is useful to assess each child and family along four parameters: (1) medical, (2) nutritional, (3) developmental, and (4) social. Problems in any or all of these areas may interact to produce growth failure. For example, a temperamentally passive child with lead poisoning may fail to receive frequent enough feedings from an exhausted mother who has other more demanding children.

  2. **Psychosocial causes**

     a. Child may fail to thrive in families of any social class **when parents' emotional and material resources are diverted from the care of the child.** This can occur because of parental depression, maladaptive parenting practices, family discord, another chronically ill family member, substance abuse, or losses (such as death of grandparent or unemployment).

       FTT does not necessarily imply parental neglect or pathology. Feeding disorders can develop when not eating serves other purposes (e.g., to express anger, to exert autonomy from overly intrusive caretakers, to gain the attention of otherwise abstracted caretakers, or to divert adults from conflict with each other).

     b. Children with **preexisting minor developmental deficits** (e.g., subtle oral motor difficulties, hypersensitivity to stimulation) may develop feeding

Table 29-1. Often inapparent medical causes of inadequate intake

Infectious
Giardiasis (other parasites, e.g., nematodes)
Chronic urinary tract infection
Chronic sinusitis
Mechanical
Adenoid hypertrophy
Dental lesions
Vascular slings
Gastroesophageal reflux with esophagitis
Neurologic
Oral-motor dysfunction (gagging, tactile hypersensitivity)
Toxic/metabolic
Lead toxicity
Iron deficiency
Zinc deficiency
Gastrointestinal
Celiac disease
Malabsorption (various causes)
Chronic constipation

---

problems that lead to nutritional FTT. Apathy and irritability associated with malnutrition may exacerbate parent-child interactional dysfunction and lead to further feeding difficulties.

   c. Children **living in poverty** are often at nutritional risk because of inadequate food supplies in the home, homelessness and overcrowding, and the inability of federal feeding programs (e.g., food stamps, supplemental food program for women, infants, and children [WIC], school meals) to reach many of the eligible families. In other cases, the benefit levels of such programs are insufficient to meet the nutritional needs of at-risk children.

3. **Medical causes**

   a. The **organic causes** of FTT encompass a whole textbook of pediatrics. Usually most are suggested by a careful history and physical examination, but some are occult (Table 29-1).

   b. **Perinatal risk factors** include prematurity and intrauterine growth retardation (IUGR). IUGR with dysmorphic features suggests a growth-retarding syndrome (genetic, congenital, or related to teratogen exposure).

D. **Long-term outcomes.** FTT is a major risk factor for later developmental and behavioral difficulties, usually reflecting both the nutritional deprivation of the developing nervous system and the environmental experiences of the child.

II. **Making the diagnosis**

A. **Signs and symptoms.** While there are no universally accepted anthropometric criteria, the following are frequently used:

   1. **Weight less than fifth or third percentile.**

   2. **Failure to maintain previously established growth trajectory,** with parameters crossing two major percentiles (e.g., seventy fifth to below twenty fifth).

   3. **Decreased rate of daily weight gain for age** (Table 29-2).

   4. **Depressed weight for height,** which always reflects inadequate nutritional intake for the child's metabolic requirements. (Short stature with a weight that is proportionate to height may reflect chronic malnutrition or may be genetic or endocrinologic in origin.)

Table 29-2. Average daily weight gain for age

Age	Median daily weight gain (g)
0–3 mo	26–31
3–6 mo	17–18
6–9 mo	12–13
9–12 mo	9
1–3 yr	7–9
4–6 yr	6

B. **Key clinical questions.** It is important first to scrutinize the growth chart to ascertain the timing of onset of growth failure:

1. *What were the changes in your family's or child's life around the time the child's growth slowed?* Perhaps a parent returned to work and the child was placed in day care at the time; perhaps there was a family loss.

2. *What, when (how often), where, why, and by whom is your child fed?* It is useful to ascertain a 24-hour dietary recall. Additionally, the child's behaviors and affect at mealtime should be elicited.

3. *How much low-calorie liquid (e.g., juice, soda, iced tea, Kool-aid) does your child drink each day?*

4. *Does your child choke on food, have trouble chewing or swallowing, vomit, or spit up?* Oral motor problems and gastroesophageal reflux usually present with these symptoms.

5. *What are your child's bowel movements like?* Frequency and nature of stools may be a clue for occult gastrointestinal disease.

6. *Do you ever run out of food?* If the clinician does not ask, the parents may never tell.

7. *Does your child snore, even when there is no cold?* Adenoidal hypertrophy is a frequently missed cause of poor oral intake.

8. *Are there any foods to which your child is allergic or which he or she is not allowed to eat for religious or other reasons (e.g., vegetarian)?*

9. *Do you and the child's other caretakers see eye to eye about the growing and eating problem?*

10. *Are there any significant stresses in the house?*

C. **Behavioral observations**

1. The clinician can **observe the child while eating or being fed** in his or her office (or ideally during a home visit by trained observer):
   • Is the child adaptively positioned to eat?
   • Are the child's cues clear, and does the caretaker respond appropriately?
   • Are there oral motor difficulties?
   • Does the caretaker permit age-appropriate autonomy and messiness?
   • What is the affective tone at the feeding interaction?
   • Is the child easily distracted during the feeding?
   • Is the child fed in front of television?

2. The clinician should also observe the **quality of the *nonfeeding* interactions:**
   • Is the caretaker irritable, punitive, depressed, disengaged, or intrusive?
   • Is the child apathetic, irritable, noncompliant, or provocative?

D. **Physical examination.** A careful physical examination should be performed to rule out apparent medical causes of the FTT. Additionally, all children with FTT should have formal developmental testing.

Try to keep mealtimes and snack times about the same each day. Children work well with schedules.

Children need to eat often, not constantly. Offer something every 2–3 hours, to allow three meals and two to three snacks per day.

Make sure your child can reach the food. Use a high chair, telephone book, or a small table.

Allow your child to feed himself or herself. Try very small amounts at first. Offer seconds later. *Expect messiness.*

No force feeding, bribing, or cajoling! This will backfire.

Variety is not important. Total *calories* and *protein* are.

Offer solids before liquids.

Limit juice, water, and carbonated drinks. Offer milk or formula instead.

Offer foods that are easy for your child to handle: "finger foods" such as Cheerios, french fries, slices of banana, cut-up burger, hot dogs, or peas.

Add margarine, mayonnaise, gravies, and grated cheese. For snacks, use peanut butter, cheese, pudding, bananas, or dried fruit.

Junk foods (soda, doughnuts, candy, etc.) have little protein and fewer calories than some other food choices. Junk foods will not help growth; they only take up valuable space in the stomach.

Eat with your child when possible, or allow your child to eat with others, so meals and snacks can be fun.

Figure 29-1. Effective feeding checklist for parents

E. Tests

1. Testing should be performed on the basis of the history and physical examination. **Basic screening laboratory tests** should include CBC, lead, FEP, urinalysis, urine culture, electrolytes, and a purified protein derivative (PPD).

2. If the child is a new immigrant or recent traveler, lives in a homeless shelter, has been camping, or is in day care and has a history of diarrhea or abdominal pain, **evaluation for enteric pathogens** (e.g., *Giardia*) should be considered.

3. If the child is short but is an appropriate weight for height, a **bone age** may be useful to distinguish the constitutionally short child (with a bone age equivalent to chronological age) from a child with endocrine or nutritional derangement (with a delayed bone age).

III. Management

A. Primary goals. The primary goal is for the child to attain catch-up growth at a rate faster than average for age in order to repair the growth deficit. This typically requires a calorically dense diet that provides one and a half to two times the recommended daily allowance of calories. In addition, other identified socioemotional difficulties must be specifically addressed.

B. Treatment strategies

1. **Instruct the parents in high-calorie/high-protein diet** (Figs. 29-1 and 29-2). This diet may violate current norms since increased fat may be necessary to provide adequate calories in small volume.

2. **Feed the child three meals and three snacks** on a consistent schedule.

3. Give a **multivitamin** with iron and zinc (and therapeutic dosages of iron if indicated).

24-calorie per ounce formula
  1 can (13 oz) formula concentrate.
  8 oz. water.

Note: Don't make the formula more concentrated than this: overconcentrating can be harmful to a child's kidneys.

Super fruit
  1 jar (4 oz) strained fruit
  1 scoop formula powder

Super milk (use instead of whole milk; 28 calories per ounce)
  1 cup dry milk powder
  4 cups whole milk

Super pudding
  2 cups whole milk
  ½ cup dry milk powder
  1 pkg. instant pudding mix
Mix whole and dry milk together. Then follow package directions for making pudding. Yield: 4 servings. (116 calories per serving)

Super shake
  1 cup whole milk
  1 pkg. Carnation Instant Breakfast
  1 cup ice cream
Mix together in blender. (430 calories)

Note: If making any of these changes causes your child to have diarrhea, stop and call your pediatrician.

Figure 29-2. Recipes for children

4. **Meet with *all* caretakers** involved in feeding the child to reduce conflict, to prevent the child from playing one caretaker against another, and to ensure consistency in the feeding regimen.

5. **Discuss optimal feeding interactions** (e.g., allowing the child to self-feed even if messy, decreasing power struggles at meals, fewer distractions in the environment). Encourage turning off the television at mealtimes, eating with other family members, and pleasant conversation not related to food. Discourage grazing and constant sipping on low-calorie liquids.

6. **Ensure access to resources** (e.g., WIC, food stamps, food pantries).

7. **Give all immunizations** (including influenza vaccine); aggressively **treat intercurrent infections; use anti-microbial prophylaxis for recurrent otitis.**

8. **Follow growth weekly to monthly,** depending on age and severity of malnutrition. Success is manifested as faster than normal rate of weight gain for age.

9. Depending on the needs of the family, **mobilize community services,** including mental health, substance abuse treatment, housing advocacy, and job training.

10. **Ensure that the child receives developmental intervention** through Head Start, early intervention, or public school programs.

C. Criteria for referral

1. Children whose **growth rate fails to respond in 2–3 months** should be referred to a multidisciplinary team in an appropriate center.

2. Children with **severe malnutrition, risk of abuse, serious intercurrent illness,** or **extreme parental impairment or anxiety** should be hospitalized.

IV. Clinical pearls and pitfalls

- Failure to correct for prematurity in plotting growth may lead to a factitious diagnosis of FTT. The chronologic age should be corrected for prematurity until 18 months for head circumference, until 24 months for weight, and until 40 months for height. Even after correcting for prematurity, very low birth weight children may remain short for corrected age, but weight for height should be proportionate.
- Children with symmetrical intrauterine growth retardation may remain short but should not be underweight for height.
- Depressed height for age may be genetic, endocrine, or nutritional, but depressed weight for height always reflects primary or secondary malnutrition.

Bibliography

Bithoney WG, Dubowitz H, Egan H. Failure to thrive/growth deficiency. *Pediatr Rev* 13:453–460, 1992.

Chatoor I, et al. Nonorganic failure to thrive: A developmental perspective. *Pediatr Ann* 13:829–843, 1984.

Frank DA, Silva M, Needlman R. Failure to thrive: Mystery, myth, and method. *Contemp Pediatr* 10:114–133, 1993.

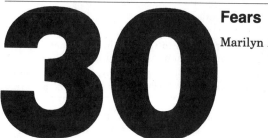

Fears

Marilyn Augustyn

I. **Description of the problem. Fear** is an unpleasant emotion with cognitive, behavioral, and physiological components. It occurs in response to a consciously recognized source of danger, either real or imaginary. From an evolutionary perspective, fear is a key to survival.

A **phobia** is a persistent and compulsive dread of and preoccupation with the feared object or event. Phobias may interfere with the child's functioning in a way that fears do not.

A. **Epidemiology**
   - Fears are present at various times in the lives of *all* children.
   - Studies of identical twins suggest a genetic predisposition to fearfulness in some children.
   - Females report fears more often than do males.
   - Phobias are seen in 7% of adults (disabling phobias in 2%); the prevalence in children is unknown.

B. **Familial trends**

   1. **Fearful, anxious parents tend to have fearful, anxious children,** through social learning.

   2. **Simple phobias appear to run in families,** although individuals rarely share the same specific phobic stimulus.

C. **Etiology/Contributing factors**

   1. **Environmental**

      a. Although fears in childhood reflect a universal developmental tendency, the **onset often relates to a triggering event.** For example, a child may become fearful of dogs following a startling experience with an unleashed large dog. The (perhaps) innate human fear of large animals is intensified by a developmental level that does not allow a nonthreatening explanation of the event.

      b. New **stimuli from the popular culture** join the roster of later childhood fears (e.g., parental divorce, physical assaults, sexual abuse, environmental toxins, terrorist attacks) even as old ones have dissipated (e.g., the communists).

      c. Significant fears may reflect an **accurate assessment of a truly harmful situation** or represent a **displacement of feeling** from another environmental stressor (e.g., physical or sexual abuse).

   2. **Developmental.** Irrational fears intensify when the child's cognitive understanding of the feared object is insufficient to allay the fears or to generate a comforting explanation of why the object has suddenly come into the child's life, if the situation is safe, and whether the event is likely to be repeated. Therefore, fears change and evolve as cognitive development becomes more sophisticated. Table 30-1 provides the timing of selected fears throughout early development.

II. **Making the diagnosis.** The most useful way to differentiate a fear from a phobia is the degree to which the fear interferes with the child's daily activities (Table 30-2). If the child is developing normally in all other aspects, most often the behavior is a

Table 30-1. Common fears in early development

Fear	Age							
	1	2	3	5	7	9	12	14
Separation	X	X			X			
Noises		X			X			
Falling	X				X		X	
Animals/insects	X		X	X				
Toilet training	X	X						
Bath	X	X						
Bedtime		X	X		X			
Monsters/ghosts			X	X				
Divorce				X				
Getting lost			X	X				
Loss of parent				X				
Social rejection						X		
War						X		
New situations						X		
Adoption						X		X
Burglars							X	X
Injections								X
Sexual relations								X

Table 30-2. Differentiation of fears and phobias

	Fears	Phobias
Response to reassurance	Yes	No
Plausible event as cause	Yes	No
Distractable	Yes	No
Impinges on play/development	No	Yes

simple fear. If the fear impinges on important activities, it may have progressed to a phobia and require specialized attention.

A. History: Key clinical questions. The primary care clinician must determine if the symptoms represent a simple fear, a response to significant environmental pathology, or a displacement of other stresses in the child's life.

   1. *Does your child's fear interrupt his or her daily schedule more than three times per day?*

   2. *Can anyone recall a specific trigger to the fear?*

   3. *How do you [the parents] usually respond to the child's fear?*

III. Management. Management will depend on whether the problem is a simple fear, a mild phobia, a debilitating phobia, or a response to environmental pathology. In most cases, simple parental support and empathy will suffice. Fears are ubiquitous throughout childhood. The goal is not to *banish* all of them but to help the child learn positive ways of coping with and transcending them. In the words of Selma Fraiberg, "The future mental health of the child does not depend upon the presence or absence of ogres in his fantasy life. . . . *It depends upon the child's solution to the ogre problem.*"

   A. Information for parents. Parents should understand that simple fears are normal and do not necessarily represent a problem in the child or in the environment.

The complexity and overwhelming nature of the world, coupled with a child's limited cognitive resources, conspire to create fears in *all* children, even those in the most secure and loving of homes.

B. **Supportive strategies.** Parents can exacerbate children's fears by using them as a threat (e.g., "The doctor is going to give you a shot if you're not good"), by humiliating the child (e.g., "Only *babies* are afraid of bugs"), by indifference to the child's distress, by unrealistic expectations to master the fear, and by over-protectiveness (thereby confirming the child's hypothesis that the stimulus is to be feared). They should follow these guidelines:

1. Parents should **respect the child's inclination to withdraw from that which is feared.**

2. **The parents and the clinician should not exaggerate the fear or belittle it.**

3. **Support should be provided to the child as he or she develops an increased mastery of the fearful object.** This may involve initial avoidance of the fearful stimulus, planned discussions about the fear with attempts to correct cognitive misconceptions, and a gradual introduction to the feared stimulus with much family support.

4. In young children, some fears can never be reasoned away. **Parents may have to resort to comprehensible and concrete actions,** such as "monster proofing" the bedroom.

C. **Criteria for referral.** The child/family should be referred to a mental health professional for a phobic condition when fears begin to generalize from the situation of origin or the fears significantly hamper the child's activities of daily living or if the fears are felt to represent a realistic response to a truly threatening environment. Mental health professionals may use such techniques as behavioral modification with systematic desensitization or psychopharmacology to treat severe phobias.

Bibliography

For Parents
Fraiberg S. *The Magic Years.* New York: Charles Scribner's Sons, 1959.

Ilg F, Ames B (eds). *Child Behavior.* New York: Harper, 1981.

Schachter R, McCauley CS. *When Your Child Is Afraid.* New York: Simon and Schuster, 1988.

For Young Children
Dutro J. *Night Light.* New York: Magination Press, 1991.

Lankton S, Wiley N. *The Blammo-Surprise Book!* New York: Magination Press, 1988.

Wineman M, Marcus I, Marcus P. *Scary Night Visitors.* New York: Magination Press, 1990.

For Professionals
Bauer D. An exploratory study of developmental changes in children's fears. *Child Psychol Psychiatry* 17:60–74, 1976.

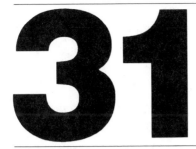

Feeding Problems

Kathleen Nelson

I. **Description of the problem.** Feeding problems include eating too much or too little, picky eating, vomiting, unusual food habits, and poor mealtime behavior. Early feeding problems are often associated with other behavioral concerns (e.g., fearfulness, aggressive behavior, or toileting disorders) and, if they persist, may lead to long-term growth disturbances or eating disorders.

A. **Epidemiology**
   - 25–35% of children experience feeding problems.
   - More serious problems, such as nonorganic failure to thrive, occur in 1–2% of children.

B. **Familial transmission/genetics.** Although there is no genetic transmission of feeding problems, it is not unusual to find parents with past personal histories of feeding problems (especially specific food avoidance) reporting similar traits in their children.

C. **Etiology.** Feeding involves complex motor and social skills. Successful feeding depends not only on the motor and digestive abilities of the child but on the child's temperament, relationship with family members, and the responses of the caregivers to the child's cues regarding hunger, satiety, and food preference.

   Factors that may contribute to feeding problems are outlined in Table 31-1. There may be disturbances in more than one area by the time a problem is brought to medical attention.

II. **Making the diagnosis**

A. **Signs and symptoms.** A feeding problem should be suspected whenever a child presents with poor weight gain, regurgitation, food refusal, diarrhea, colic, or obesity. In addition, parental concerns about feeding (including those about overeating or eating "too little," objectionable behaviors during meals, bizarre food habits, or difficulty weaning) should alert the primary care clinician to ask more pointed questions about the feeding process.

B. **History: Key clinical questions**

   1. *What is your current way of feeding your child (including the amount and type of food, timing of meals, and feeding environment)? Does your child feed herself or himself? Choose her or his own food?* These questions elicit specific information about the quantity and appropriateness of feeding, the social interactions around feeding, and the consistency of the caregiver responsible for feeding the child.

   2. *Tell me about your child's past feeding history.* It is important to know the antecedents to the problem.

   3. *What is your child's general state of health?* The response may alert the primary care clinician to health issues related to feeding difficulties or to parental perceptions of the child's vulnerability or special needs.

   4. *Is your child developing as well as other children the same age?* Feeding problems may be an early sign of development disability.

   5. *Do you try to force your child to eat? What happens then? Do you punish the child for not eating? Are there struggles between you at other times during the day?* Feeding problems may represent just one area of autonomy struggles and behavioral concerns for families.

Table 31-1. Potential etiologies of feeding problems

Environmental
   Feeding on a schedule rather than on demand
   Multiple caregivers
   Nonengaged caregiver (e.g., bottle propping)
   Nonstructured mealtime
   Inappropriate feeding environment (e.g., no infant seat or high chair)
   Multiple distractions (e.g., television blaring)
Organic
   Delay in introduction of oral feeding because of significant illness (e.g.,
      bronchopulmonary dysplasia)
   Motor impairment of swallowing
   Neurologic disease
   Gastrointestinal disease (e.g., gastroesophageal reflux)
   Poor intrinsic appetite ("picky eater" for unknown reasons)
Developmental
   Developmental delay
   Developmentally specific issues (intolerable for some parents)
      8–12 mo—messy eater
      18–24 mo—picky eater
      24–36 mo—pica
               bad manners
Transactional
   Parents who do not recognize signs of child's hunger or satiety
   Forcing child to eat when not hungry (e.g., overly intrusive parent)
   Not allowing child to touch food or self-feed (e.g., overcontrolling parent)
   "Overmanaging" feeding situation (e.g., overly concerned with neatness)

---

6. *What is the importance of food in the context of your family's cultural and social values?* Pressure to eat is frequently accentuated in some cultures. Some parents experience considerable pressure from relatives about their feeding ability.

7. *Is there a family history of feeding problems?* Frequently there is a familial pattern of feeding problems.

C. **Behavioral observations.** The primary care clinician may have the opportunity to observe the parent and child in a feeding situation. Important observations include parental sensitivity to the child's cues of hunger and satiety, the feeding technique, and the emotional tenor of the feeding interaction.

D. **Physical examination.** The physical examination may demonstrate associated physical findings that indicate the severity of the feeding problem (e.g., poor growth) or potential organic causes of the problem (e.g., significant neurologic dysfunction).

E. **Tests.** Unless there is significant evidence of inadequate nutrition or a history suggestive of organic reasons for the feeding problem, no specific diagnostic tests are routinely indicated. Often a developmental screening test may be helpful in demonstrating the child's competencies to both parent and provider. A videotape of a mealtime can be especially revealing of problem areas.

III. **Management**

A. **Primary goals.** The most important goals for the family and child should be to:
   • Promote age-appropriate feeding behaviors.
   • Ensure optimal physical growth and emotional development of the child.
   • Enhance parental feelings of competence.
   • Improve the parent-child relationship.

B. **Treatment strategies.** Families need to know that feeding problems are common and that their concerns about feeding their child are of interest to the primary care provider. Providers need to recognize parental concerns that may not be verbalized. For example, some parents may inquire about vitamins when their real concern is a stubborn, picky eater.

Families also should be made aware of the effect (or lack of effect) of the child's feeding problem on his or her growth. As much as possible, parents should be informed of what information is available to assist in the management of the problems.

The common feeding problems, their presenting complaints, signs and symptoms, and management strategies are detailed below.

1. Overfeeding in infancy

    a. Presenting complaint: "Always hungry"; "spitting up"; "will cry if not fed."

    b. History: Child ingests more calories than appears needed for growth (e.g., much more than 100 cal/kg/day).

    c. Signs and symptoms: Weight gain is too rapid (more than 1 oz/day or crossing percentiles on weight for height curve); vomiting; loose stools.

    d. Management
- Demonstrate excessive growth to parents using growth chart.
- Limit feedings to appropriate amount.
- Encourage parents to offer alternatives to feeding for comforting infant (e.g., pacifier, holding and talking to baby, music).

2. Underfeeding in infancy

    a. Presenting complaint: "Sleeps through feedings"; "never cries"; "nurses briefly or infrequently."

    b. History: Child ingests fewer calories than are needed for growth (less than 80 cal/kg/day) or nurses less than every 4 hours.

    c. Signs and symptoms: Poor weight gain, somnolence.

    d. Management
- Demonstrate poor growth on growth chart to parent.
- Evaluate formula preparation technique.
- Evaluate the child's health status to rule out organic etiology (e.g., oral motor dysfunction).
- Increase caloric intake by waking the child to feed (e.g., by placing cool compress on forehead) at least every 4 hours.
- If the child is unable to ingest appropriate calories because of limited strength, caloric content of milk should be increased.
- Encourage breast milk production by increasing maternal caloric and fluid intake.
- Examine the child's ability to suckle and if necessary refer to lactation consultant.
- Contact the family frequently over the first several weeks after this problem is identified to ensure recommendations are effective and to support parents' efforts.

3. Overfeeding in childhood

    a. Presenting complaint: "Always hungry"; "eats constantly"; "eats most in household"; "too fat"; sometimes no complaint.

    b. History: Child has voracious appetite.

    c. Signs and symptoms: Weight excessive when plotted on growth chart.

    d. Management
- Evaluate the family for a history of obesity (strong family history makes early identification and management critical).
- Attempt to limit caloric intake by giving high volume–low calorie foods (vegetables, air-popped popcorn). Review diet with nutritionist for recommendations.
- Examine the context of eating. Is it the only time the child has the parents' attention?

- Have specific snack time and mealtime, with limited access to food in between.
- Limit portion size (a smaller plate for child makes small portion seem larger).

4. Underfeeding in childhood

a. **Presenting complaint:** "Won't eat"; "too thin"; "needs vitamins."

b. **History:** Does not eat much during meals; may drink large quantities; does not like to sit at the table; ingests fewer calories than needed for growth.

c. **Signs and symptoms:** Poor weight gain or inadequate linear growth on growth chart.

d. **Management**
- Increase caloric intake by increasing caloric density of foods.
- Limit fluid ingestion, especially 1 hour prior to meals.
- Offer snacks and involve the child in food preparation activities.
- Show pleasure when the child increases intake. Never nag.
- Put only small amounts on the plate initially with expectations that all be eaten. Gradually increase the amount.
- Make feeding situations pleasant with conversation and other social interaction.
- Use star charts for good intake.

5. Picky eater

a. **Presenting complaint:** "Child won't eat"; "wants same thing to eat all the time"; "only eats _____"; "needs vitamins."

b. **History:** Child's intake is restricted to a few favored foods. Refuses to try new foods. May have a behavioral style that does not adjust well to new situations in general.

c. **Signs and symptoms:** Usually demonstrates adequate growth when plotted on growth charts.

d. **Management**
- Demonstrate adequacy of growth to parents.
- Prescribe a vitamin and tell parents that now they do not have to worry if the child does not eat vegetables.
- Decrease power struggles around intake.
- Reassure parents that over the course of several days, children select a well-balanced diet.
- Evaluate adequacy of the diet.
- Encourage parents to provide a varied diet and offer the child choices.
- Offer positive reinforcement and praise for trying new foods.
- Limit portions of new foods initially so the child only needs to taste them and offer new food before giving preferred food.
- Serve nonpreferred foods often and make sure other family members enjoy eating them (this modeling behavior is often a very positive influence).

6. Unacceptable mealtime behavior

a. **Presenting complaint:** "Disrupts meals"; "throws tantrums"; "has no manners."

b. **History:** Child uses mealtimes as occasions for behaviors deemed inappropriate by parents.

c. **Signs and symptoms:** Child may show other behavioral problems.

d. **Management**
- Parents may need guidance on setting appropriate limits for the child. Often this complaint is one manifestation of a child's need for guidance from parents on acceptable behaviors. Since family meals may represent the only opportunity for the family to meet together during the day, it is often an ideal time for a child to demand attention (albeit negative).

• Determine if the parents' expectations are developmentally appropriate (e.g., 1 year olds do not eat neatly; 2 year olds need to be fed promptly).
• Are mealtimes too close to bedtime, and is the child tired?
• Praise appropriate behaviors and use strategies such as time-out or limiting dessert unless behavior improves.

7. Bizarre food habits

a. **Presenting complaint:** "Child frequently eats from garbage."

b. **History:** Child approaches meals with much gusto but also is found to seek food in trash and stash food in closets and furniture.

c. **Signs and symptoms:** Child may be growing poorly; family may be dysfunctional.

d. **Management**
   • Obtain psychological history from family and evaluate appropriateness of other child behaviors. Often children with bizarre feeding habits have not formed close attachment to family and other caregivers. Family evaluation and treatment by a mental health professional is often required.

8. Food phobia

a. **Presenting complaint:** "Absolutely refuses to eat _____"; "gets upset/ physically ill when she sees _____."

b. **History:** Child experiences severe physical and emotional reaction (significantly worse than that experienced by children with "picky eating" or specific food preferences).

c. **Signs and symptoms:** Child may exhibit other behavioral concerns, especially other phobias or anxiety reactions.

d. **Management**
   • Unless the child is nutritionally at risk, it is acceptable to avoid the food that elicits phobic response. However, if there are other behavioral concerns or if the phobias are interfering with general well-being, refer to a mental health professional.

9. Pica

a. **Presenting complaint:** "Puts everything in her mouth"; "eats dirt"; "eats ice."

b. **History:** Child may have a history of toxic ingestions requiring a call to the poison center or visits to the emergency room; may have lead poisoning or iron deficiency.

c. **Signs and symptoms:** Pallor, irritability, developmental delay.

d. **Management**
   • Evaluate development. Pica may be "appropriate" for children less than ages 2–3 years. If it occurs beyond that time, it may be a manifestation of developmental delay.
   • Determine lead and iron levels.
   • "Child-proof" the house.
   • Evaluate parenting ability. Is the child receiving positive attention? Do child and parent interact appropriately?

10. Rumination

a. **Presenting complaint:** "Spits up"; "vomits frequently."

b. **History:** Child exhibits frequent regurgitation beyond early infancy; may have chronic disease or be in a chaotic household.

c. **Signs and symptoms:** Child gags self with tongue or by putting hand in throat. This often occurs when the child is not engaged in interpersonal activity.

d. Management
- Evaluate the psychosocial milieu. If appropriate, limit caregivers to one or two.
- Thicken liquid feedings with cereal.
- Provide increased interpersonal contact during the day and at mealtime.

Bibliography

For Parents
Satter EM. *How to Get Your Child to Eat—But Not Too Much.* Palo Alto CA: Bull Publishing, 1987.

For Professionals
American Academy of Pediatrics. *Guidelines for Health Supervision II.* Chicago: AAP, 1989.

Finney JW. Preventing common feeding problems in infants and young children. *Pediatr Clin North Am* 33:775–788, 1986.

Hammer LD. The development of eating behavior in childhood. *Pediatr Clin North Am* 39:379–394, 1992.

Satter EM. The feeding relationship: Problems and interventions. *J Pediatr* 117:S181–S189, 1990.

Fetal Alcohol Syndrome

Barbara A. Morse and
Lyn Weiner

I. **Description of the problem.** Fetal alcohol syndrome (FAS) is a specific cluster of physical and neurobehavioral birth defects associated with maternal alcohol abuse during pregnancy. FAS represents the most severe end of possible damage; fetal alcohol effects (FAE) represent less severe forms of damage.

A. **Epidemiology**
- FAS occurs in 0.33/1000 live births.
- Among alcohol-abusing mothers, 10% will deliver a child with FAS and as many as 30–40% will deliver a child with FAE.
- FAS/FAE occur in all races and at all socioeconomic levels.
- The risk for FAS/FAE may increase with greater parity or poor nutrition.
- Higher rates (1/250) are seen among certain ethnic groups (e.g., Native Americans).

B. **Etiology/contributing factors**

1. **Dosage.** The more alcohol that is consumed, the greater the risk for FAS. Conversely, when consumption is reduced, so is risk.

2. **Pattern.** Drinking patterns that produce very high blood alcohol levels, whether daily or weekly, pose the greatest risk.

3. **Timing.** Effects vary by gestational stage of exposure. First trimester exposure poses risks to structural development; third trimester exposure may impair CNS development.

4. **Genetic sensitivity.** Dizygotic twins have demonstrated differential effects. There may also be racial or ethnic differences in the metabolism of and sensitivity to alcohol exposure.

5. **Maternal metabolism.** Chronic heavy alcohol use impairs maternal hepatic function and reduces the mother's capacity to metabolize alcohol. Elimination of alcohol is slowed, acetaldehyde levels rise, and the potential for damage is increased.

6. **Maternal nutrition.** Poor diet influences outcome. Chronic maternal alcohol use can deplete minerals and vitamins available to the fetus (notably magnesium, zinc, and folic acid).

7. **Parity.** FAS is uncommon in a first pregnancy. The effects of alcohol become more severe with each child born.

II. **Making the diagnosis**

A. **Signs and symptoms.** Signs should be evident in each of these areas:

1. **Pre- and/or postnatal growth retardation.** Weight, length, and/or head circumference are below the tenth percentile. Growth retardation persists throughout childhood, with weight more affected than height. Expected adult growth potential is seldom achieved, although adolescent girls often become plump.

2. **CNS involvement.** CNS problems may range from subtle to severe. Microcephaly, diminished cognition, developmental delays, neurobehavioral disorders, perceptual dysfunction, memory loss, and hyperactivity are common. Development may proceed erratically, appearing normal at times and delayed at others.

About 10% of affected children have very low IQs. The 40–50% with IQs greater than 85 have fewer morphologic anomalies but have persistent neurobehavioral problems, including sleep disorders, sensory integration difficulties, and information processing difficulties.

3. **Characteristic facial dysmorphology.** This may include microophthalmia and/or short palpebral fissures, a poorly developed philtrum, a thin upper lip, and flattening of the maxillary area. A "scooped" nose, wide nasal bridge, and low-set ears are also commonly seen. These characteristics are most easily seen in severe cases and may be subtle in newborns, making diagnosis difficult. Sometimes these features become apparent only at age 2 or 3 years. They often diminish in adolescence.

B. **Signs of FAE.** FAE is diagnosed when there are one or two of the signs noted for FAS in the presence of maternal alcohol abuse. Growth and neurodevelopmental problems such as hyperactivity and learning disabilities are most typically seen in FAE.

C. **Differential diagnosis.** A careful history that includes maternal alcohol use is needed to differentiate the effects of alcohol from those of other teratogens. The combination of growth retardation, facial dysmorphology, and CNS disturbance is not unique to FAS and may also be seen in other disorders (e.g., fetal hydantoin syndrome, Cornelia de Lange syndrome, maternal phenylketonuria, Noonan syndrome).

D. **History: Key clinical questions**

1. *During this pregnancy, how many times a week did you drink beer, wine, or liquor? How many cans, glasses, or drinks each time?* (Or in the case of a foster or adopted child, *Do you know how much alcohol was consumed during this pregnancy?*). FAS/FAE is associated with high blood alcohol concentrations and can be ruled out in children born to women known to have consumed small amounts.

2. *Does your child show unusual sensitivity to touch (overreaction to injury, tags in the back of clothes, hugs), light, or sound (says things are too bright or too loud)?* Sensory hypersensitivity is a frequent but poorly recognized feature of FAS.

3. *How does your child relate to peers?* Many children with FAS read social cues very poorly and have few friends their own age. They may appear excessively friendly or fearless and exhibit poor judgment or impulse control.

4. *Does your child understand cause and effect?* Although their verbal skills make them *appear* to understand cause and effect, they are often unable to link consequences with their actions.

5. *How does your child react to a change in routine, such as a substitute teacher?* Children with FAS rely on consistency. When a change occurs without sufficient preparation, they may react with frustration, aggression, or perseveration.

6. *Does your child seem to "learn" and "forget" the same piece of information over and over?* A child's ability to retrieve cognitive information is often impaired in FAS/FAE.

E. **Physical examination**

1. **Assessment** of growth, CNS functioning, and facial dysmorphology is critical.

2. **Associated pathology** may be found in the following areas: cardiac (e.g., septal defects), renal (e.g., hypoplasia, hypospadias), ocular (e.g., intraocular abnormalities, strabismus, ptosis), ear (e.g., recurrent otitis media, deafness), skeletal (e.g., radioulnar synostosis, retarded bone growth), oral (e.g., poor suck, cleft palate) or immune system (increased infections, nonspecific neoplasms).

F. **Tests.** There are no specific diagnostic tests for FAS. Neuropsychological assessment and sensory integration assessment may assist in planning appropriate treatment and interventions.

III. Management

A. Information for the family

- Symptoms are not the result of "poor parenting" or "a bad personality." The child is "unable," not "unwilling."
- Children with FAS depicted in the media are often uniquely severe cases and do not represent the majority of children with FAS.
- FAS/FAE is permanent but not degenerative. Some problems persist, while others improve. Intervention and treatment improve outcomes.
- FAS results from chronic maternal alcoholism, not "a single drink before knowledge of conception."

B. Treatment

1. **Sensory integration.** Sensory integration therapy (by specialized occupational therapists) can desensitize the child to tactile, auditory, and proprioceptive stimulation. Adaptations in the environment (e.g., nonrestrictive clothing, placement at end of line, sunglasses to reduce glare) help to avoid overstimulation and improve the child's ability to pay attention. Preparing the child for physical contact, loud noises, or bright lights can reduce overreactions.

2. **Social skills training.** The ability to read social cues is improved by teaching the child (using photographs and television) how to interpret facial expressions. Another strategy is to have the child practice specific expressions and communicative gestures in front of a mirror or on videotape.

3. **Teaching cause and effect.** Repetition is the most effective way to teach cause and effect. Role playing the appropriate interpretation of ambiguous situations and appropriate reactions will also increase understanding. Children learn more quickly when external cues, such as pictures, are used.

4. **Adapting to transitions.** Adaptation to transitions is best achieved with explanations and ample warnings of an impending change in the routine or environment.

5. **Improving memory.** Learning can be improved by going beyond auditory and visual teaching methods and using tactile and kinesthetic strategies. Typewriters, computers, and tape recorders can compensate for poor memory. Learning may be reinforced by singing information to simple tunes.

IV. Clinical pearls and pitfalls

- For many affected children, facial features are subtle and may only be observed *after* the diagnosis has been suggested from other signs.
- Normal or average IQ is not a disqualifier for FAS/FAE, since the range of IQ is broad and at least 40% of those with FAS/FAE have IQs greater than 85. Severe mental retardation is rare.
- Sensory hypersensitivity is often misread as aggression or emotional lability; learning disabilities are misconstrued as behavioral problems.
- Many children with FAS suffer from low self-esteem due to their disabilities. Referral to a supportive therapist may be useful in such cases.
- The clinician who suspects continuing addiction must be prepared to refer a parent for substance abuse evaluation and treatment. He or she can join with the parent's desire to help the child.
- The clinician can help the biologic mother to understand that she did not drink during pregnancy out of malice or with intent to damage and that both she and her child are victims of the disease of alcoholism.

Bibliography

For Parents

Fetal Alcohol Network Newsletter (FANN), 158 Rosemont Avenue, Coatesville, PA 19320-3727; (215) 384-1133

Growing with FAS (newsletter), 7802 Southeast Taylor, Portland, OR 97215.

Kleinfield J, Wescott S (eds). *Fantastic Antone Succeeds: Experiences in Educating Children with Fetal Alcohol Syndrome.* Fairbanks AK: University of Alaska Press, 1993.

Morse BA, Weiner L. *FAS: Parent and Child—A Handbook for Parents Raising Children with FAS*. Available from the Fetal Alcohol Education Program, Boston University School of Medicine, 7 Kent Street, Brookline, MA 02146. (617) 739-1424

For Professionals

Clarren SK. Fetal alcohol syndrome: Diagnosis, treatment and mechanisms of teratogenesis. In Bellisario R, Mizejewski GJ (eds). *Birth Defects Symposium XIX: Transplacental Disorders*. New York: Alan R. Liss, 1990.

Rosett, HL, Weiner L. *Alcohol and the Fetus: A Clinical Perspective*. New York: Oxford University Press, 1984.

Weiner L, Morse BA. Facilitating development for children with fetal alcohol syndrome. *Brown Univ Child Adoles Behavior Lett*, November, 1991.

Fragile X Syndrome

Randi Hagerman

I. **Description of the problem.** Fragile X syndrome (FXS) is the most common inherited form of mental retardation. It causes a spectrum of developmental problems, ranging from learning disabilities and emotional problems in those with a normal IQ through all levels of mental retardation.

A. **Epidemiology**
- Causes mental retardation in approximately 1 in 1250 males in the general population and 1 in 2500 females.
- Responsible for 30–50% of all cases of X-linked mental retardation.
- Approximately 1 in 409 females in the general population carries the mutation.
- No known racial or ethnic differences; identified in all racial groups tested.
- Both males and females can be unaffected carriers.

B. **Genetics.** FXS is caused by a mutation in the fragile X mental retardation-1 gene (FMR-1), which is located on the bottom end of the X chromosome. The mutation causes a fragile site or break in the chromosome at that location. The FMR-1 gene was identified and sequenced in 1991. An unusual expansion of a cytosine, guanine, guanine (CGG) nucleotide repetitive sequence was found to be the mutation. Within the FMR-1 gene, normal individuals have a nucleotide CGG sequence that repeats up to 50 times, carriers have an expansion of the CGG sequence between 50–200 times, and individuals affected with FXS have a CGG repeat number greater than 200 (termed a full mutation). When this occurs, the gene usually becomes methylated or turned off so that no FMR-1 protein is made, and the full fragile X syndrome occurs.

A carrier male will pass his only X chromosome to all of his daughters, who will be obligate carriers and pass the mutation to 50% of their offspring. A significant expansion of the mutation will often occur in their children so that retarded male and significantly learning disabled female offspring are common. A detailed family tree must be drawn to sort out possible carriers and other extended family members who may be affected by FXS.

II. **Making the diagnosis.** Both behavioral and physical features are included in the fragile X checklist (Fig. 33-1), which serves as a reminder for clinicians of the signs and symptoms of fragile X.

A. **Signs and symptoms in males**

1. **Early signs and symptoms.** Infants with FXS may appear to be normal, although temperamental and feeding difficulties have been described. Recurrent otitis media begins in the first year of life for the majority of males affected by this syndrome. Hypotonia is also notable in young boys, with subsequent mild delays in motor milestones. Many fragile X boys and significantly affected fragile X girls are delayed in the onset of language. Phrases or short sentences are usually delayed until age 3 years or older. The language delays in addition to hyperactivity or tantrums are the typical initial concerns leading to medical consultation.

Prominent ears with occasional ear cupping, hyperextensible finger joints, double-jointed thumbs, flat feet, and soft skin are seen in the majority of fragile X boys in early childhood. These physical findings are considered to be part of a connective tissue dysplasia that is related to the absence of the FMR-1 protein. Young boys with FXS may also have a broad or prominent forehead and a large head circumference.

SCORE:	0	1	2
		Borderline or present	
	Not present	In the past	Definitely present
Mental retardation			
Hyperactivity			
Short attention span			
Tactilely defensive			
Hand flapping			
Hand biting			
Poor eye contact			
Perseverative speech			
Hyperextensible finger joints			
Large or prominent ears			
Large testicles			
Simian crease or Sydney line			
Family history of mental retardation or autism			

TOTAL SCORE _____

A score > 15 has a 45% chance of FXS

Figure 33-1. Fragile X checklist. Modified from Hagerman RJ, Amiri K, Cronister A. Fragile X checklist. *Am J Med Genet* 38:283–287, 1991.

2. **Later signs and symptoms.** Macroorchidism becomes prominent in males with fragile X during the early stages of puberty. Usually the testicular volume is at least twice normal size, with an adult range in FXS of 40–100 cc. Although the spermatic tubules are tortuous by histological studies, fertility has been reported in several males with FXS. Additionally, a long face and prominent jaw are often noted after puberty. Other diagnoses such as Soto's syndrome, Tourette's syndrome, Pierre Robin sequence and other congenital defects such as cleft palate or hip dislocation may be associated with FXS because of the connective tissue problems and behavioral difficulties that occur in this disorder.

B. **Behavioral problems in males.** Behavioral problems are a common presenting complaint in young boys with FXS. These include hyperactivity; impulsivity; an extremely short attention span; perseveration in speech and actions; hand flapping with excitement; hand biting with anger or frustration; oversensitivity to touch, noises, and textures of food or clothing; shyness; poor eye contact; and tantrums. These behaviors are often described as autistic-like, and a diagnosis of pervasive developmental disorder or attention deficit hyperactivity disorder (ADHD) may be in accurately made.

C. **Signs and symptoms in girls.** Approximately 50% of females who carry the full mutation will have a borderline or retarded IQ. The other half will have a normal IQ but may have significant learning disabilities, including attentional problems

Table 33-1. Associated medical problems in fragile X syndrome in males

Medical problem	Frequency in males
Flat feet	80%
Scoliosis	<20%
Mitral valve prolapse	50–80% in adulthood
Recurrent otitis	60%
Strabismus	30%
Nystagmus	occasional
Refractive errors	20%
Seizures	15%
Macroorchidism	80% after puberty

(with or without hyperactivity), math deficits, and language delays. Significant shyness is very common, often accompanied by poor eye contact. FXS females may be given a psychiatric diagnosis of avoidant disorder or autism because of their social deficits. Schizotypal features (i.e., oddness in social interactional skills and appearance), depression, mood lability, anxiety, impulsive behavior, or emotional problems have also been reported in women affected by FXS.

D. **Tests.** If the diagnosis is suspected in a retarded or autistic child, cytogenetic studies for FXS are recommended since they can detect not only the fragile site but other cytogenetic abnormalities. If a learning disabled or carrier individual is suspected, DNA testing should be undertaken because it is more accurate than cytogenetic studies for fragile X, especially in mildly affected or unaffected carriers. Once a proband is diagnosed with FXS, other family members should be assessed with DNA testing, including all siblings of the proband and of the carrier parent.

III. Management

A. **Goals and initial treatment strategies.** The goals of the primary care clinician are to provide appropriate medical therapy and to coordinate a team of professionals who will provide optimal treatment for the fragile X child. Speech and language therapy and occupational therapy are essential for all young children affected by FXS. A developmental preschool setting can usually provide these therapies, in addition to special education. Whenever possible, mainstreaming or full inclusion with normal peers is preferable since children with FXS usually model their behavior after their peers.

B. **Follow-up.** Medical follow-up includes recognition and treatment of connective tissues problems and associated complications of fragile X syndrome (Table 33-1). Since ophthalmological problems are common, referral to an ophthalmologist prior to age 5 years will facilitate early treatment. Orthopedic referral is appropriate if scoliosis or joint dislocations occur. Mitral valve prolapse is usually noted in the older child or adult, so referral to a cardiologist for evaluation and echocardiogram is necessary if a murmur or click is heard in auscultation. Vigorous treatment of recurrent otitis media in early childhood is indicated and usually includes the use of pressure equalizing (PE) tubes, so that a fluctuating hearing loss does not interfere with optimal language development.

C. **Psychopharmacology.** The most common behavioral problem is hyperactivity, which is seen in approximately 80% of affected boys and 30% of affected girls. Therefore treatment of ADHD symptoms in these children is a main focus of intervention (see Chapter 24). Folic acid in a dosage of 10 mg/day may be somewhat helpful for approximately 50% of young children. However, it is not as effective as stimulant medication, which is helpful for over 60% of children with FXS who are age 5 years or older.

A common concern of families of adolescent children with fragile X syndrome is treatment of outbursts or aggression, a significant problem in approximately 30% of male adults and adolescents with FXS. Episodic dyscontrol usually occurs during or after significant environmental overstimulation (such as shopping in a busy store), or it may be precipitated by anger or frustration. A variety of medications have been used with anecdotal success (including carbamazepine, lithium, thioridazine, and fluoxetine), but controlled studies have not yet been performed. Serotonin reuptake blockers such as fluoxetine, sertraline, and buspirone show the most promise; they have fewer side effects than antipsychotic medication and help to stabilize mood and improve obsessive-compulsive behaviors and anxiety. Fluoxetine has also been helpful to the majority of carrier females who have had significant problems with depression and mood lability.

D. **Other therapies.** Sensory integration therapy by an occupational therapist with a specific focus on calming techniques may be helpful. Significant behavioral problems may also respond to a behavioral modification program organized by a psychologist who can also provide support and guidance for the parents.

E. **Criteria for referral.** All families with fragile X syndrome should be referred to a geneticist or genetics counselor for a detailed discussion regarding the inheritance of this gene and an assessment of other family members, who require DNA testing to clarify their carrier status.

Bibliography

For Parents
National Fragile X Foundation, 1441 York Street, Suite 215, Denver CO; (800) 688-8765.
Has produced many educational pamphlets, books, and videotapes regarding FXS; has compiled a list of over 50 resource centers associated with parent support groups in the United States and internationally; and organized conferences for parents and professionals.

For Professionals
National Fragile X Foundation, (800) 688-8765 or (303) 333-6155.
Identifies laboratories that carry out DNA testing.

Hagerman RJ. Medical follow-up and pharmacotherapy. In RJ Hagerman, AC Silverman (eds), *Fragile X Syndrome: Diagnosis, Treatment and Research.* Baltimore: Johns Hopkins University Press, 1991.

Hagerman RJ, Amiri K, Cronister A. Fragile X checklist. *Am J Med Gene* 38:283-287, 1991.

Rousseau F, et al. Direct diagnosis by DNA analysis of the fragile X syndrome of mental retardation. *New Eng J Med* 325(24):1673–1681, 1991.

Simko A, Hornstein L, Soukup S, Bagamery N. Fragile X syndrome: Recognition in young children. *Pediatrics* 83:547–552, 1989.

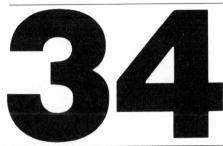

Gay, Lesbian, and Bisexual Youth

Clifford W. Sells and
Gary Remafedi

I. Description of the issue. *Homosexuality* is defined as "a persistent pattern of homosexual arousal accompanied by a persistent pattern of absent or weak heterosexual arousal." *Sexual orientation* encompasses sexual fantasies, emotional and romantic attractions, sexual behavior, and self-identification. The heterosexual or homosexual direction of any of these dimensions may not be consistent, defying the simple categorization of individuals as heterosexual, homosexual, or bisexual. Sexual orientation, rather, should be viewed as a continuum between absolute heterosexuality and homosexuality.

A. Epidemiology
- In a survey of more than 36,000 junior and senior high school students, the percentage of youth reporting predominantly homosexual attractions steadily increased with age, with a peak of 6.4% among 18 year olds.
- In various studies the prevalence of same-sex experiences has ranged from 1–37%.

B. Familial transmission/Genetics. Increasing evidence suggests that homosexuality is genetically influenced. The occurrence of homosexuality in family pedigrees often exceeds that of the general population. Various studies have found a higher concordance for homosexuality among monozygotic twins than dizygotic twins. A recent study genetically links one form of male homosexuality (preferentially transmitted through the maternal side) with a region of DNA on the X chromosome.

C. Etiology/Contributing factors

1. **Environmental.** There is no scientific evidence that environmental stressors lead to a homosexual orientation. Additionally, it is now generally accepted that homosexual orientation is not due to parental influences, as had been suggested by the early "dominant mother–passive uninvolved father" theories.

2. **Organic.** A biologic model involving hormonal influences and homosexuality has been postulated. However, assays of androgens, estrogens, and other hormones have not shown consistent differences between adult homosexual and heterosexual persons. Interestingly, an increased incidence of homosexuality in women with congenital adrenal hyperplasia (despite early detection and correction of androgen excess) has been observed. Neuroanatomic differences between homosexual men and heterosexual men and women have been noted in sexually dimorphic regions of the brain. These observations support the hypothesis that factors operating early in development may have differentiated structures and functions of the brain that influence sexual orientation.

3. **Developmental.** The development of a homosexual identity occurs in four stages:

   a. **Stage I: Sensitization.** During childhood there is often a sense of being different from same-sex peers.

   b. **Stage II: Identity confusion.** Homosexual feelings create confusion and uncertainty about sexual identity. The adolescent may respond by trying to ignore homosexual impulses and activities or to view these behaviors as temporary.

    c. Stage III: Identity assumption. When the adolescent or young adult's confusion about sexual orientation is resolved, he or she is often able to share his or her identity with others ("coming out"). Close friends are usually informed before parents or professionals.

    d. Stage IV: Commitment. Stage IV is generally reached during adulthood when the individual experiences self-acceptance, emotional intimacy, and an unwillingness to alter sexual orientation.

II. Making the diagnosis

A. Recognizing gay, lesbian, and bisexual youth.
Homosexual youth have many of the same medical concerns and needs as heterosexual teenagers. However, they are at greater risk for both psychosocial and medical problems because of the experience of growing up gay, lesbian, or bisexual.

1. Psychosocial issues

a. Homophobia is an irrational, distorted fear of homosexuality or homosexual individuals. This fear may be manifested as discomfort, prejudice, verbal abuse, or psychological or physical hostility. In the face of disapproval from friends or family, the teenager may internalize feelings of guilt and shame, contributing to poor self-image.

b. Depression and suicidality are common consequences of the teenager's sense of isolation in an openly hostile environment. In two separate large samples, 30% of homosexual male youth reported a suicide attempt.

c. Homelessness and prostitution. Many gay or lesbian adolescents leave their homes each year because of parental abandonment or rejection (or fear of rejection). The teenager's desperation, poor self-esteem, lack of education or job skills, and social isolation without adult or peer role models may leave few options for survival other than prostitution.

d. Substance abuse may represent an attempt to decrease the pain of isolation, condemnation, and rejection. In a cohort of gay and bisexual males less than age 20 years, more than half reported substance abuse.

2. Medical issues.
Gay youth who have multiple partners and engage in high-risk behaviors are at greatest risk for sexually transmitted diseases (STDs). Lesbian teenagers with only same-sex partners are at lower risk for STDs than either gay or heterosexual youth.

B. Differential diagnosis

1. Transient sexual orientation ambiguity.
Given appropriate information and support, **individuals generally will resolve uncertainty about sexual orientation by late adolescence** through self-exploration of feelings, fantasies, and experiences.

2. A transvestite
is a person who derives pleasure by dressing in clothing of the opposite sex. Typically, this person's sexual orientation is heterosexual.

3. Transsexual individuals
feel that their anatomic gender does not correspond to psychological gender identity.

C. History: Key clinical questions

1. *Have you ever dated?*
Asking "Do you have a girlfriend?" of a gay male teenager may suggest that the health provider is not open to a discussion of the youth's boyfriend.

2. *There are many different ways of being sexual with another person: hugging, kissing, touching genitals, intercourse. Have you ever been sexual with another person?*
It is important to understand the extent of the teenager's sexual activity.

3. *Many teenagers are attracted to individuals of the same sex; are you attracted to boys, girls, or both?*
Although the teenager may not discuss his or her homosexual behaviors or feelings, the patient now knows that there are others with similar feelings and that the health provider is approachable.

4. **Have you ever been sexual with boys, girls, or both? Have you ever had oral sex? Vaginal intercourse? Rectal intercourse?** Once an individual has acknowledged homosexual sexual behaviors, it is important to explore his or her specific sexual experience. Defining sexual experience and participation (e.g., receptive versus insertive) will help assess risk factors for STDs.

5. **How do you protect yourself against sexually transmitted diseases (including AIDS)?** It is important to determine the teenager's knowledge of pregnancy, STDs, and AIDS in order to help the youth with risk reduction.

6. **Do you consider yourself heterosexual (straight), bisexual, gay, or lesbian?** Sexual activity alone may be a poor indicator of sexual orientation.

7. **Do you have any concerns about your sexual feelings, attractions, or the things you are doing?** The youth should know that it is permissible to discuss his or her concerns.

8. **Have you discussed your sexual attractions with your friends? Parents? Other adults?** It is important to know if the teenager has a support system with whom he or she can discuss openly these very personal feelings.

D. **Behavioral observations.** Observation of gender-atypical behaviors is not a reliable indicator of sexual orientation. The health care provider should avoid stereotyping the effeminate male and "tomboy" female.

III. Management

A. **Primary goals** include the promotion of healthy physical, sexual, social, and emotional development. The teenager must develop a positive gay, lesbian, or bisexual self-image in which he or she is seen as a respectable, lovable, and competent person with the ability to enjoy emotional and safe physical intimacy with persons of the same gender. Many youths will experience significant confusion, guilt, fear, and anxiety as they raise questions about their sexual orientation. These feelings are common and need to be discussed and understood. There is no need for the youth to make an immediate decision concerning sexual orientation; over time sexual orientation will become clear.

B. **Information for the family.** Parents of homosexual teenagers may experience a multitude of emotions, including anger, guilt, grief, and fear. It is important to explore these feelings. In many cases, the primary care provider may help the family view homosexuality as an acceptable variation of sexual orientation. The child's potential for a happy, healthy, and productive life need not be limited by his or her sexual orientation.

C. **Specific care**

1. **Initial strategies** emphasize patient and parent education concerning development and sexuality, including AIDS prevention information. Healthy adult and peer role models, in addition to social support groups, are extremely important to youth. Support groups for parents are also very useful.

2. **Anticipatory guidance** is extremely important for gay and lesbian youth. Many youth will have difficult and extremely complicated questions (e.g., with whom, how, and when to discuss their sexual orientation).

3. **Psychosocial development** should be carefully monitored. Both the teenager's and the family's adjustment should be followed. Additional services and support may be needed, including alternative schools, gay or lesbian sensitive mental health and social services, foster home placement, prostitution diversion programs, special programs for adolescents with human immunodeficiency virus (HIV), and gay and lesbian community clinics.

4. **High-risk behaviors.** The clinician should assess the patient's symptoms and high-risk behaviors, inquiring about depression, suicidality, conflict with family and peers, faltering academic and job performance, substance abuse, and unsafe sexual behaviors.

D. **Criteria for referral** include severe psychiatric symptoms (e.g., suicidal ideation, depression), serious social problems (e.g., prostitution, homelessness, school dropout, chemical dependency), or problems of personal or family adjustment that do not respond to education and social support.

IV. Clinical pearls and pitfalls

- When coming out, isolated adolescents may exhibit severe psychiatric symptoms (e.g., extreme anxiety, depression, cognitive impairment, emotional lability), which may resolve quickly when appropriate information and social support are provided.
- Most teenagers are aware of their attractions before having sex. Discourage sexual experimentation as a litmus test for sexual orientation.
- In order to avoid embarrassment and judgment, gay and lesbian adolescents often tell health care providers that they are unsure of their sexual feelings or that they are "experimenting" with bisexuality.
- When a professional says that an adolescent is confused about sexual orientation, more often than not it is the professional who is confused because of lack of information or misinformation.
- Regardless of sexual orientation labels, young men who have unsafe sex with men require intensive HIV prevention services, which should not await the determination of sexual identity.
- Because of the risks of rejection and discrimination, the clinician should encourage careful forethought and planning prior to disclosure of homosexuality to family and friends.
- Even if initially vitriolic, parents' first reactions to a child's homosexuality often temper with time.
- Young lesbians and gay men often experiment with partners of the opposite sex. The clinician should inquire about heterosexual experience and the need to protect against pregnancy and HIV/STDs.

Bibliography

For Parents

National Organizations, Support Groups
Federation of Parents and Friends of Lesbians & Gays, Inc. (P-FLAG), 1012 14th Street, NW, Suite 700, Washington DC 20005; (202) 638-4200.

International Gay Youth Information Pool (IGYIP), P.O. Box 1305, Vika N-0112; Oslo 1, Norway.

National AIDS Hotline, (800) 342-2437.

National Gay and Lesbian Task Force, 1724 14th Street, NW, Washington DC 20009-4309; (202) 332-6483.

Publications
Borhek MV. *Coming Out to Parents: A Two-Way Survival Guide for Lesbians and Gay Men and Their Families.* New York: Pilgrim, 1983.

Fairchild B, Hayward N. *Now That You Know: What Every Parent Should Know about Homosexuality.* San Diego: Harcourt Brace Jovanovich, 1979.

Rench JE. *Understanding Sexual Identity: A Book for Gay Teens and Their Friends.* Minneapolis: Lerner, 1990.

Scanzoni L, Mollenkott VR. *Is the Homosexual My Neighbor?* San Francisco: Harper and Row, 1978.

For Professionals
Neinstein, LS, Cohen, E. Homosexuality. In LS Neinstein (ed), *Adolescent Health Care: A Practical Guide.* Baltimore: Urban & Schwarzenberg, 1991.

Remafedi G. Fundamental issues in the care of homosexual youth. *Med Clin North Am* 74:1169–1179, 1990.

West JC, Remafedi G. When your patient is gay. *Contemp Pediatr* 6:125–138, 1989.

35

Gender Identity Issues

Susan Coates and
Sabrina Wolfe

I. **Description of the problem.** Children with disturbances in gender identity wish to be the other sex (or insist that they *are* the other sex), have strong and persistent preferences for cross-sex roles in fantasy play, have an intense desire to participate in the stereotypical activities of the other sex, and have a strong preference for playmates of the other sex. Cross-gender interests occur in both normal development and when developmental processes are disrupted. At times, cross-gender behavior is a brief passing phase, particularly in the 2-year-old child. At other times it is an indicator of gender nonconformity. At still other times, it is a signal of intense psychological suffering and can mark the beginning of significant emotional difficulties, culminating in enduring disturbances in gender identity. When a child's cross-gender preoccupations are *intense, persistent, and pervasive,* the condition is defined by the DSM as a **childhood gender identity disorder (GID).**

A. **Epidemiology**
- The prevalence of childhood GID has not yet been systematically assessed. Clinical experience suggests that it is a rare disorder but occurs in all socioeconomic, ethnic, and racial groups.
- Boys are referred for childhood GID more often than girls. This may be because boys are more vulnerable to this disorder or because cross-gender behaviors are more readily tolerated in girls than in boys.
- The onset of GID is usually between ages 2–4 years in boys. In girls, it is not yet clear whether the disorder emerges at the same time as it does for boys or a year or two later.

B. **Familial transmission/Genetics.** There is no current evidence of familial transmission or a genetic contribution to this disorder.

C. **Etiology/Contributing factors**

1. **Environmental.** Cross-gender behavior in boys frequently emerges in the context of significant familial stress, such as loss of a loved one, severe physical illness in the child or parent, severe marital stress, or parental depression or anxiety that disrupts the parent-child relationship. Boys who develop GID often have fathers who are emotionally unavailable to the mother and son. Girls with GID often devalue their mothers and both fear and overidolize their fathers.

2. **Organic.** No genetic or hormonal contributions to childhood GID have yet been identified; however, *temperament* appears to be a contributor to the development of GID. For example, boys who develop GID are usually avoidant of rough-and-tumble play, are less physically active than other boys, and are often shy and anxious in new situations. Many of the boys who have GID also have a variety of sensory sensitivities that are reflected in both an increased capacity to derive pleasure from particular sensory modalities (such as odors, colors, textures, or sound) and in a heightened vulnerability to the negative aspects of sensory experience. For example, a mother may report that her child will spontaneously remark on good odors, such as cookies baking in the oven, but will gag when a garbage truck passes. Girls who develop GID often have a high energy level and are skilled at athletic pursuits.

3. Developmental

a. **Gender categorization.** Children's understanding of gender is constructed and reorganized as they move through Piagetian cognitive-developmental stages. By age 12 months, infants can distinguish between female and male faces, smells, and voices. By ages 16–20 months toddlers can correctly label adult females and males. By age 2½ years a majority of children can accurately label themselves and others according to gender, but not until age 3 years do all children make this *gender categorization* accurately and consistently. Once children are able to label gender for peers and for themselves reliably, there is a marked increase in stereotypically same-sex interests, a marked increase in playing primarily with one's own gender, and (for girls) a marked decrease in aggression.

b. **Gender understanding.** Between ages 3–6 years, the child gradually acquires gender constancy, gender stability, and the understanding that genitals define gender.

c. **Gender stability** refers to the understanding that one's gender was the same when one was born and will remain the same when one is grown up.

d. **Gender constancy** refers to the understanding that a change in one's external appearance, such as when a boy puts on a dress, does not change one's gender.

e. These cognitive differentiations in turn become integrated with the understanding that the **defining attribute of gender is one's genitals** and not one's culturally determined outward appearance. Children with GID have more difficulty in developing a solid cognitive understanding of gender.

4. **Transactional.** Although the etiology of GID in children is under active investigation, most believe that it occurs in the context of cumulative risks. For example, the following risk factors in boys are hypothesized:
   • A shy, reactive temperament
   • Significant family stress during the sensitive period of gender development (18 months–3 years)
   • Initial reinforcement of cross-gender behavior.

   For girls with GID, some hypothesize that the girl has "disidentified" with the mother due to a highly conflictual mother-child relationship. Another theory, particularly when there has been an abusive father, is that the girl identifies with the aggressor.

D. **Long-term correlates.** Although it is not possible to predict the sexual orientation of any individual child, longitudinal studies of boys with GID have shown that a majority grow up to be homosexual or bisexual. (However, only a small minority of adult homosexual men have had a childhood history of GID.) Boys who continue cross-dressing and experience intense gender dysphoria into adolescence may be on a transsexual course. Longitudinal follow-up studies of the sexual orientation of girls with GID have not been conducted.

II. Making the diagnosis

A. **Signs and symptoms.** Table 35-1 contains the behaviors that should alert the primary care provider to the possibility that the child may have difficulty with his or her gender development, particularly if they have *continued for more than 3 months.*

B. **Differential diagnosis**

1. **Normal developmental variability.** It is not uncommon for 2–3-year-old children to dress up and make believe that they are the other gender. This ordinarily will be manifested by children *flexibly* imitating parents, siblings, the baby, or even the family pet. If the child is *compulsively* and continuously interested in cross-gender pretend play, it is very atypical, even at age 2 years.

Table 35-1. Behaviors consistent with possible gender identity difficulties

Insists that he or she is the other gender

Expresses dislike for his or her own gender

Persistently wishes to be the other gender

Has a strong and persistent preoccupation with or preference for cross-sex roles in fantasy

Has an intense desire to participate in stereotypical activities of the other sex

Has a strong preference for playmates of the other sex

In boys

A preference for dressing up in girls' clothes or in simulating female attire

A persistent repudiation of male anatomic structures (a dislike of his penis or testes and/or a wish to be rid of either).

Insistence on urinating only while sitting down or pushing the penis between his legs and pretending that he has a vagina

In extreme cases, trying to harm their penis physically

In girls

An insistence on wearing only stereotypically masculine clothing and experiencing significant distress if they are required to wear a dress for a specific occasion

A persistent repudiation of female anatomic structures, manifested in behaviors such as asserting the belief that she has a penis or will grow one, rejection of urinating sitting down, and repeated insistence that she does not want to develop breasts or menstruate

---

2. **Gender nonconformity in boys.** Children who have gender-nonconforming interests (such as boys who have marked artistic interests, who avoid rough-and-tumble play, who prefer solitary intellectual activities like reading or listening to music, or who enjoy cooking) *do not,* based on these behaviors, have gender identity problems.

3. **Tomboyism.** It is essential to differentiate GID in girls from tomboyism. Girls who prefer wearing pants, who enjoy rough-and tumble play, and who prefer boys as playmates but do not dislike being female are likely to be "tomboys." Girls who exhibit these behaviors in the context of persistent dislike of their gender and sexual anatomy and who are extremely upset if they have to wear female clothing even for a special event are likely to have gender identity problems.

4. **Transvestism.** Boys who cross-dress in women's undergarments are different from boys with GID, as the latter cross-dress in outer female attire to enhance the illusion of being female. Although the former group should be referred because of the compulsivity of their transvestitic behavior, their identifications and behaviors (aside from dressing in female undergarments) are almost invariably masculine.

C. **History: Key clinical questions**

1. *Does your child wish that he or she is or will grow up to be the other sex?*

2. *Does your child dislike being his or her own gender?*

3. *Are his or her main fantasy or make-believe identifications with heroes or heroines of the other sex?*

4. *Does your child have a marked preference for playing with children of the other sex?*

5. *Does your son have a strong interest in cross-dressing or in simulating female attire?*

6. *Does your son sometimes pretend that he doesn't have a penis?*

7. *Does your daughter become very upset if she has to wear a dress on a special occasion?*

8. **Does your daughter refuse to urinate sitting down?**

9. **Has this been going on for more than 3 months?**

D. **Behavioral observations.** The child's cross-gender preoccupations may not be at all evident during a routine pediatric examination. Direct questioning of the child is often not very productive because the child may have become aware of the parent's discomfort and will therefore deny these interests.

III. **Management**

A. **Goals of treatment**

1. To help the child **develop a range of coping mechanisms** for managing the conflicts underlying the cross-gender fantasies.

2. To **develop social skills with same-sex peers.**

3. To **repair the derailed attachment relationship to the mother and the father** if it is problematic.

4. To **increase self esteem** and to restore his or her creativity.

B. **Discussing the issue with parents**

1. **Effect of punishment.** Parents need to know that attempting to stamp out the cross-gender behavior with punishment is not a constructive solution and rarely is effective in altering the child's cross-gender identifications and wishes. It is more likely to make the child hide the behavior and does not solve the underlying issues.

2. **Referral.** Patients should be referred for psychological counseling. They should be informed that not seeking professional help is also not in the child's best interest because such behaviors are often an indication of developmental difficulties and psychological suffering that warrant professional attention.

   The child needs to be evaluated to determine whether his or her cross-gender behavior is a passing preoccupation, or whether it may be linked to more significant difficulties. If parents resist professional help, they should be reminded that no matter what their own attitudes may be, persistent cross-gender behavior is invariably associated with the loneliness and the humiliation of peer ostracism.

3. **Timing of treatment.** Time is of significance in treating children with GID because, for reasons that are not yet understood, cross-gender fantasies may become fixed as enduring cross-gender identifications during the sensitive period of gender development. The optimal time of referral is between ages 2–4 years.

Bibliography

Coates S. The ontogenesis of boyhood gender identity disorder. *J Am Acad of Psychoanal.* 18:414–438, 1990.

Coates S, Wolfe S. Gender identity disorders in toddlers and preschool children. In J. Noshpitz (ed), *The Handbook of Child and Adolescent Psychiatry.* New York: Wiley (in press).

Zucker KJ, Green R. Gender identity disorders. In M Lewis (ed), *Child and Adolescent Psychiatry: A Comprehensive Textbook.* Baltimore: Williams & Wilkins, 1991.

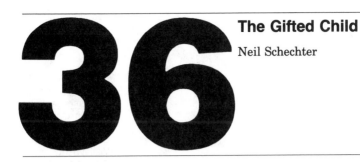

The Gifted Child

Neil Schechter

I. **Description of the issue.** The definition of giftedness—even, in fact, its very existence as an entity—is controversial. Initially giftedness was thought to be synonymous with high IQ: early work in this field defined a child with an IQ in the top 1% as gifted. However, a linear relationship between high IQ and eventual societal contribution and productivity has not been found, and creativity and task persistence, among other factors, have also been deemed important. The definition of gifted children has been expanded to include the interaction of three basic clusters: above-average intellectual ability, high levels of creativity, and high levels of task commitment (Fig. 36-1). In this model gifted children are viewed as those with unusual potential in a broad range of areas that leads to "gifted products" (high academic achievement, scholarly or creative writing, art work, community leadership, etc.).

The vagaries of these definitions allow for significant discrepancies in identification. It is difficult, for example, to separate truly gifted children from unduly pressured, overly scheduled, continuously taught middle-class children. Because socioeconomically advantaged children tend to have higher IQs than poorer children and because some schools rely exclusively on IQ to define giftedness, children of higher socioeconomic status are more likely to be classified as gifted. Current recommendations avoid this bias by suggesting that giftedness is a relative construct and that each community should create its own standards to determine who qualifies for programs aimed at such children. In most school systems and communities, about 5–10% of children are considered to be gifted.

II. **Making the diagnosis**

A. **Signs**

1. **Early childhood.** Parents may raise the issue of giftedness in infancy and early childhood if their children appear precocious at mastering developmental milestones. Retrospective studies of gifted children suggest that early language development and early reading were frequently present. For example, in one study, nearly half of the group later identified as gifted had learned to read before entering first grade; 20% could read before age 5 years.

Prospective studies, however, suggest that, for a given child, there is no relationship between milestone acquisition or developmental testing before age 4 years and the IQ score achieved at age 7 years. Precocious infants do not necessarily become precocious children. There is, in fact, no single measure that accurately predicts giftedness.

2. **School age.** Giftedness among school-aged children is less likely to be recognized by the primary care clinician and more likely to be identified by the school system. Occasionally parents may wonder whether their child's behavioral or academic problems in school stem from his or her boredom with the curriculum. Intelligence testing is a part of the comprehensive evaluation of any school program. If testing reveals very high intellectual potential, then perhaps gifted programming may help.

B. **Characteristics.** Children with extraordinarily high IQs (those over 180 or developmental functioning at twice their chronologic age) often have social difficulties. The disparity between their intellectual acumen, their social development, and their chronologic age poses enormous problems. For example, they

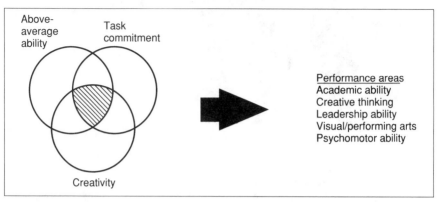

Figure 36-1. Three-ring concept of giftedness. (Reprinted with permission from Levine, Carey, and Crocker. *Developmental-Behavioral Pediatrics,* 2d ed. Philadelphia: Saunders, 1992.) p. 591.

Table 36-1. Responsibilities of primary care clinicians to gifted children and their families

Identification
    Awareness of margins of normal development and appreciation of markers of
        developmental precocity
    Identifying resources within the community to help evaluate gifted children
    Helping children and families understand the concept of giftedness
Management
    Home
        Helping parents prevent creating excessive vulnerability or privilege in the
            identified child
        Helping family deal with sibling(s) of identified child
        Helping family avoid overstimulation of child
        Awareness of enrichment and supportive resources in the community
    School
        Advocacy of appropriate educational resources in the school system
        Awareness that gifted children may have behavioral and learning problems
            that require intervention
        Fostering communication between the school and the family

often have a difficult time identifying an appropriate peer group or engaging in age-appropriate activities.

III. **Management.** For the primary care clinician working with a potentially gifted child and family, a number of issues are relevant. They are outlined in Table 36-1.

A. **Identification.** If questions are raised whether an infant or young child is gifted, it is important to explore what such a diagnosis would mean to the parents. It should be explained to the parents that testing in infancy or early childhood will not accurately predict subsequent academic high achievement and, in fact, may result in the inappropriate labeling of the child.

In older children, intellectual testing may be more helpful. Schools are not obligated to test or provide services for gifted children, but many school systems may be willing to evaluate such children and offer specialized services for those identified as gifted and talented.

Because of the inherent ambiguity in the definition of giftedness and because many parents want to bask in the reflected glory that accompanies such a label, pressure may be brought to bear on schools to label the child as gifted. The clinician should attempt to help parents separate their own desires, goals, and aspirations for their child from the child's actual abilities and potential.

B. Home

1. **Parents may be prone to overstimulate their child,** either to foster giftedness or to meet its challenges. Parents need not feel pressured to provide an elaborate intellectual enrichment program for their child in fear that his or her "gifts" will wither if not appropriately stimulated. In fact, undue pressure may prove injurious to the child's long-term development. Stimulation for children identified as academically talented and gifted should be individualized and focus on activities of the child's choosing.

2. **Siblings of children who are academically precocious often feel inferior,** especially if they are chronologically older but academically less capable. The label "gifted" should not be flaunted in front of siblings nor should siblings continuously be compared to the gifted child. All children should be treated similarly (e.g., with age-appropriate expectations for chores) and encouraged to cultivate their own areas of uniqueness.

3. **Friendships may be problematic for some gifted children,** especially for children who are extremely intellectually advanced. Attempts should be made to encourage gifted children to play with same-age peers so that social skills will develop appropriately. However, there may be specific friendships that emerge with older children who have interests or expertise in similar areas to the gifted child. Parents of gifted and talented children may benefit from support groups for gifted children and their parents.

C. School. There remains significant controversy about how to educate gifted and talented children. Some school systems urge acceleration and place children in advanced grades that parallel the child's ability rather than chronologic age. Other systems cluster academically advanced children in substantially separate classrooms in which they receive an advanced program. More typically, gifted and talented programs exist within school systems and not as a separate curriculum. Such programs provide a designated period for children to focus on a specific area in greater depth and in a more creative way than typically allowed by the curriculum.

Resources

For Parents

Advocacy Groups

Council for Exceptional Children, 1920 Association Drive, Reston VA 22091-1592; (703) 264-9471.

National Association for Gifted Children, 1155 15th Street NW, Suite 1002, Washington DC 20005; (202) 785-4268.

Publications

Gifted Child Today, P.O. Box 6448, Mobile AL 36660-0448.

Smutney JR, Veenker K, Veenker S. *Your Gifted Child.* New York: Facts on File, 1989.

For Professionals

Gifted Child Quarterly, National Association for Gifted Education, 1155 15th Street, NW, Suite 1002, Washington DC 20005.

Journal for Education of the Gifted, Council for Exceptional Children, UNC Press, 116 South Boundary Street, PO Box 2288, Chapel Hill NC 27515-2288.

National Research Center on the Gifted and Talented Newsletter, University of Connecticut, 362 Fairfield Road, U-7, Storrs CT 06269-2007.

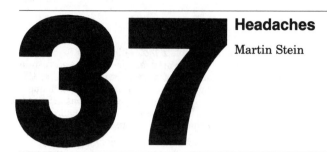

Headaches

Martin Stein

I. Description of the problem

A. Epidemiology
- Headaches represent the most common recurrent pain pattern in childhood and adolescence.
- 40% of children and 70% of adolescents have experienced a headache at some time.
- Chronic recurrent headaches occur in 15% and migraine headaches in 2–5% of all children by age 15 years.

B. Etiology.
Children experience headaches from many causes, but only a few pathologic mechanisms induce head pain:
- Inflammation, traction, and direct pressure on intracranial structures.
- Vasodilation of cerebral vessels.
- Sustained contractions, trauma, or inflammation of scalp and neck muscles.
- Sinus, dental, and orbital pathologic processes.

The brain parenchyma, most of the dura and meningeal surfaces, and the ependymal lining of the ventricles are insensitive to pain. CNS causes of headache result from stretching or inflammation of a limited number of pain-sensitive intracranial structures.

II. Making the diagnosis.
Most headaches are brief and do not significantly alter a child's life. Recurrent headaches may be accompanied by fears and anxieties about brain tumors and other life-threatening diseases. The diagnostic challenge for the primary care clinician is multifaceted:
- To differentiate benign, self-limited headaches from those that suggest a serious organic disease.
- To explore the potential relationship between headaches and a child's home, school, and social environment.
- To recognize patients with headaches secondary to internal stressors (depression, anxiety, phobias) and those with environmental causes.
- To develop a therapeutic plan consistent with the cause, severity, and significance of the headaches for the child and family.

A. Differential diagnosis.
A useful clinical model to differentiate the large variety of headaches in children and adolescents focuses on four categories: (1) tension headaches, (2) migraine headaches, (3) extracranial headaches, and (4) intracranial headaches (Table 37-1). Tension-related headaches occur the most frequently, but their symptoms and signs are often nonspecific compared to the less common causes. Headaches in younger children, especially infants and toddlers, are more likely to have a specific organic cause. A focused clinical interview, coupled with age-appropriate behavioral observations and a comprehensive physical examination, will result in the probable diagnosis at the initial office visit for most patients.

B. History: Key clinical questions.
Whenever possible, questions should be directed to the patient, inquiring of the parent only after the child or adolescent has had an opportunity to describe the headache to the clinician. With the knowledge that most recurrent forms of pediatric headaches are associated with a behavioral diagnosis (in the presence or absence of migraine), the astute provider should guide the clinical interview in a manner that raises questions simultaneously about both organic and behavioral causes. An open-ended question ("Tell me about your headaches") will allow the child and parent to explore what seems

Table 37-1. Classification of headaches

	Mechanism	Features/etiology
Tension headaches (muscle contraction headaches)	Contraction of scalp and neck muscles	Sensation of tightness or pressure over frontal, temporal, occipital regions, or generalized Life-event change/stress: home, school, social relations, activity overload, depression Normal physical examination (occasional tightness or tenderness of posterior cervical muscles)

Migraine headaches	Vasoconstriction and/or vasodilation of cerebral vessels	Family history (70–80%)
		Paroxysmal attacks
		Gender: in childhood, boys and girls equally; in adolescence, girls more than boys
		Common migraine
		  Unilateral or generalized
		  Throbbing or aching
		  Nausea/vomiting
		  No aura
		Classic migraine
		  Aura (visual)
		  Nausea/vomiting
		  Unilateral
		  Throbbing
		Complex migraine
		  Ophthalmoplegia
		  Hemiparesis
		  Acute confusional state
		  Cyclic vomiting
		  Paroxysmal vertigo

Extracranial sources	Inflammation or trauma of structures or sustained contracture of scalp and neck muscles	Typically regional pain in area of pathology but often generalized in young children Otitis media and mastoiditis Sinusitis (chronic purulent rhinorrhea and/or nocturnal cough) Dental infection Tonsillopharyngitis (streptococcal) Refractive errors and strabismus Cervical spine osteomyelitis or discitis Systemic infection with fever Temporal-mandibular joint syndrome Severe malocclusion
Intracranial sources	Inflammation	Meningitis, encephalitis, cerebral vasculitis, subarachnoid hemorrhage
	Traction	CNS tumor Cerebral edema Abscess Hematoma Postlumbar puncture Pseudotumor cerebri
	Toxic substances	Lead Alcohol Carbon monoxide Hypoxia Foods and food additives (nitrates, nitrites, monosodium glutamate, phenylethylamine) Paint, glue (including model glue) Oral contraceptives Renal disease

Table 37-1. (continued)

Mechanism	Features/etiology
Direct pressure	Hydrocephalus
	Trauma
Vascular (non-migraine)	Hypertension
	Arteriovenous malformation
	Fever
Miscellaneous	Noise
	Sensory overload

important to them and may lead to further exploration in the direction of either organic or behavioral etiologies. At some point, focused questions that may suggest common (sinusitis, migraine) or uncommon (increased intracranial pressure, chronic infection) organic etiologies should be directed to the patient or parent.

The history should begin, when possible, with a description of the headache pattern. In infants and toddlers, nonspecific symptoms may reflect a headache (e.g., irritability, inconsolability, sleep disturbances, poor appetite, head banging, or repetitive placing of a hand to the head or face). In older children and adolescents, an open-ended question may yield important information about the location, quality, onset, duration and frequency of the headache.

The clinical interview begins the therapeutic process. Detailed, focused, and empathic questions give the child and family a sense of security that the symptoms are being evaluated by a concerned, knowledgeable clinician. It also gives the child and parents the opportunity to explore the interpersonal, educational, and family aspects of their lives that may provide insight into the headache formation.

1. *Tell me about your headaches. What do they feel like?* The child who has difficulty describing the headache can be asked to "draw a picture of what the headache feels like." The drawing may be concrete (a person or family) or abstract with designs or color. The child's description of the drawing, as well as the parents' and clinician's emotional responses, may provide useful information about the nature of the pain.

2. *What seems to bring on a headache?* [or] *What are you doing when the headache starts?* The emotional or physical environment in which the headache occurs may provide a clue to etiology.

3. *What do you do to stop the headache?* Common migraine typically resolves with sleep. Tension headaches resolve gradually during an awake state.

4. *Do others in your family experience headaches?* A history of episodic throbbing headaches in adults will suggest familial migraine headaches.

5. *What is a headache?* [To the preschool child:] *Where do headaches come from?* [School-aged child:] *What causes your headache?* [Adolescent:] *Why do you think you get headaches?* These developmentally appropriate questions give a clue to the child's explanatory model of headache formation. Responses provide clinical insight into a patient's development, a clue to cognitive adaptation to the headache, and a source for improved communication between clinician and child through empathic connections.

6. *Why do you think that your headaches are more frequent or more severe?* For most children who experience headaches, it is helpful to explore the child's developmental understanding of headaches. A perceived cause of a headache will be linked to the child's cognitive and developmental stage (Table 37-2). The child is given an opportunity to reflect on the symptoms. The response may provide a clue to self-esteem, ego integration, superego formation, and interpersonal relationships.

7. *How are things going at school . . . at home . . . with your friends?* The structure of the family (and a family medical history), friendships, and the

Table 37-2. Developmental conceptions of headache

Cognitive stage	Answer to "How do people get headaches?"
Prelogical (3–6 yr)	
Phenomenism	"From God" or "From the weather"
Contagion	"From foods, like chocolate"
Concrete-logical (7–12 yr)	
Contamination	"From running and getting hot"
Internalization	"Eating or doing certain things that make inside your head hurt" or "From thinking too hard in math class"
Formal-logical (> 13 yr)	
Physiological	"From things happening to you that cause too much blood flowing to your head; that's why it feels like a hammer pounding in your head"
Psychophysiological	"When people get nervous or do too much, this causes their body to react with a headache"

Source: Modified with permission from Marcon RA, Labb EE. "Assessment and treatment of children's headaches from a developmental perspective. *Headache* 9:586–592, 1990.

school environment are critical to understanding the etiology of and response to the headache, and potential therapeutic interventions.

a. **Family stress.** Is the child living with someone who experiences headaches? The family constellation should be explored for recent changes in parental relationships, a new sibling, emotional illness in family members, economic stress (lost job, homelessness, and child support), and family violence.

b. **Social stress.** When factors such as inherent shyness, bullies, class and racial differences, and physical or mental dysfunction affect social relationships, psychophysiologic reactions are common. Recurrent frontal, generalized, or temporal headaches (both with and without associated symptoms of pallor, malaise, nausea, and vomiting) are seen in these situations. Importantly, common migraine headaches as well as tension headaches may be associated with social or familial stress.

c. **School stress.** Stress that originates in the classroom may be associated with headache formation. The school may act as an environmental stressor by placing demands on both cognitive achievement and social behavior. Children's adaptive potential to a variety of school pressures varies significantly.

   The clinical interview should explore the nature of the classroom (number of students, where the child sits), the relationship between the child and the teacher, the quality and quantity of academic work, the child's response to homework, and the parents' attitudes about learning. Parents can be asked when they last spoke to the child's teacher, the content of the conference, whether the child is learning, and if the child is happy at school.

8. *What do you think we can do together to help the headaches go away?* This question engages the child in a therapeutic alliance and opens the possibility of managing the problem together.

C. **Physical examination and further testing.** Narrating normal physical findings to the child during a comprehensive physical examination is reassuring and helps to demystify the medical evaluation. Organic causes for a child's headaches are usually apparent after a complete history and physical examination. Appropriate blood, urine, or imaging studies confirm a suspected organic diagnosis. Specialty consultation will suggest the next therapeutic step. When the signs and symptoms of organic causes of headache are vague or subtle and a specific diagnosis remains elusive, a specialty consultation may be useful.

III. **Management**

A. **Primary goals.** The clinician's goals for management should be to provide a developmentally appropriate understanding of the cause of headaches for both parent and child. The working assumption is that through a greater understanding of the physical and behavioral causes and triggers for headaches, both the child and the parent will be able to cope with and adapt to the pain as well as collaborate in recommended therapies.

B. **Treatment strategies**

1. **Information.** When migraine or tension headaches are present, the anatomic mechanisms of pain should be illustrated by means of a descriptive narrative and schematic drawings. Visual images of the abnormal anatomic structures may help some children to gain control over the symptoms. Simple drawings of a blood vessel contracting and dilating with an explanation of pain-sensitive nerve endings within the blood vessel illustrates the physical nature of migraine headache and the associated symptoms.

2. **Relaxation exercises.** For tension headaches, children may respond to a progressive relaxation exercise that teaches them to relax specified areas of the body. The exercise may be followed by teaching the child to focus on a pleasant image of his or her choosing. Other children respond to an explanation directed at "tight muscles around the head" that cause pain at times of stress and tension ("worry," "nerves," and "daily hassles"). The clinician can demonstrate this phenomenon by tensing her or his biceps and asking the child to mimic that maneuver. This should be followed by an explanation that the biceps muscle is similar to the thin muscles around the head, which tighten at the point where the headache occurs. The child can learn to image—through visual imagination—the tense, painful cranial muscles' relaxing gradually and voluntarily as the pain diminishes.

These forms of voluntary relaxation follow the principles of self-regulation that have been successful in the elimination of migraine and tension headaches in school-aged children and adolescents (Chapter 13). Controlled studies of children with headaches have shown that relaxation therapy and imaging (with or without biofeedback) decrease headache frequency up to 88% with lasting effects. It is a safe and simple intervention that can be practiced by the primary care clinician.

3. **Headache diary.** A headache diary may be a useful adjunct intervention. The older child or parent is asked to chart the headaches (time of day, intensity on a 1–10 scale, associated symptoms, intervention, and duration) and record any stressful events that occur in the life of the child or family around the time of the headache. This exercise may encourage parents and children to talk about environmental triggers for headaches specifically and improve parent-child communication in general. Following an initial treatment period, it may be useful to shift the emphasis of the diary to headache-free days, which can shift family focus to successes rather than failures.

4. **Medication.** A pharmacologic approach to acute, chronic, and recurrent headaches may be beneficial for pain relief and prevention. Most children and adolescents with occasional migraine and tension-related headaches respond to acetaminophen when the pain is of mild to moderate severity. Parenteral medication is available for the very severe migraine. More severe recurrent headaches respond to prophylactic suppression therapy along with the treatment of the acute headache when it occurs. The primary care clinician will rarely need to resort to suppression therapy because episodic, severe headaches are uncommon in children and adolescents.

C. **Follow-up.** In general, a child with recurrent headaches should always be followed up within 2–4 weeks after the initial office evaluation. Support for behavioral interventions, monitoring of headache frequency and functional severity, and reviewing the parent-child understanding of the symptoms are the goals for the follow-up visit. New information or clinical observations may either alter the initial diagnosis or provide a new direction for management.

Bibliography

Duckro PN, Cantwell-Simmons E. A review of studies evaluating biofeedback and relaxation training in the management of pediatric headache. *Headache* 29:428–433, 1989.

Igarashi M, May WN, Golden GS. Pharmacologic treatment of childhood migraine. *J. Pediatr* 120:653–657, 1992.

Marcon RA, Labbe EE. Assessment and treatment of children's headaches from a developmental perspective. *Headache* 9:586–592, 1990.

Olness KN, MacDonald JT. Recurrent headaches in children: Diagnosis and treatment. *Pediatr Rev* 8:307, 1987.

Singer HS, Rowe S. Chronic recurrent headaches in children. *Pediatr Ann* 21:369–373, 1992.

Welsh JB. The use of drawings by children in the pediatric office. In SD Dixon, MT Stein (eds), *Encounters with Children: Pediatric Behavior and Development* (2nd ed). St. Louis: Mosby Year Book, 1992.

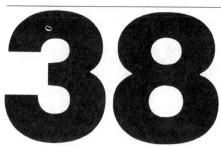

Hearing Loss

Hilde S. Schlesinger

I. **Description of the condition. Hearing loss** refers to a reduced ability to hear in the so-called speech range of 125–8000 hertz (Hz) (Table 38-1).

Deafness is a severe to profound hearing loss that precludes the ability to understand speech through the ear alone, with or without the use of a hearing aid.

Hearing loss can be classified in five ways: (1) age of onset, (2) type (dependent on the part of the auditory system that is affected—conductive, sensorineural, mixed, or central), (3) degree (from mild to profound), (4) configuration (the decibel [dB] loss at different frequencies), and (5) by parental hearing status.

A. **Epidemiology**
   - Nearly 21 million Americans have some degree of hearing loss, and 500,000 are deaf.
   - The estimated incidence of hearing impairments in newborns is 1–2 per 1000.
   - 20–30% of bilateral significant hearing loss occurs after the neonatal period.
   - Among all deaf children, 54% are boys and 46% are girls.
   - Among American schoolchildren, 135,000 have hearing losses that can be a major source of limitation in school.
   - 30% of deaf schoolchildren have an additional handicap (8% have mental retardation, 7.5% have learning disabilities, 6% have emotional problems, 4.4% have behavioral problems, and 4.4% have uncorrected vision problems).

B. **Outcomes of hearing loss**

   1. Failure to identify hearing loss early (by age 6 months is a reasonable goal) and to provide early intervention (amplification, speech therapy, and/or language interchanges via sign language) will affect **language development** far beyond the effect of the hearing loss itself.

   2. **A postlingual onset of mild hearing loss will have less impact than a profound, congenital, sensorineural loss.**

   3. Recent findings suggest that even a mild (25–40 dB) loss or an intermittent conductive loss (e.g., with repeated bouts of otitis media) can adversely affect the child's **perceptual, cognitive, psychological, language, and/or academic development.**

   4. **Impact on parent-child relationship.** There are many risks to parental caregiving in raising a deaf child.

      a. **Overcontrolling caregiving.** Early childhood deafness has a strong impact on most hearing parents. Many have been noted to interact with their children more with the intent to "control" than to "converse." They use fewer open-ended questions, more imperatives, more attention-getting devices, more negative actions and verbalizations, more rapid topic changes, more monologue, and less dialogue than do parents who want to converse rather than control. Such interactions may further impede language development.

      b. **Less sensitive interactions.** Preliminary reports indicate that many hearing parents are less responsive, contingent, and sensitive to their deaf infants than are hearing parents with their hearing infants or deaf parents with their deaf infants. It may be that deafness creates emotional, as well as communicative, barriers that can be difficult for parents to breach without professional intervention.

Table 38-1. Classification of hearing loss

Loss in decibel and severity	Usual age at identification	Impact of loss on speech reception	Impact of loss on spoken language
< 25	Late or not known	Virtually none	Probably insignificant
25–40: mild	Age 3 yr (if unilateral, not until age 5 yr)	Difficulty with whispers or faint speech; may benefit from hearing aid (only 50% use them)	Increasing evidence of school problems at first grade, with greater difficulty at fourth grade
41–55: moderate	22 mo	Difficulty hearing normal speech	Increasing evidence of school problems at first grade, with greater difficulty at fourth grade
56–70: moderately severe	22 mo	May understand loud conversation	Difficulties acquiring spoken language
71–90: severe	18 mo	May hear a loud voice 12 in. from ear	Difficulties acquiring spoken language
> 90: profound	16 mo	Usually cannot understand even amplified speech	Uses primarily visual channel for communication

5. **Child outcomes.** Despite many advances, the average deaf adolescent's reading is at about a fourth-grade level and is only slowly rising. Thirty percent who graduate from high school are unable to continue their education or to obtain a job. They may show emotional immaturity, lowered autonomy, impulsivity, and a lack of social cognition. However, with optimal intervention and caretaking, deaf youngsters can and do achieve at grade level with normal behavioral adjustment.

On average, deaf children with deaf parents achieve at higher levels and demonstrate better adjustment than their deaf peers with hearing parents. Their deaf parents are more accepting of them and tend to use a language system that is perceptually more available.

C. **The Deaf community.** It is estimated that 500,000 individuals in America form the Deaf community and share a Deaf culture.

1. **Language.** American Sign Language is at the core of the Deaf community and is perpetuated not only through dialogue but through poetry, the theater, the arts, and numerous national and international organizations for the deaf. It is a complex and rich language, expressed through visual-motoric rather than vocal means and is unique in its phonological, syntactic, and semantic structure.

2. **Marriage.** Among deaf individuals, 85–95% marry other deaf individuals.

3. **Attitudes.** Historically, the Deaf community has been both oppressed and ignored. Deaf teachers were not permitted to teach deaf children, and forbidden to use American Sign Language in schools. It has only been since the 1970s that some localities began recruiting deaf teachers to work with young deaf children. Currently, the Deaf community is split: some deaf individuals continue to object to the very existence of the Deaf community and to the use of sign language. They promote the adage, "Act hearing at all costs." Others promote separatism and dichotomize the options for deaf individuals (e.g., "Do you want to live in the deaf world or the hearing world?"). They use the expression "thinking like the hearing" pejoratively and question the ethics of using cochlear implants for deaf children. Still others accept the riches of both the hearing and deaf world.

Table 38-2. Risk factors/etiology of sensorineural hearing loss

Neonates
  Family history of congenital or delayed hearing loss
  Congenital (silent) infections: toxoplasmosis, syphilis, rubella, cytomegalovirus, and herpes
  Craniofacial and neck anomalies (e.g., premature closing of cranial suture lines, auditory meatus atresia)
  Birthweight < 1500 g
  Bilirubin levels requiring transfusions
  Ototoxic drugs (especially the aminoglycosides or more than 5 days on loop diuretics, such as furosemide with aminoglycosides)
  Bacterial meningitis
  Severe depression at birth; Apgar 0–3 at 5 min; failure to initiate respiration; hypotonia for more than 2 hr
  Prolonged mechanical ventilation (10 days or more)
Infants
  Parental concern regarding hearing, speech, language, and/or developmental delay
  Conditions leading to progressive hearing loss (e.g., cytomegalovirus, genetic)
  Head trauma associated with fractures of the temporal bone
  Neurodegenerative disorders (e.g., neurofibromatosis)
  Childhood infectious diseases (e.g., mumps, measles)
All children
  Excessive exposure to loud noise (e.g., rock music on personal radio, hearing aids that may produce excessive amplification)

D. Genetics. Between 46–60% of severe childhood hearing loss is genetically determined. Autosomal dominant genes are responsible for 20% and autosomal recessive genes for 80%. Less than 2% are the result of sex-linked or sex-influenced genes.

   One-third of genetic-linked hearing loss occurs as part of about 150 syndromes. Finally, 5–10% of deaf children have deaf parents, and 10% of deaf parents have deaf children.

E. Etiology/Risk factors (Table 38-2). An awareness of risk factors can lead to a more accurate and prompt diagnosis of hearing loss. Knowledge of these factors, however, has not proven sufficient for the identification of hearing loss during infancy. This has prompted the National Institutes of Health to issue a position statement in 1993 recommending universal screening for all infants within the first three months of life.

II. Making the diagnosis

A. Parental concern. Parents and other caregivers are the first to suspect deafness in up to 86% of deaf children. Unfortunately, parental concerns are often dismissed; false reassurance leads, on the average, to a 12-month delay between the parents' suspicion and referral to an audiologist.

B. Language delay. The most immediate and obvious impact of hearing loss is on spoken language acquisition. Any deviation from normal language development or poor academic functioning should raise the index of suspicion.

C. History: Key clinical questions

1. *Has anyone in your family had difficulty hearing?*

2. *Has anyone in your family had difficulty speaking clearly?*

3. *Does your child wake up with a loud noise?*

4. *Does your baby pay attention to your speech?*

5. *Does your baby babble?* Deaf babies babble normally until age 6 months.

6. *Is your child's language as good as others her or his age?*

D. **Behavioral observations.** The diagnostic usefulness of behavioral observations during history taking, physical examination, or with noisemakers is disappointing. Children, especially alert ones, use visual adaptive maneuvers to "outwit" examiners who use screening noisemakers. A standardized testing kit such as the Hearkit has been found useful by trained professionals and nonprofessionals (around $60 at Merrimedics 303-762-8971).

E. **Physical examination.** Sensorineural hearing loss is usually invisible. However, some hereditary syndromes (e.g., Waardenburg, Usher's, Klippel-Feil, and Treacher Collins' syndromes) produce anomalies related to the embryological development of the auditory system (e.g., the neural crest, the surface ectoderm, and the first two branchial arches). These are characterized by craniofacial abnormalities and pigmentary changes of hair, skin, and eyes. Any structural abnormality of the external ear should also heighten the index of suspicion for hearing loss.

Careful evaluation of the middle ear (e.g., lack of mobility, bulging, opaqueness of the tympanic membrane) may be pathognomonic for the diagnosis of intermittent conductive loss.

F. **Tests** (most of which are to be performed by specialists)

1. **Not requiring cooperation of the child**

   a. **BAER** (brainstem auditory evoked responses) measures the variations in the electric activity as caused by brief tones (e.g., clicks or tone pips) measured through two scalp electrodes. The tones are repeated up to 100 times and averaged by computer. Auditory thresholds obtained through this test are quite close to those obtained through routine audiometry.

   b. **OAE** (otoacoustic emissions) is a new test that is likely to replace the BAER. OAE are sounds measured in the external ear canal through a miniature microphone. These sounds are produced by the motile, outer hair cells of the cochlea. This movement produces mechanical energy, which is transmitted through the middle ear and tympanic membrane and is converted into an acoustic signal in the ear canal. OAE are absent when the hearing thresholds are greater than 30–40 dB and in the frequency regions of the hearing loss. This test can help differentiate hearing problems caused by the brain from those caused by the ear.

   c. **Behavioral audiometry with young infants.** This technique relies on the detection of a behavioral response (cessation of activity, eye widening, subtle changes of facial expression, crying, and gross startle response) when a high-intensity auditory stimulus is presented to the baby. There is general concern about the effectiveness of this technique.

   d. **Tests of immitance.** These refer to either admittance (how easily energy flows through a system) or impedance (the opposition to the flow of energy). They are used in conjunction with hearing tests since there may be significant ear disease with little hearing loss.

      (1) **Tympanogram.** The tympanometer is most likely to be used by the primary care clinician. It measures the electrophysiology of external and middle ear functioning. An impedance probe is placed in the ear canal (after thorough otoscopic examination), and a seal is obtained at the canal opening. Air pressures are varied, which produces graphic representations that can be compared with normative graphs of differently functioning ears. This test can be normal despite a nonfunctioning acoustic nerve and is useful for diagnosis of conductive losses that may require medical intervention.

      (2) **Acoustic reflex.** This test measures the time lock change produced by the contraction of the stapedius or the tensor tympani muscle activated by auditory, electric pneumatic, or tactile stimuli in a healthy middle ear.

2. Requiring cooperation of child

    a. Play audiometry for young children. Through conditioning, the child learns to engage in some activity when she or he hears the signal. The test is widely used among clinicians, but, as in the case of behavioral audiometry, questions remain as to its accuracy.

    b. Pure-tone air conduction. Pure tones at different frequencies from 125–8000 cycles/second travel through air to the ear's conductive mechanism, which stimulates the auditory nerve. The child indicates when she or he hears the sound.

    c. Pure-tone bone conduction. Pure tones at the same frequencies vibrate the skull and thus the cochlea, thereby bypassing the air conduction pathway.

    d. Speech audiometry. Pure-tone tests tell the nature and extent of hearing loss but do not reveal the extent of communication problems. Speech audiometry determines the lowest level the child can hear and repeat standardized two-syllable words (*airplane, cowboy, birthday*) and at what level the child can discriminate between standardized single-syllable words.

III. Management

A. Communication. All management of hearing loss consists of providing access to the communicative riches of the environment.

    1. Accessibility to the auditory aspects of spoken language through hearing aids, auditory training, amplified phones, and assistive listening devices (e.g., audio loop, FM, and infrared transmitter).

    2. Accessibility to the visual aspects of language.

        a. Favorable seating in school.

        b. Speech-reading training for spoken language.

        c. Acquisition of sign language in English or in American Sign Language.

        d. TTD-teletypewriter for the Deaf, which permits an exchange of written messages replacing the vocal interchanges on phones.

        e. Cued speech, a sound-based communication system in which English is represented through hand shapes that accompany the natural mouth movements.

        f. Interpreters for English or American Sign Language.

        g. Closed captions on television (now required on all new television sets) and real-time captioning for live events.

    3. Accessibility to important environmental sounds alerting the deaf individual to the sounds of danger, knocks at doors, telephone ringing, and others through the use of household devices designed for this purpose or a certified hearing dog.

B. Educational growth. Most of the management of children with sensorineural deafness resides in the hands of specialists—audiologists, otologists, teachers of special education, and language specialists—who often have conflicting approaches to the deaf child's education. Some emphasize the skills involved in all aspects of spoken language—speech or lip reading, hearing aids, auditory training, and an emphasis on English. Some emphasize the skills required in American Sign Language. Others reject the dichotomy and emphasize both skills.

C. Primary care clinician's role

    1. Provide a realistic but optimistic picture of the achievement and adjustment of deaf children and adults.

    2. Help parents to understand and respect the culture of Deafness, to meet deaf adults, and to help the child acquire the skills to live in both cultures: the hearing and the Deaf.

3. **Help parents with the acquisition of knowledge regarding the new technology of deafness,** especially that which is helpful to children.

4. **Establish a team relationship with other professionals and parents** in order to facilitate the coordination of overwhelming, conflicting, and often incompatible advice.

IV. **Clinical pearls and pitfalls**
- Screening procedures are not diagnostic procedures. They only identify youngsters who need more sophisticated diagnostic evaluation.
- Take parental suspicions of hearing loss seriously, and respect their educational and communicational choices for their children.
- Resist reassuring parents that "everything will be all right" during their mourning period following the diagnosis of deafness.
- Differentiate between the reaction of hearing and of deaf parents. For example, many deaf parents do not consider having a deaf child as a problem, a fact that must be considered when genetic counseling is proposed by the professional or requested by the parent.
- Deaf children live up or down to their parents' and teachers' expectations. The attitude of the primary care clinician may greatly influence the deaf child's academic achievements and social adjustment.

Bibliography

For Parents

Organizations
A. G. Bell Association for the Deaf, Volta Place, NW, Washington DC 20007; (202) 337-5220 (Voice/TDD)

American Society for Deaf Children, 814 Thayer Avenue, Silver Spring MD 20910; (301) 585-5400 (Voice/TDD).

SEE Center for the Advancement of Deaf Children, PO Box 1181, Los Alamitos CA 90720.

Tripod, 2901 North Keystone Street, Burbank CA 91504; (800) 352-8888.

Publications
Benderly BL. *Dancing without Music: Deafness in America.* Garden City NY: Anchor Press, 1980.

Freeman RD, Carbin CF, Boese RJ. *Can't Your Child Hear?* Baltimore: Baltimore University Park Press, 1981.

McCarthur S. *Raising Your Hearing-Impaired Child: A Guideline for Parents.* Washington DC: Alexander Graham Bell Society, 1982.

National Information Center on Deafness. *Growing Together: Information for Parents of Hearing Impaired Children.* Washington DC: Gallaudet University Press.

Ogden P, Lipsett S. *The Silent Garden.* New York: St. Martin's Press, 1982.

For Professionals
Bess FH (ed). *Hearing impairment in children.* Parkton, MD: York Press, 1988.

Coplan J. Deafness ever heard of it? Delayed recognition of permanent hearing loss. *Pediatrics* 79:206–213, 1987.

Gannon J. *Deaf Heritage.* Silver Spring, MD: National Association of the Deaf, 1981.

Joint Committee on Infant Hearing. *1990 position statement. Am Speech Hearing Assoc* 33 (Suppl. 5), 3–6.

Marschak M. *Psychological Development of Deaf Children.* New York: Oxford University Press, 1993.

Hospitalization

Abraham Joseph Avni-Singer and
John M. Leventhal

I. **Description of the problem.** Hospitalization is an inherently stressful experience, although there is wide variability in the nature and intensity of that stress for any given child. Table 39-1 lists many of the common stressors for children during a hospitalization.

II. **Factors affecting the child's response**

   A. **Child factors**

      1. **Cognitive level.** A child's cognitive level has a profound effect on his or her ability to understand and cope with a hospitalization. Since the preverbal child cannot comprehend adult explanations, the hospitalization may be experienced as an unexplainable abandonment. Preschoolers, who lack a sophisticated understanding of causality, may view the hospitalization and treatments as punishment for bad behavior. Even with older children, their understanding of the reasons for the hospitalization may be erroneous and lead to maladaptive responses.

      2. **Temperament.** Shy children who are slow to adapt to new situations and have difficulty with transitions may have greater problems coping with the hospitalization. The intense child may manifest more overt behavioral problems for the staff, who, in turn, may not treat the child as positively as they do an inhibited (but equally anxious) child.

      3. **Experience.** Previous experience with hospitalization or illness can profoundly influence the child's response to hospitalization. The child may associate hospitals with death, for example, particularly if he or she experienced the loss of a loved one who was chronically ill. An episode of abdominal pain in a 13 year old admitted to rule out appendicitis will have a special meaning for a child and family that recently lost a grandparent to colon cancer. When a child's or parent's reaction seems disproportionate to the severity of the illness, questions about family history can be revealing.

   B. **Parental/Familial factors**

      1. **Anxiety.** One of the best predictors of how a child will cope with a hospitalization is the parents' level of anxiety about it. Anxious parents beget anxious children. These families should be identified in advance of elective hospitalizations and preventive interventions offered.

      2. **Attitudes toward illness, death, and health care.** Children adopt the illness behaviors of their family and culture. A child from a family that views hospitalization as tantamount to incarceration will respond very differently from the hospitalized child whose family views hospitalization as a healing interval.

      3. **Parenting experience.** Inexperienced parents have more difficulty helping their children cope with the stress of hospitalization. The parents may be insecure and less open to the advice of staff or, alternatively, acquiesce to every suggestion and exude a pervasive sense of powerlessness.

      4. **Parents' emotional adjustment.** Parents may be emotionally unavailable for their children if they are struggling with their feelings of fear, grief, depression, or exhaustion.

Table 39-1. Stressful aspects of hospitalization for pediatric patients

Loss of control
Painful procedures
Separation/isolation from family and friends
Infantilization
Incomprehensibility of the experience
Fear of death
Loss of privacy
Altered body image
Being ill

Note: Any of the stressors may be operative for a given child, regardless of the age, although they take on different meanings at different developmental stages.

III. Strategies for management

A. Goals. Short term goals are to (1) prevent or reduce anxiety, pain, and discomfort; (2) facilitate cooperation and participation in care; and (3) hasten recovery.

Long-term goals are to (1) enhance coping skills, (2) improve self-control, (3) foster positive attitudes toward health care, and (4) minimize the potentially disruptive effects of hospitalization on normal developmental processes.

B. Separation from parents. In most cases, it is ideal for a parent to accompany the child through as much of the hospitalization as possible. However, the needs of the child should be carefully balanced with the needs of the family. Some parents, for example, should be encouraged to leave the hospital in order to attend to siblings or to their own emotional and physical needs.

Considerable research has documented the benefits of having parents present during painful medical procedures (although their presence can also increase the child's anxiety when the parent is particularly anxious). Parental presence can also be helpful at other times, such as during elective induction of anesthesia.

As staff encourage parental involvement in the child's daily care, they must foster relationships with parents that are noncompetitive.

C. Anticipatory guidance

1. To provide effective preparation for children for the experience of hospitalization, it is helpful to know the **strengths and vulnerabilities of the parents and child** that will affect the response to the experience.

2. **Children should be prepared** in advance of an elective hospitalization. *When* to do so, however, is less certain. Certainly the age and personality of the child should be considered. For example, a preschool or anxious child should only be given 2–3 days notice between preparation and procedure, since longer intervals increase tension.

3. In the case of **surgery,** children need to know that the surgery itself will not be painful. They should be told what to expect postoperatively. This means that if a Foley catheter or chest tube will be in place when they awaken, they should be forewarned. They should be told to expect some discomfort following the surgery but should be reassured that effective medication will reduce their pain.

D. Continuity of care

1. **Coping.** Multiple hospital caregivers can needlessly exacerbate stranger anxiety. The use of the primary nurse and physician allows the child to develop a relationship with the staff characterized by predictability and trust. Other techniques to minimize disruption of the child's routine should be used. These include the use of transitional objects (such as a favorite blanket or toy) and, for older children, the use of ward-based school programs. Ideally, these services should be integrated into a comprehensive child-life program at the hospital that is designed to facilitate coping at each stage of the hospitalization experience.

2. **Staff.** Staff should be educated to engage in responsive, interactive social play rather than intrusive, interrupting play. This play must be geared to the individual needs of the child. Some hospitalized children are passive and lethargic or irritable, and therefore are less competent at engaging caregivers in meaningful interactions. These children require extra effort by the staff to address their emotional needs. Other patients are lively and adorable and soon become the "favorites" of the hospital staff. These children are at risk of being treated (unintentionally) as mascots, with frequent, brief, highly stimulating interactions that do not facilitate healthy relationships. Without continuity, it is difficult for the staff to understand the individual child's needs. A foster grandparent program may be helpful in this regard.

3. **Daily routine.** The child's day should be as structured as possible, with medical treatments bunched together to provide long, uninterrupted blocks of time for play or naps.

E. **Pain management.** An emphasis on diminishing physically painful experiences is a hallmark of sensitive care during a hospitalization. This involves careful attention to adequate analgesia, parental support, anticipatory guidance, and sympathetic care.

F. **Cognitive/behavioral techniques**

1. **Information**

   a. **Providing developmentally appropriate and accurate information** helps effective coping by correcting misconceptions, reducing fears, and facilitating active participation in care. The child's understanding can be determined with a few simple questions such as, "Why do you think you got sick?" and "How does the medicine work to make you better?" Explanations should then be carefully geared to the child's developmental level, medical jargon should be avoided, and unfamiliar terms should be explained.

   b. For the child whose level of cognitive understanding is still very concrete, **explanations should be very basic** and supplemented with concrete actions. For example, the use of an *oral* medication to reduce itching of a *skin* rash may bewilder the preschool child and can be supplemented with concrete interventions such as cool compresses. A strategy to increase the efficacy of pain medications might involve using two 15-mg pills instead of one 30-mg pill, as a young child reasons that two small pills are twice as effective as one larger one.

   c. **It is especially important for parents and professionals not to reinforce the concept of immanent justice,** particularly prevalent among preschoolers: the child's idea that the hospitalization and illness are direct consequences of his or her previous "bad" behavior or breaking of the rules. Hospitalized children need to know that they may get sick and need treatment even if they follow all the rules, and that they are not being punished for real or imagined misdeeds.

   d. **Preparation for painful procedures** should also be cognitively appropriate. Preschool children might be told about what the room will look like and who will be with them, whereas older children can be provided with more detailed descriptions of the procedures and their mechanisms of action. The child who reacts anxiously to preparatory information, however, should not be forced to listen.

2. **Special techniques**

   a. A variety of techniques have been developed to facilitate the **active participation of the child and parent in the care,** thereby reducing the feelings of loss of control. Whenever feasible, *allow the child some kind* of choice within the mandated rules and procedures. Something as simple as allowing the child to choose the site for the venipuncture can enhance the child's sense of autonomy.

   b. The **use of medical toys and dolls** in play can be a way to provide information and allow the child to develop mastery over the situation. By playing with teddy bears or dolls that have the same stitches or cast, children gain a better understanding of their own experience. Children may benefit from handling the objects to be used in procedures and practicing the procedure on a doll or puppet. Role play with puppets has been useful to facilitate self-care management of a chronic illness such as asthma.

   c. **Modeling** refers to the use of a live or filmed peer model undergoing a procedure and can provide the child with a vicarious exposure to the stressor under controlled circumstances. Videotapes have been used successfully to prepare children for elective procedures and surgery, while providing examples of appropriate and adaptive behaviors for inexperienced children. To be effective, the model should demonstrate how children might feel during a stressful event rather than simply providing details of the event. Anxious children who view film models have greater reduction in anxiety if the model exhibits initial anxiety and overcomes it than when the model shows no initial fear whatsoever.

   d. **Hypnosis, relaxation, and imaginal distraction** are valuable techniques that help children to cope with medical procedures. These techniques are particularly helpful when the parents are enrolled as coaches (see Chapter 13).

G. Parental support

   1. **Parents who cope well are much better equipped to help their children deal with the stress of hospitalization.** These stressors can best be addressed by anticipating the problem, giving parents opportunities to voice their concerns, and sharing information with them in an open and consistent manner. Additionally, parents may need to be encouraged to meet their own personal needs for food and rest. By taking an interest in the parents' needs, clinicians can foster better communication with them.

   2. **Support groups** can provide a framework for parents to share their emotions and concerns in a caring and safe environment. An unstructured format allows parents to initiate discussion. Topics often include death and dying, guilt, experiences with hospitalization, financial concerns, behavioral problems, and lack of support from spouses or other family members. Through empathic problem solving, these groups can decrease a parent's sense of isolation and helplessness.

H. Support for the clinician.
One of the first steps to greater sensitivity to the emotional needs of pediatric patients is for clinicians to gain an awareness of their own feelings and responses to the child and family. Clinicians may find themselves identifying with the children and feeling rage against the hospital system. Alternatively, they may seek to distance themselves from their own reactions, especially when they need to perform painful procedures repeatedly. Thus, the clinicians and parents may subconsciously collude in a conspiracy of silence that makes them emotionally unavailable to the children. There is no easy solution, but the best approach is to create an atmosphere of communication and mutual support between children, parents, and professionals where feelings can safely be discussed.

Bibliography

For Parents
Baznik D. *Becky's Story.* 1981.
Encourages siblings of hospitalized children to explore and understand their own reactions, needs, and emotions.
For Teenagers: Your Stay in the Hospital (2nd ed). 1991.

Krementz J. *How It Feels to Fight for Your Life.* Boston: Little, Brown, 1990.
A collection of 14 case histories of children coping with serious illness and disabilities.
Preparing Your Child for the Hospital: A Checklist (2nd ed). 1990.

All these titles and others may be ordered through Association for the Care of Children's Health, 7910 Woodmont Avenue, Suite 300, Bethesda MD 20814; (301) 654-6549.

For Professionals

Granger RH. Psychologic aspects of physical trauma. In R. Touloukian (ed), *Pediatric Trauma*. St. Louis: Mosby, 1990.

Melamed BG, Ridley-Johnson R. Psychological preparation of families for hospitalization. *Dev Behav Pediatr* 9:96–101, 1988.

Parmelee AH Jr. *Children's Illnesses and Normal Behavioral Development: The Role of Caregivers, Zero to Three* 13:4–10, 1993.

Schonfeld DJ. The child's cognitive understanding of illness. In M Lewis (ed), *Child and Adolescent Psychiatry: A Comprehensive Textbook*. Baltimore: Williams & Wilkins, 1992.

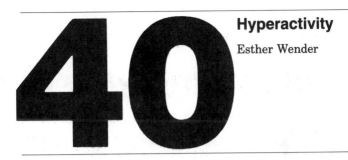

Hyperactivity

Esther Wender

I. **Description of the problem.** Attention-deficit hyperactivity disorder (ADHD) is a cluster of behaviors (a behavioral syndrome) that appears early in the child's life. The behaviors typically persist throughout childhood and adolescence, though the manifestation of those behaviors changes over the span of development. The defining behaviors fall under the general categories of hyperactivity, inattentiveness, and impulsivity (Table 40-1). These clusters of behaviors in the recently revised nomenclature of the *Diagnostic and Statistical Manual of Mental Disorders* (4th ed.) are separated into two groups. Group 1 contains behaviors often described as **inattentive.** Group 2 behaviors include **hyperactivity** and **impulsivity.** This nomenclature recognizes that some children with ADHD behaviors may be primarily inattentive, others may be primarily hyperactive or impulsive, and yet others may have both types of behavior.

Additionally, the symptom clusters known as ADHD often coexist with other behavioral and cognitive syndromes (Table 40-2). More than one of these additional syndromes can be (and often are) identified in the same child.

A. **Epidemiology**
- ADHD is the most common, significant behavioral syndrome in childhood, with an overall prevalence of 4–6% of elementary school-aged children.
- Prevalences of up to 20% have been cited in children of lower socioeconomic status.
- Male to female ratio is about 6:1.

B. **Etiology.** Just as the syndrome of ADHD is complex, so too are speculations regarding etiology. Most experts agree that there are multiple causes.

1. **Genetic factors.** Studies of first- and second-degree relatives (parents, siblings, and grandparents) of children with ADHD reveal a much higher incidence of the disorder than in the population as a whole.

2. **Differences in the brain.** Animal studies and the effects of psychoactive medications have led to speculations of altered neurotransmitter profiles in persons with ADHD. Recent positron emission tomography (PET) scan studies suggest underactivity in portions of the cerebral cortex, especially the frontal lobes. Finally, a variety of insults to the CNS system (prematurity, prenatal drug exposure, infections) have also been associated with ADHD.

3. **Environmental factors.** Environmental issues, such as parental psychopathology and low socioeconomic status, play a role in the etiology or exacerbation of ADHD. A family environment that includes poor monitoring of behavior and a punitive approach to discipline, for example, may magnify the symptoms of ADHD.

II. **Making the diagnosis.** The diagnosis of ADHD is based primarily on a report of the characteristic behaviors by multiple observers, occurring in a variety of different settings, over an extended period of time. The behaviors themselves may not be abnormal, but they occur with greater intensity and frequency than is typical for other children of the same developmental age. Information obtained from teachers is especially important because teachers are often the best judge of what is normal behavior at different ages and because the typical behaviors of ADHD are most obvious in a school classroom environment.

Table 40-1. Diagnostic criteria for attention-deficit hyperactivity disorders

A. Inattention or hyperactivity-impulsivity

1. *Inattention:* At least six of the following symptoms of inattention have persisted for at least 6 mos to a degree that is maladaptive and inconsistent with developmental level:
   • Often fails to give close attention to details or makes careless mistakes in schoolwork, work, or other activities
   • Often has difficulty sustaining attention in tasks or play activities
   • Often does not seem to listen to what is being said to him or her
   • Often does not follow through on instructions and fails to finish schoolwork, chores, or duties in the workplace (not due to oppositional behavior or failure to understand instructions)
   • Often has difficulties organizing tasks and activities
   • Often avoids, expresses reluctance about, or has difficulties engaging in tasks that require sustained mental effort (such as schoolwork or homework)
   • Often loses things necessary for tasks or activities (e.g., school assignments, pencils, books, tools or toys)
   • Is often easily distracted by extraneous stimuli
   • Often forgetful in daily activities

2. *Hyperactivity-impulsivity:* At least five of the following symptoms of hyperactivity-impulsivity have persisted for at least 6 mo to a degree that is maladaptive and inconsistent with developmental level:
   Hyperactivity
   • Often fidgets with hands or feet or squirms in seat
   • Leaves seat in classroom or in other situations in which remaining seated is expected
   • Often runs about or climbs excessively in situations when it is inappropriate (in adolescents or adults, may be limited to subjective feelings of restlessness)
   • Often has difficulty playing or engaging in leisure activities quietly
   • Is always "on the go" or acts as if "driven by a motor"
   • Often talks excessively

   Impulsivity
   • Often blurts out answers to questions before the questions have been completed
   • Often has difficulty waiting in lines or awaiting turn in games or group situations
   • Often interrupts or intrudes on others (e.g., butts into other's conversations or games)

B. Some symptoms that caused impairments were present before age 7 yr.

C. Some symptoms that cause impairment are present in two or more settings (e.g., at school, work, and at home).

D. There must be clear evidence of clinically significant impairment in social, academic, or occupational functioning.

E. Does not occur exclusively during the course of a pervasive developmental disorder, schizophrenia, or other psychotic disorder and is not better accounted for by a mood disorder, anxiety disorder, or a personality disorder.

Code based on type*
314.01   Attention-deficit/Hyperactivity Disorder, Predominantly Inattentive Type: If criterion A(1) is met but not criterion A(2) for the past 6 mo
314.01   Attention-deficit/Hyperactivity Disorder, Predominantly Hyperactive-Impulsive Type: If criterion A(2) is met but not criterion A(1) for the past 6 mo
314.01   Attention-deficit/Hyperactivity Disorder, Combined Type: If both criteria A(1) and A(2) are met for the past 6 mo

Source: American Psychiatric Association, *Diagnostic and Statistical Manual of Mental Disorders* (4th ed) Washington DC: American Psychiatric Association, 1994.
* For individuals (especially adolescents and adults) who currently have symptoms that no longer meet full criteria, "in partial remission" should be specified.

Table 40-2. Other diagnoses frequently co-occurring with attention-deficit hyperactivity disorder

Comorbid disorders	Range of prevalence from several studies*
Specific developmental disorders (academic skills disorders, language and speech disorders, motor skills disorder)	20–60%
Mild mental retardation	3–10%
Oppositional defiant disorder	30–60%
Conduct disorder	20–30%
Anxiety disorders of childhood or adolescence (separation anxiety disorder, avoidant disorder, overanxious disorder)	20–30%
Other neurologic disorders	<10%

* Percentage of children diagnosed as ADHD who also qualify for this disorder.

A. Signs and symptoms (see Table 40-1).

   1. Inattention. A child with a short attention span in school may daydream, be easily distracted, and fail to complete tasks. At home the child does not follow instructions well or listen to what is being said to him or her. However, children with ADHD may pay attention well and even become totally absorbed in activities of their own choosing, such as video games or television shows. The inattentiveness is not so much an inability to pay attention as it is an unwillingness to do so when not interested in the activity.

   2. Overactivity. Children with ADHD are typically overactive. From an early age (2–3 years) the child will be described as being in constant motion. Often the activity is poorly directed, such as moving aimlessly from one toy or game to another. The motor activity, combined with inattention, leads these children to trip over or run into objects. They may talk excessively and ramble in their speech. Often the overactivity is seen in the form of restless, fidgety behavior, especially when attempting to sit still. The child may watch television but be unable to do so without fiddling with toys or other objects.

   3. Impulsivity. Children with ADHD are impulsive. If there is something they want, they touch or grab it even when told not to. When asked to complete a chore or school work, they will do a sloppy job or write down any answer rather than work at the task systematically. They frequently interrupt or disrupt others in their pursuit of a desired object and act without thinking of the consequences.

   4. Other. Because ADHD often co-occurs with other syndromes, other inappropriate or excessive behaviors may be seen. The child may be oppositional, defiant, or negativistic or show excessive anger and aggression. Later, the child may engage in antisocial behaviors such as lying, stealing, and hurting others. If a learning disability is present, the child may have difficulty learning and retaining certain academic skills, such as reading, writing, and spelling. Children with ADHD may also have symptoms of excessive anxiety.

B. History: Key clinical questions

   1. *Are the behaviors more intense, and do they occur more frequently than in other children of the same age?* Since the behaviors characteristic of ADHD are seen in all children occasionally, the key is their severity rather than their presence or absence.

   2. *Do the behaviors change in different settings and with different kinds of activities?* Behaviors that occur only in the context of certain kinds of school work suggest the presence of a specific learning problem rather than ADHD.

Table 40-3. Conditions that may look like attention deficit hyperactivity disorder but are not

Pervasive developmental disorder
Major affective disorder
Reactions to stress (e.g., post-traumatic stress disorder)
Hyperthyroidism
Iron deficiency anemia
Lead toxicity
Hearing loss

Inattention is typically worse when pursuing activities that the child is required to do but dislikes and in settings with many distractions and excessive stimulation.

3. *When did you first begin to notice and be concerned about the behavior?* This question often reveals that the behavior had its onset early in the child's life even though diagnostic evaluation is being pursued much later.

4. *Are there several people who notice the characteristic behaviors?* True ADHD behavior is seen by multiple observers. A negative answer to this question may indicate that the child's behavior is not due to ADHD but is produced by a particular situational or interpersonal interaction problem or by a biased observer.

C. **Differential diagnosis.** Table 40-3 lists conditions that should be considered in the differential diagnosis of ADHD. Pervasive developmental disorder (autism and autistic-like disorder) and major affective disorder (depression) can be confused with ADHD since inattentiveness and restless overactivity, which are major components of ADHD, may also be seen in autism and depression.

Any kind of stress in children can result in the temporary appearance of ADHD behaviors. The stress can range from the serious (e.g., separation or divorce in the parents, abuse and neglect) to the trivial (e.g., fatigue or hunger). The diagnosis may be complicated in these situations because ADHD behaviors can both result from and contribute to family stress.

The clinician should be particularly wary of diagnosing ADHD in the child whose unrecognized learning disability or below-average cognitive ability has resulted in an inappropriate school placement. In such cases, proper classroom placement or the provision of appropriate remedial services may result in a dramatic improvement in the ADHD-like behaviors.

Making the diagnosis of ADHD is ultimately an issue of clinical judgment in which the clinician must weigh all of the evidence. The decision whether to diagnose ADHD and to embark on a program of treatment should depend ultimately on how much the child's functioning is impaired by his or her symptoms.

D. **Behavioral observations.** The behaviors typical of ADHD may be observed by the clinician in the health care setting, although children with ADHD are often able to control themselves in the one-to-one setting of a brief office examination. The typical manifestations of the syndrome are much more likely to occur in the waiting room or when sustained effort and attention are required, such as during a soft-sign neurologic examination or cognitive testing.

E. **Examination**

1. **Physical examination.** The physical examination should focus on the conditions included in the differential diagnosis (see Table 40-3). There should also be a systematic search for possible genetic syndromes (e.g., fragile X syndrome, neurofibromatosis) or neurologic disorders (e.g., Tourette's syndrome, fetal alcohol syndrome, seizures) that are known to be associated with a higher-than-normal incidence of ADHD.

2. **Soft signs.** ADHD is frequently associated with nonspecific neurologic soft signs, indicating associated neurologic immaturity or poor coordination. Such neurologic soft signs are not diagnostic of ADHD since they are associated

Table 40-4. Questionnaires that may be useful in the diagnosis of attention deficit hyperactivity disorder (ADHD)

Questionnaire	Strengths and limitations	Source
Conners Parent Rating Scale-Revised (48-item) Conners Teacher Rating Scale-Revised (28-item) Conners Abbreviated Parent-Teacher Questionnaire	Some standardization; easy scoring and norms available In use since 1960 with greatest experience among questionnaires Very sensitive to medication effects Identifies ADHD plus conduct problems	Multi-Health Systems, 908 Niagara Falls Boulevard, North Tawanda, NY 14120
Child Behavior Checklist (CBCL) Teacher Report Form (TRF)	Both scales well standardized; computer scoring available Not specifically constructed to measure ADHD symptoms; results difficult to interpret	TM Achenbach, University of Vermont, 1 South Prospect Street, Burlington, VT 05401
ADHD Rating Scale for Parents and Teachers	Some standardization; easy scoring and norms available Based on DSM III-R criteria for diagnosis of ADHD, and therefore easy to interpret and apply* Limited experience with measure in clinical settings	George J. DuPaul, Department of Psychiatry, University of Massachusetts, Medical Center, 55 Lake Avenue North, Worcester, MA 01655
ADD-H Comprehensive Teacher's Rating Scale (ACTeRS)	Standardized, with easy scoring and norms available For teacher evaluation only Separates attention problems from conduct problems	Metri Tech, 111 North Market Street, Champlain, IL 61820

* DSM III-R-*Diagnostic and Statistical Manual of Mental Disorders* (3rd ed, rev).

with many other conditions and are seen in otherwise normal children. A systematic neurologic soft-sign examination can, however, be clinically useful for two reasons. First, identifying problems with motor coordination may lead to helpful treatment strategies. Second, the neurologic soft-sign examination, which requires persistence and attention, may reveal typical ADHD behaviors when other aspects of the physical examination have not.

F. Tests

1. **Diagnostic tests.** Laboratory tests are relevant to the diagnosis of ADHD only to rule out possible differential diagnoses suggested by the history and physical examination. Specific neurologic studies such as an electroencephalogram or MRI of the head are indicated only if there are symptoms or signs of neurologic disorder. There is no role for the use of computer-based studies of sustained attention (e.g., the Continuous Performance Task) outside the research setting.

2. **Psychological testing.** If academic problems are suspected, psychological testing and educational diagnostic or speech and language testing should be performed. Such testing is required either to rule out or adequately identify a learning problem.

3. **Questionnaires.** The ADHD history should be supplemented by questionnaires completed by the parents and the teacher(s). Table 40-4 lists some of the most useful of the many questionnaires available and the limitations of each. The value of questionnaires lies in their standardization, which allows the clinician to compare the responses of teachers to that of parents and to

quantify changes over time. However, the questionnaires should not be considered objective; they are as prone to observer bias as an interview.

III. Management

A. **Primary goals.** Preservation of good self-esteem is the ultimate goal of all treatment strategies. Additionally, therapies should be aimed toward optimal academic, emotional, and vocational outcomes. Although the short attention span and impulsivity diminish over time, self-esteem may be increasingly impaired, largely as the result of negative reactions from peers, siblings, parents, and teachers. Peer acceptance and sibling relationships are often especially poor because these children frequently have poor social skills and tend to misinterpret the motives and behaviors of others. These problems are often exaggerated because children with ADHD feel victimized by the criticism of peers and adults and then act out in ways that provoke more criticism. Parents and teachers should recognize the source of this vicious circle.

B. **Information for the family.** It is critical for the family to understand the reasons for the behavior of children with ADHD. Without the fundamental understanding that *biological* factors lead to the child's behavior, his or her actions are interpreted as willful and manipulative and may provoke an angry response, which then aggravates the child's feelings of being misunderstood and picked on. Limit setting should be accomplished sympathetically and without deprecating criticism. Parents learn to anticipate the child's reaction to specific situations and to motivate and control the child's behavior without injuring his or her self-esteem.

C. **Treatment**

1. **Medication.** There is only one treatment that consistently improves the primary behaviors of ADHD: medication, especially CNS stimulant medication. The effects of these medications can be seen on all of the fundamental behaviors of ADHD: attention span may be increased, activity level normalized, and impulsivity reduced. If the child is also oppositional and defiant, compliance is often increased, emotional liability reduced, and antisocial behaviors decreased. Therefore, when symptoms of ADHD have a significant negative effect on the child's ability to function academically and socially, medication should be prescribed, at least as an initial treatment trial.

   a. **Limitations.** The limitations of stimulant medications are many, however, even when the response is optimal. Medication is effective only during the relatively brief period of optimal blood concentration. In addition, there may be significant side effects that may limit the dosage and the hours of administration. And although 70–80% of children with ADHD experience some positive effects, 20–30% do not.

   b. **Pharmacologic agents.** The three most useful stimulant medications are methylphenidate, dextroamphetamine, and pemoline. Table 40-5 contains information concerning their use. All three can be effective, but some children may respond to only one. When problems arise with one drug or it is ineffective, another in this group should be tried.

   c. **Dosage.** These medications must be titrated by starting with the lowest possible dosage and gradually increasing until the optimal response is seen. Side effects can usually be minimized by altering the dosage, timing, or form (short or long acting) of medication. Table 40-6 lists the common side effects and how they can be managed. Throughout treatment, height and weight should be monitored. Although some children experience short-term suppression of growth, long-term effects are rarely seen. Even short-term effects can be modified by altering the timing of medication and the time when eating is allowed.

   Once the appropriate dosage is established, it should be reevaluated and adjusted upward as tolerance develops or as the child's growth necessitates a larger dosage. The decision to treat only on weekdays or during the school year should be made only when the child's symptoms do not affect his or her behavioral control in situations outside of school and when there are no difficulties getting along with peers and family.

Table 40-5. Stimulant medication: dosage and techniques of administration

Pharmacologic agent	Form of medication and duration of effect	Initial dosage and incremental increase	Frequency of administration	Effects and how to respond
Methylphenidate (Ritalin)	Short acting: 5-mg, 10-mg, and 20-mg tablets; duration: 2½–4 hr Long acting: 20-mg sustained release (SR); duration: 4–8 hr	0.3 mg/kg/dose; increase by 0.15 mg/kg/dose Use only when A.M. plus noon dose in tablet form reaches or exceeds 20 mg	Twice daily, A.M. and noon; add 4 P.M. dose as needed In A.M. only; may add 4 P.M. dose as needed	No effect: Increase dosage Wear-off effects: (1) add 4 P.M. dose; (2) switch to long-acting form Slow onset: Add tablet to A.M. dose Wear off in early P.M.: add 4 P.M. tablet
Dextroamphetamine (Dexedrine)	Short acting: 5-mg tablets; duration: 4 hr Long acting: 5-mg, 10-mg, and 15-mg spansules; duration: 8 hr	0.15 mg/kg/dose; increase by 0.15 mg/kg/dose Add up total daily dosage in tablet form and give this as one dose in A.M.	Twice daily (A.M. and noon); add 4 P.M. dose as needed In A.M. only; also combined with tablets in A.M. or P.M.	Same as for methylphenidate Slow onset: Add tablet to A.M. dose
Pemoline (Cylert)	Tablets: 18.75-mg, 37.5-mg, and 75-mg; chewable tablets 37.5 mg; duration: 8 hr	<age 8 yr: 37.5 mg in A.M. >age 8 yr: 37.5 mg plus 18.75 mg in A.M. Increase by 18.75 mg/dose	A.M. only at first; add 4 P.M. dose as needed	At any one dose, effects may not be seen for 1–2 wk No effect: Increase A.M. dose Wear off in early P.M.: Add 4 P.M. dose

Table 40-6. Stimulant medication: Common side effects and management strategies

Common side effects	Management strategies
Decrease in appetite	Administer medication with or shortly after meals Encourage eating after school and/or before bedtime When severe, institute short periods off medication
Difficulty falling asleep	Omit 4 P.M. dose; if child is restless and overactive at bedtime, may add a P.M. dose Add a mild hypnotic such as an antihistamine prior to bedtime
Dazed and/or withdrawn behavior	Reduce dosage
Rebound hyperactivity or emotional overactivity when medication wears off	Switch from short-acting to long-acting form of medication Add a 4 P.M. dose if behavior occurs at this time
Gradual return of hyperactive behaviors	Increase dosage
Gradual onset of symptoms of depression during periods of effective medication dose	Discontinue medication and refer
Development of tics that were not present prior to starting medication	Discontinue medication and refer

    d. Duration of treatment. Treatment should continue into and through adolescence (except in the 20% of children with ADHD who completely outgrow the problem). The decision to end treatment should be based on brief periods off medication (usually 2–4 weeks) during times of low stress.

  2. Psychological therapy. In addition to medication, several psychological and social treatments should be considered (Table 40-7).

    a. Parent training in behavioral management should be given the highest priority. This treatment aims to teach parents how to set limits, provide incentives for appropriate behaviors, and minimize emotionally destructive responses. Though this approach seems simple, parents find such discipline difficult to achieve. What is required is a complete change in instinctive responses to negative behaviors. A great deal of energy must be devoted to the observation of and response to those behaviors. The school should also develop an appropriate and effective response to the ADHD child's behavior that is consistent with the approach at home.

      Training adults (either parents or teachers) in behavioral management skills usually requires referral. For parents, treatment may be done in small groups, which have the advantage of providing support as well as training. The clinician should recognize that the goal of behavioral management therapy is improvement in the environment in which daily living takes place, not to change the child's fundamental nature. However, when the typical behaviors occur, the discipline exerted will be more effective and free of the negative emotion that often accompanies ineffective discipline.

    b. Additional therapies may be needed depending on the circumstances of the family and the child. The primary care clinician should note that there is a limited role for traditional, individual psychotherapy for the child with ADHD. The goal of such therapy should be to improve self-esteem. There is no evidence that individual psychotherapy improves the

Table 40-7. Attention-deficit hyperactivity disorder: psychological treatment strategies

Treatment	Goals
Teaching effective behavioral management skills to parents and teachers	Aimed at adults, and only indirectly to children with ADHD Improve effectiveness of discipline Minimize harmful adult-child interaction
Child or parent counseling	Improve understanding of ADHD Directive approach, teaching alternative ways of behaving/responding to daily incidents
Group social skills training	Provide a "laboratory" for interactions between children Model appropriate responses Promote self-awareness
Family therapy, dynamic	Help dysfunctional families become aware of and repair dysfunctional relationships
Family therapy, communication skills	Teach families improved communication skills Apply those skills to parent-child problem solving
Child psychotherapy	Improve child's self-awareness Help child understand strengths, despite problems (improve self-esteem)

child's ability to pay attention or reduces impulsiveness. As the child gets older and becomes more self-aware, however, psychotherapy may facilitate an understanding of how his or her own behavior affects others. Family dynamic psychotherapy should be reserved for families that display disturbed functioning outside the limited context of the child's ADHD behaviors. Family communication skills training has a more limited focus, which may be especially helpful when the child with ADHD is approaching adolescence. The focus of this type of therapy is establishing rules and enforcing those rules in the family setting.

D. Criteria for referral. Most primary care clinicians will be involved in two aspects of treatment: (1) explaining the condition to the child and the family and (2) prescribing and following medication. Psychosocial treatments will be given by others, though the clinician should be familiar with each type of treatment and the goals of each treatment strategy. The clinician should develop resources for referral and establish including ongoing communication with those resources. When the child fails to respond to stimulant medication or develops unacceptable side effects, referral to a specialist, such as a developmental-behavioral pediatrician or child psychiatrist, is indicated.

Bibliography

For Parents
A.D.D. Warehouse, 300 Northwest 70th Avenue, Suite 102, Plantation FL 33317; (800) 233-9273.
A catalog of books, videos, and other products to help children with ADHD and their families to understand and manage ADHD problems. Contains an excellent annotated bibliography.

CH.A.D.D. (Children with Attention Deficit Disorders), 499 Northwest 70th Avenue, Suite 308, Plantation FL 33317; (305) 587-3700.
National organization with local chapters throughout the country. Provides support to families, formation regarding local laws and school policies and an avenue for advocacy.

For Professionals

Barkley RA. *Attention-Deficit Hyperactivity Disorder: A Handbook for Diagnosis and Treatment*. New York: Guilford Press, 1990.

Shaywitz SE, Shaywitz BA. Diagnosis and management of attention deficit disorder: A pediatric perspective. *Pediatr Clin North Am* 31:429–457, 1984.

Wender EH, Solanto MV. Attention-deficit hyperactivity disorder. In RA Hoekelman et al. (eds), *Primary Pediatric Care* (2nd ed).

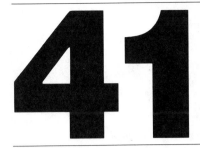

Language Delays

James Coplan

I. Description of the problem. Language can be defined as a symbolic system for the storage or exchange of information. **Expressive language** refers to the ability to generate symbolic output. This output may be either visual (writing, signing), or auditory (speech). **Receptive language** refers to the ability to decode (i.e., extract meaning from) the language output of others. Receptive language encompasses visual (reading, sign language comprehension) and auditory (listening comprehension) skills. **Speech** refers to the mechanical aspects of sound production (not the content). **Language disorders** encompass any defect in the ability to encode or decode information through symbolic means.

A. Epidemiology

- Delayed speech or language development is the most common developmental disorder of childhood, occurring in 5–10% of preschool children.
- Developmental language disorders (DLD) are rarely transmitted as a simple autosomal dominant trait. More commonly, DLD occurs in multiple members of a kindred without falling into a simple Mendelian pattern.

B. Development of language

1. **Language acquisition** results from a complex interplay of innate biological capabilities and environmental stimulation. Infants acquire language through observation and through listening to speakers in their environment. Early efforts at imitation tend to be stimulus driven (i.e., automatic or unconscious), but by the latter half of the first year of life, infants appear capable of deliberate imitation of others' language. Parents and caretakers usually strongly reinforce and model linguistic behavior in order to create a *linguistically enriched environment.*

2. **By age 12 months,** normal infants have grasped the notion that an arbitrary set of sounds (a word) symbolically represents a specific object or action. Likewise, a 12 month old knows that he or she can signify a desired object by pointing to it rather than reaching for it. This ability to represent objects or actions in symbolic form constitutes the central feature of language.

3. **Language proficiency** correlates closely with overall cognitive development in normal children and in children with global developmental delay (mental retardation). Some consider language development to be a special aspect of overall cognitive development. Alternatively, language acquisition may represent the emergence of a parallel but independent set of skills, which develop at the same time as general cognitive ability.

C. Etiology

1. **Environmental.** Although language delay is frequently observed in association with various social or emotional risk factors, many risk factors that at first appear to be purely social in origin or related to the degree of environmental stimulation are confounded by organic variables such as nutritional status, low-level lead exposure, or low-grade iron deficiency. In an average home with average parents, "lack of stimulation" is seldom, if ever, a cause of language delay. Suggestions that such parents become "more stimulating" may do more harm than good, either by inspiring misplaced parental guilt or by delaying a search for an underlying organic disorder as the basis for the child's delay.

Table 41-1. Patterns of language delay

	HL	MR	DLD	Autism
Auditory expressive				
Vocabulary size	X	X	X	X
Linguistic complexity	X	X	X	X
Intelligibility	X	X[a]	X	
Prosody				X
Pragmatics				X
Auditory receptive	X	X	X[b]	X
Visual		X		X

Source: Reprinted with permission from Coplan J. *The Early Language Milestone Scale* (2nd ed). Austin, TX: Pro-Ed, 1993.
HL = hearing loss; MR = mental retardation; DLD = developmental language disorder.
[a] Intelligibility is usually normal for the child's developmental level rather than chronological age.
[b] Variable.

2. **Organic.** Developmental language disorders are due to impairment of those portions of the brain that serve language. A critical period for the postnatal maturation of brainstem auditory pathways has been established in animal models and is strongly suggested in the first 12 months of life in human infants. Fluctuating mild to moderate conductive hearing loss during the first 12–24 months of life (e.g., from otitis media) has been associated with subtle delays in language development and may be attributable to disruption in maturation of these pathways. Early postnatal maturation of sensory pathways may be accompanied by a similar critical period (or, at least, optimal period) for cerebral acquisition of language. Failure to provide adequate language input during this period may produce changes in brain function that irrevocably compromise cerebral competence for language, over and above the effects of hearing loss per se.

3. **Developmental.** "Laziness," birth order, twinning, and "tongue tie" do not cause language delay, nor does bilingual rearing. The bilingual child may intermix the vocabularies of both language, but total vocabulary size and length of utterance should be normal by age 2–3 years.

"Constitutional delay" implies a normal long-term developmental outcome. Although such an entity exists, this is a diagnosis that can be established only in retrospect. If a preschool child's speech pattern is deficient based on comparison with age norms, then action is called for. Adopting a wait-and-see attitude in a speech-delayed preschooler in the hope that his or her delay will prove to be "constitutional" is rarely justifiable.

II. Making the diagnosis

A. **Signs and symptoms.** The pattern of language delay, coupled with an appraisal of development in other domains (fine motor, adaptive, play, personal/social), will often suggest a specific developmental diagnosis (Table 41-1). Note the value of visual language development as a distinguishing feature: visual language development (see Appendix E) is delayed in mental retardation and autism but normal in hearing loss and DLD.

B. **History.** A well-taken history of language development is the most important diagnostic measure. It should encompass auditory expressive, auditory receptive, and visual language milestones. The **Early Language Milestone Scale** (2nd ed.) (ELM Scale-2; see Appendix E) provides guidelines for normal language milestones to age 3 years and can be used to direct the history taking.

C. **Physical examination.** Elements of the history and physical examination pertinent to the assessment of the child with language delay are listed in Table 41-2.

Table 41-2. Assessing the child with language delay

Medical history
Teratogenic exposure (alcohol, drugs; risk factors related to the human immunodeficiency virus)
Fetal growth (weight, length, head circumference, and percentile values)
Neonatal intensive care unit
Recurrent otitis media
Developmental history
Oromotor
Problems with sucking, swallowing, chewing, excess drooling?
Fine motor/adaptive
Age at acquisition of tool use (spoon, crayon; normal = 12 mo)?
Language
Auditory expressive, auditory receptive, visual*
Play
Banging and mouthing (9 mo); casting (12 mo); stacking and dumping (14 mo); scribbles with crayons (16–18 mo); imitative play ("helps" with housework; 24 mo); make-believe (36 mo); rule-based play (board games; 48 mo)
Personal/social
Eye contact; cuddly? rigid behavior patterns? "fascination" with certain objects?
Family history
Educational attainment of parents and siblings
Language delay, hearing loss, or other developmental disability in extended family?
Physical examination
Length, weight, head circumference, and percentile values
Dysmorphic features
Neurocutaneous lesions

* See Table 41-1.

D. Tests

1. **Language testing.** The ELM Scale-2 covers language development from birth to age 36 months and intelligibility of speech from ages 24–48 months. It is designed for child care professionals with varying degrees of expertise in early child development and demonstrates excellent test-retest and interobserver reliability.

2. **Auditory testing.** Screening audiometry procedures used by physicians are prone to yield false-negative results or are inappropriate for the very young child. Therefore, all language-delayed children should have their hearing tested by a certified audiologist, regardless of the clinician's subjective impression of how well the child seems to hear.

3. **Developmental testing.** Language and global cognitive function should be formally assessed. Language delay is often the first indication of a global problem (most commonly, mental retardation). Two questions must be addressed: (1) Is the child's language significantly delayed relative to age norms? and (2) Is language significantly delayed relative to the child's present level of overall cognitive function?

4. **Referral.** The primary care clinician should not hesitate to refer children with suspected language delays for evaluation and treatment. If the results are negative, everyone will be appropriately reassured; if the results are positive, developmental intervention can be implemented in a timely fashion.

E. Prognosis

1. **Children with DLD** initially manifest impaired intelligibility of speech and delayed emergence of phrases and sentences. Comprehension often appears

Table 41-3. Tips for parents to promote language development

Don't try to force your child to speak; it's unhelpful and demoralizing.

Read books aloud to your child.

Don't use complicated language. Expand a little bit on whatever your child says (e.g., *Child*: "Cookie!"; *Parent*: "Oh, you want a cookie.")

Talk a lot to your child. Narrate concrete daily events as you do them (e.g., "O.K. now I'm cleaning the floor. Oh, it's dirty. Can you see the dirt? . . .").

Respond whenever your child speaks. It's important to reward every utterance.

Ask your child a lot of questions (e.g., "What's that? Where should we put that?").

Accompany your words with gestures to make them more comprehensible.

Don't criticize grammatical errors.

Find a play group of children with language a little better than your child's.

---

normal, at least initially. Speech is usually improved by the time of school entry and often becomes normal with the passage of time.

2. **Children with language delay as preschoolers** are more likely to manifest problems with auditory comprehension, short-term auditory memory, reading, or other signs of academic impairment.

3. **Children with constitutional delay** may be virtually indistinguishable from children with mild DLD as preschoolers and can be differentiated from DLD only in hindsight (after speech has normalized and academic problems have failed to surface).

III. Management

A. **Primary goals.** The primary goal of management is to minimize frustration for the child and his or her parents, while promoting optimal development of language. Table 41-3 lists suggestions for parents to provide a linguistically enriched environment for their child when linguistic stimulation is not considered optimal.

B. **Reading aloud.** Information on reading-aloud programs is usually available through the local public library. Not infrequently, a recommendation that the parent read aloud with his or her child will lead the clinician to discover that the parent is semiliterate or illiterate. A remedial reading program for the parent can sometimes be instituted in conjunction with the reading-aloud program for the child.

C. **Information for the family.** The parents should be informed of the organic etiology if known. If the specific underlying etiology is unknown, the parents can still be given an explanation of the biological basis of their child's language delay (for example, in DLD, "Your child's language is delayed because the part of his or her brain that controls language is developing differently from other children").

The clinician should not rush to judgment, giving parents either false reassurance ("Don't worry, he'll grow out of it") or needless anxiety ("Johnny will never be able to do . . ."). On the other hand, the clinician should not procrastinate once the outcome seems clear ("Why didn't our doctor tell us before now?" is a common complaint). Following identification, the primary care clinician serves a key role by ensuring that the consultants who are involved have appropriately explained the issues and by regularly monitoring the child and the family's progress.

D. **Treatment**

1. If hearing loss is present, **amplification** may be indicated.

2. **Pressure equalization tubes and/or antimicrobial prophylaxis** may be indicated for the child with conductive hearing loss due to otitis media with effusion.

3. The treatment of language delay is primarily **educational**. Infants and toddlers up to age 36 months are typically served in home-based programs. Enrollment in a special education program administered by the child's school

district is often the best option for children age 36 months or older, since a classroom setting will provide not just language instruction but practical experience in the use of language in a social setting.

For children with DLD, the emphasis will often be on speech sound production. For children with autism, the emphasis will often be on *pragmatics* (the use of language as a medium for social interchange). Language therapy for the child with mental retardation will be integrated into an overall program stressing adaptive, play, and social development, in addition to language. Therapy for the child with hearing loss will vary, depending on the degree of hearing loss, but may commonly include some combination of orally based speech therapy plus sign language.

IV. Clinical pearls and pitfalls

- Parents will often say, "My child's speech is delayed, but he understands everything." On the contrary, the child with delayed language often does not understand everything that is being said but relies instead on contextual cues or repetition of set routines or depends on the parents to break everything down into a series of one-step commands. While these strategies may be highly adaptive for the child, they imply a receptive language level of age 18 months, regardless of how many one-step commands the child has mastered.
- Clinical detection of hearing loss, even severe to profound loss, is astonishingly difficult on physical examination, since children "cheat" by observing visual cues. If the child's language is delayed or if the parents question hearing loss, the clinician should get an audiogram, no matter how well the child seems to hear in the office.

Bibliography

For Parents

Beginning with Books, Carnegie Library of Pittsburgh, Homewood Branch, 7101 Hamilton Avenue, Pittsburgh PA 15208; (412) 731-1717.
Information on reading aloud.

For Professionals.

Coplan J. *The Early Language Milestone Scale* (2nd ed). Austin TX: Available from Pro-Ed, 1993.

Coplan J, and Gleason JR. *Test-Retest and Interobserver Reliability of the Early Language Milestone Scale* (2nd ed). *J. Pediatr Health Care* 7:212–219, 1993.

Silva PA, Williams S, McGee R. A longitudinal study of children with developmental language delay at age three: Later intelligence, reading and behavior problems. *Dev Med Child Neurol* 29(5):630–640, 1987.

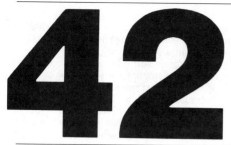

Masturbation

Ilgi Ertem and
John M. Leventhal

I. **Description of the problem.** Sexual health has been defined by the World Health Organization as the "integration of the somatic, emotional, intellectual, and social aspects of sexual being, in ways that are positively enriching and that enhance personality, communication and love." Childhood sexuality is as much a part of a child as are physical health, growth, and other aspects of development. It is within this framework that the clinician should address parental concern with masturbation, one of the early manifestations of the sexual development of the child.

The term *masturbation* is derived from the Latin words for "hand" (*manus*) and "defilement" (*stupratio*). It is defined as a deliberate self-stimulation that results in sexual arousal. At least since the time of Hippocrates (400 B.C.), masturbation has evoked negative attitudes within societies. For example, during the eighteenth century, two-thirds of all human illnesses were attributed to masturbation. Various treatment regimens, such as disciplining the patient, mechanical preventions, cautery of genitals, clitorectomy, and castration, were established and practiced until the mid-twentieth century. It is still true that parents' responses to sexual behavior in their children are largely influenced by cultural patterns. Some societies condone and encourage self-stimulation during childhood; others condemn it. In general, Western societies take a more restrictive view of masturbation.

A. **Epidemiology.** Masturbation is universal and intentional in children of both sexes by age 5–6 years. Almost all boys and 25% of girls have masturbated to the point of orgasm by age 15 years.

B. **Environmental, developmental, and transactional factors in etiology.** Masturbatory activity has been observed in the male fetus in utero. In the first months of life, infants of both sexes learn to experience the sensations associated with diapering and the cleansing of genitals. A developmental progression toward adult erotic responsiveness proceeds from these early pleasurable sensations and includes the differentiation and appreciation of genitals, inclusion of sexual parts in the body concept, "exhibitionism" to test adult reactions, mastery of a variety of self-elicited sensations, and the integration of sexual function into the emerging self-concept.

C. **Signs and symptoms.** Most commonly, masturbatory activity in infants and toddlers involves a particular posturing, tightening of the thighs, handling of the genitals, and symptoms of sexual arousal (e.g., flushing, rapid or irregular breathing). Masturbation may also involve less obvious acts such as leaning the suprapubic region on a firm edge, stiffening of the lower extremities, or rocking movements in various positions. These may be accompanied by brief bouts of crying or sweating and may last from minutes to hours at a time. In some cases, these manifestations may simulate symptoms of organic disease (such as seizures).

II. **Making the diagnosis**

A. **Differential diagnosis**

1. **Masturbatory actions may be misdiagnosed as seizures** because of the abrupt onset of the episodes, the tonic posturing, facial flushing, irregular breathing, and the child's preoccupation. During masturbation, there may also be blank stares or tremulous movements. The child may resume his or her previous play or activity after the event or may appear drowsy and fall asleep, mimicking children in the postictal phase.

2. **The symptoms of masturbation also have been confused with abdominal pain or the "retentive" posturing that occurs in children who withhold stool.** This is manifested as episodic tightening of the buttock and thighs, often accompanied by facial flushing and grunting.

3. **The clinician should consider the diagnosis of sexual abuse** in children with compulsive masturbation, especially if accompanied by other sexualized behaviors.

B. **History: Key clinical questions.** A thorough history is key to an appropriate diagnosis and effective management. Since masturbation is not harmful, it should be considered a problem only when it causes distress to the child, parental anxiety, or social condemnation.

1. *Tell me what you've noticed about your child's touching his or her genitals. Where does this happen? In school? At home?* This elicits the method the child uses and the frequency and the context in which the child engages in masturbation and other sexualized behaviors.

2. *Parents have different thoughts and feelings when their children touch their own genitals. Can you tell me how it is for you? What do you do when this happens?* The meaning of masturbatory behavior to the parents and their responses to the behavior should be understood.

3. *When you respond like that, how do you think he or she feels?* The parents' perceptions of the consequences of their responses and the outcome of the behavior are important.

C. **Physical examination.** Clinical circumstances may dictate exploration of a more pathologic interpretation of the masturbatory behaviors. This could include the possibility that the child has been sexually abused (especially if the behavior is especially compulsive and of acute onset), significant stressors for family and/or child, and developmental delays.

Masturbation may begin with genital irritation or discomfort. A child who has been sexually abused may have physical findings suggestive of or consistent with genital trauma. Also, children may insert objects in their genitalia during sex play. Therefore, the anus, genitalia, and perineum should be examined as part of a general physical examination.

D. **Tests.** Laboratory tests are almost never required during a work-up for masturbation. However, causes of irritation such as pinworm infestations or urinary tract infections will require appropriate diagnosis and treatment.

III. **Management**

A. **Anticipatory guidance.** A clinician who, from the beginning of a relationship with parents, is open to discussing issues of sexuality is more likely to receive questions about sexual development, behaviors, and problems as the child grows older. Parents are less likely to be anxious, confused, or scornful of masturbatory behavior in their child if they have been told in advance that this behavior is normal, universal, and healthy. Such anticipatory guidance should be offered early in life, when infants begin to explore their bodies. During a review of developmental milestones or during a genital examination, parents can be asked in a matter-of-fact manner whether their child has discovered his or her genitals and whether he or she plays with them. Parental feelings and attitudes can then be explored and information on how they would react to the situation can be obtained.

B. **When masturbation is viewed as a problem behavior.** The clinician should not simply dismiss parental concerns about the issue by flatly stating that "masturbation is normal." Rather he or she should attempt to understand the level of parental discomfort and the social and psychological consequences of the behavior for the child, with the goals of alleviating parental anxiety and diminishing feelings of fear, anxiety, guilt, and shame in the child.

A detailed history will not only establish the diagnosis but also give the parents a chance to discuss their fears and worries. Examples of parental concerns include fear that their child has an organic disease, has been sexually abused, is experiencing conflict with a family member or teacher/caretaker, will develop promiscuity, or will be mentally handicapped. The masturbatory behavior may evoke a parent's own conflicts about sexuality, and the parent may withdraw attention and/or affection from the child. In the majority of cases, after such concerns and attitudes are explored, reassurance will be sufficient.

Parents should be advised not to overreact to the child's behavior. It should be emphasized that punishing and scolding can be harmful to the child's self-esteem and long-term sexual development.

Parents can tell their preschool child that masturbation is a private behavior that is best not done in public (e.g., "There are some things that we do around other people. This is one of the things that we do in private").

Behavioral modification techniques, such as positive reinforcement, have been helpful in cases of compulsive masturbation (especially in children with mental retardation).

C. Criteria for referral

1. When appropriate counseling by the clinician elicits complaints by the parents that the **child is in psychologic distress.**

2. When **unusual manifestations or excessive masturbation impede self-esteem** and adaptive functioning of the child and/or cause social problems.

3. When **other family or interpersonal pathology** is recognized by the clinician to contribute to the problem.

4. When there are accompanying **developmental/behavioral or affective disturbances** in the child.

Bibliography

For Parents
Sex Education: A Bibliography of Educational Materials for Children, Adolescents, and Their Families. Available from American Academy of Pediatrics, Department of Publications, 141 Northwest Point Blvd., P.O. Box 927, Elk Grove Village, IL 60009.

What Kids Want to Know about Sex and Growing Up. From Children's Television Workshop, One Lincoln Plaza, New York, NY 10023.

For Professionals
Friedrich WN et al. Normative sexual behavior in children. *Pediatrics* 88(3):456–464, 1991.

Haka-Ikse K, Milan M. Sexuality in children. *Pediatr Rev* 14(10):401–407, 1993.

Yates A. Childhood sexuality. In M Lewis (ed), *Child and Adolescent Psychiatry: A Comprehensive Textbook.* Baltimore: Williams & Wilkins, 1992.

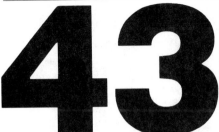

Mental Retardation: Behavioral Problems

Theodore Kastner and
Kevin Walsh

I. Description of the problem

A. Epidemiology
- The incidence of behavioral disorders in children with mental retardation is greater than in nonretarded children because any brain damage or dysfunction appears to increase the likelihood of behavioral or psychiatric disorders.
- 40% of people with mental retardation experience a period of disturbed behavior and function at some time in their lives.
- The epidemiology of behavioral problems among children with mental retardation is unknown because of their cognitive and communicative limitations and because appropriate diagnostic tools are not yet available.
- It is estimated that diagnosable psychiatric disorders exist in 5–10% of children with mental retardation.

B. Etiology.
There are four major causes of severe, challenging behavior in children with mental retardation: adaptive dysfunction, psychiatric disorders, medication side effects, and organic causes. In many cases, the etiology is of multiple origin (e.g., a psychiatric disorder accompanied by family dysfunction).

1. **Adaptive dysfunction** is a mismatch between the needs, abilities, and goals of the child and that of the environment (usually the school and/or family unit). In this model, the potential *communicative* nature of the behavior is often considered. For example, does a behavioral outburst always accompany a request to accomplish difficult tasks? In this case, the behavioral problem may be due to unrealistic environmental expectations. Adaptive dysfunction can often be distinguished from mental illness or an organic cause by a lack of vegetative signs (weight loss or sleep problem) and a consistent relationship between the behavior and antecedent events.

2. **Psychiatric disorders** are more common in children with mental retardation than in the general population. The most common psychiatric disorders associated with mental retardation in children may be the mood disorders, such as depression and bipolar disease (often in atypical forms, e.g., rapid cycling and chronic mania). Mood disorders in children with mental retardation can often be recognized by the presence of a sleep disturbance, change in weight or eating habits, overactivity or motor restlessness (sometimes confused with the hyperactivity of attention deficit hyperactivity disorder) [ADHD], mood lability (crying or laughing), and a behavioral history of cycling. Less commonly, anxiety disorders, psychosis, Tourette syndrome, ADHD, and obsessive-compulsive disorder are seen.

3. **Medication side effects** are a common cause of behavioral morbidity among children with mental retardation. For example, in a study of 209 people with mental retardation who presented with behavioral complaints, undiagnosed medication side effects were noted in 7%. These included akasthisia, tardive dyskinesia, and other side effects typically associated with the use of major tranquilizers.

4. **Organic causes.** Occult medical illnesses have been found in about 20% of behaviorally disordered children with mental retardation. The high prevalence is due to their greater health care needs, communication barriers around symptomatology, and a lack of effective health care services. Perhaps the most common medical cause of disturbed behavior is unrecognized or

Table 43-1. Formulating a diagnostic and treatment plan for children with mental retardation and behavioral problems

1. Rule out the presence of a medical disorder.
2. Evaluate the presence of environmental supports and stressors.
3. Look for a complex of behavioral symptoms.
4. Establish a psychiatric diagnosis using standard or modified criteria.
5. Develop treatment goals.
6. Monitor treatment with a predetermined methodology.
7. Establish a treatment end point.

poorly treated epilepsy, especially partial complex seizures. Interictal irritability, for example, can exacerbate aggressive or self-injurious behaviors. Other undiagnosed medical causes of behavioral problems include thyroid dysfunction, premenstrual syndrome, and cardiac disease.

II. Making the diagnosis

A. Signs and symptoms. Behavioral problems in children with mental retardation include aggression, self-injury, overactivity, and sleep disturbances. In addition, rumination, elopement, property destruction, and other behaviors are occasionally seen.

B. Behavioral questionnaires. Inventories or behavioral scales are available to facilitate the evaluation of behavioral problems in children with mental retardation. These include the Reiss Scale for Maladaptive Behavior, the Reiss Scales for Children's Dual Diagnosis, the Psychopathology Instrument for Mentally Retarded Adults (PIMRA), and the Aberrant Behavior Checklist. It is frequently of benefit to use two or more inventories and to have more than one caregiver complete the instrument.

C. Physical examination. The physical examination should be comprehensive and thorough. If an organic cause of behavioral problems (e.g., hypothyroidism in a child with Down syndrome) is missed by the clinician, it is unlikely that the disorder will be recognized by another child care provider. Laboratory testing should be based on clinical suspicions aroused by the history and physical examination. Even when these produce no clues, however, the clinician should remain ever vigilant to the possibility of an occult medical problem.

D. Diagnostic hypotheses. The clinician should formulate a psychiatric diagnosis or etiologic hypothesis before prescribing a treatment. For example, in a child with epilepsy who is treated with phenobarbital and is noted to be overactive, the presence of vegetative signs should alert the clinician to the possibility of depression or mania. The clinician might then consider changing the anticonvulsant medication to carbamazepine, which can have a mood-stabilizing effect. Steps needed to develop a diagnosis and treatment plan for children with mental retardation and behavioral problems are outlined in Table 43-1.

Strict diagnostic criteria for psychiatric disorders may not be met due to a number of features related to mental retardation, especially cognitive and communicative deficits. Frequently, a clear diagnosis cannot be made, and the clinician may resort to empirical trial-and-error treatments. For example, some children with mental retardation, irritability, sleep problems, aggressive or self-injurious behavior, and behavioral cycling respond to treatment with valproic acid or carbamazepine. The general points in Table 43-2 should be noted when considering the use of psychotropic medication in children with mental retardation.

III. Treatment. The treatment of behavioral problems in children with mental retardation may require changes in the caretaking environment, psychoactive medications, medical interventions, or any combination of the three.

A. The environment. If the social milieu is nonoptimal, the behavior of the child with mental retardation may represent an attempt to control or alter that environment. Behavioral problems may then be reduced or eliminated as the child

Table 43-2. Clinical concerns when using psychopharmacology in children with mental retardation and behavioral problems

The diagnosis should guide treatment.

The more severe the behavior or the degree of mental retardation, the more likely it is that the problem is biologically based and will respond to appropriate medication.

Anticonvulsants (such as carbamazepine and valproic acid), and antihypertensives (such as beta-blockers) are powerful psychotropic agents.

Treat multiple diagnoses with a single medication if possible (e.g., treat epilepsy and depression with carbamazepine; treat attention deficit hyperactivity disorder and anxiety with a tricyclic antidepressant).

The end point in a trial of medication is behavioral remission or intolerable side effects.

Table 43-3. Behavioral symptoms suggesting psychiatric diagnoses and treatment

Behavioral symptoms	Possible diagnoses	Potential psychoactive therapy
Overactivity, decreased sleep, poor attention, self injury, aggression	Bipolar disorder	Carbamazepine, valproate, lithium
Overactivity, poor attention, autism, self injury, aggression	Anxiety disorders	Propranolol, buspirone,
Poor attention, fragile X syndrome	Attention deficit hyperactivity disorder	Methylphenidate, tricyclic antidepressant, clonidine
Stereotypic behavior, self injury, aggression	Obsessive compulsive disorder, depression	Sertraline, fluoxetine
Social withdrawal, abnormal sleep pattern, poor attention, self injury, aggression, rumination	Depression	Carbamazepine, lithium, antidepressants

is taught appropriate replacement behaviors that can serve the same function. This intervention, called *functional analysis,* is best conducted as part of a comprehensive diagnostic process that includes traditional medical and psychiatric evaluations.

B. Psychoactive medications. Given the vast number of psychoactive medications on the market, it is wise to be familiar with one or two drugs in each of the major classes of medications. This is generally sufficient to allow the clinician the flexibility to make appropriate choices between treatments. Specifically, the clinician should be comfortable using anticonvulsants (carbamazepine, valproic acid), antimanic drugs (lithium carbonate), tricyclic antidepressants (desipramine and imipramine), stimulants (methylphenidate and dextroamphetamine), antianxiety drugs (propranolol and buspirone), serotonin reuptake inhibiting antidepressants (sertraline and fluoxetine), and major tranquilizers (thioridazine and haloperidol). The general indications for use of many of these medications are included in Table 43-3.

Many of the medications have multiple effects. Carbamazepine is an effective anticonvulsant with antidepressant, antimanic, and neuralgic effects. It is an excellent first choice in the treatment of aggression and/or self-injury, particularly in the presence of overactivity or a sleep disorder. In addition to depression, tricyclic antidepressants are valuable in the treatment of anxiety disorders and ADHD. The major tranquilizers are often a good first choice of treatment during an acute problem, although every effort should be made to find alternative treatments because of long-term side effects.

C. The family. The level of family stress and the family's ability to use the resources of the extended family or obtain alternative community supports are important predictors of outcome. For example, a recent study of children with epilepsy noted that family function was one of the most important predictors of behavioral problems. The primary care provider should always remember that a strong family is a more effective treatment partner.

D. Follow-up. Interventions for children with mental retardation and behavioral problems should be accompanied by careful follow-up. The behavioral response to the treatment plan should receive careful scrutiny. Children taking psychoactive medication may require periodic screening for drug levels, side effects, and behavioral changes, depending on the medication used. In addition, the diagnosis may need to be reconsidered in the light of the response to treatment. For example, when a trial of stimulant medication causes a worsening of behavior or ever-increasing dosages are required to maintain therapeutic effect, the diagnosis of bipolar disorder should be considered.

Bibliography

For Parents

Batshaw M, Perret Y (eds). *Children with Disabilities: A Medical Primer.* Baltimore: Brookes 1992.

For Professionals

Kastner T. Health care and mental illness in persons with mental retardation. *Habilitative Ment Healthcare Newslett* 9:17–24, 1990.

Matson J, Mulick J. *Handbook of Mental Retardation* (2nd ed). New York: Pergamon, 1991.

O'Neill R et al. *Functional Analysis of Problem Behavior: A Practical Assessment Guide.* Sycamore IL: Sycamore Publishing Co., 1990.

Rubin L, Crocker A (eds). *Developmental Disabilities: Delivery of Medical Care for Children and Adults.* Philadelphia: Lea & Febiger, 1989.

Sovner R. Limiting factors in the use of DSM-111-R criteria with mentally-ill mentally-retarded persons. *Psychopharmacol Bull* 22:1055–1059, 1986.

Newsletters, Reviews

Exceptional Health Care, Developmental Disabilities Publications, 100 Madison Avenue, Morristown NJ 07960-9886.
Monthly reviews of selected mental retardation articles.
Habilitative Mental Health Care Newsletter, P.O. Box 57, Bear Creek NC 27207.
Addresses psychiatric and behavioral aspects of care.

Behavioral Questionnaires

Aberrant Behavior Checklist, Slosson Educational Publications, PO Box 280, East Aurora NY 14052; (800) 828-4800.

Reiss Screen for Maladaptive Behavior, Reiss Scales for Children's Dual Diagnosis, and Psychopathology Instrument for Mentally Retarded Adults, International Diagnostic Systems, PO Box 389, Worthington OH 43085; (800) 876-6360.

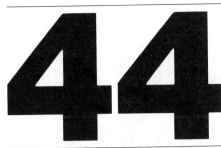

Mental Retardation: The Diagnostic Workup

David L. Coulter

I. **Description of the problem.** The definition of mental retardation underwent a dramatic change in 1992:

> Mental retardation refers to substantial limitations in present functioning. It is characterized by significantly subaverage intellectual functioning, existing concurrently with related limitations in two or more of the following applicable adaptive skill areas: communication, self-care, home living, social skills, community use, self-direction, health and safety, functional academics, leisure and work. Mental retardation manifests before age 18. (Luckasson et al. 1992)

Thus, classification of individuals with mental retardation is no longer based on the IQ score, and categories of mild, moderate, severe, and profound mental retardation (which were based solely on the IQ score) are no longer used. Instead, *classification is based on the types and intensities of supports and services needed by the individual.* These are categorized as:
- Intermittent.
- Limited.
- Extensive.
- Pervasive.

A. **Etiology.** Mental retardation may be the end result of one or more of the following categories of risk:

1. **Biomedical.** These are factors that have had a deleterious impact on the child's CNS (e.g., genetic disorders, environmental toxins, infections).

2. **Social.** Inadequacies in the social and/or family environment (e.g., inadequate stimulation, social unresponsiveness) can diminish cognitive and social growth and functioning.

3. **Behavioral.** The damaging behavior of others (e.g., trauma, maternal substance abuse) can lead to mental retardation.

4. **Educational:** The availability and quality of educational and training programs, under the new classification, can determine whether a child functions in the range of mental retardation.

5. **Multiple factors.** In any given case, many of these risk factors may play a significant role. This concept reflects the transactional approach to human development, in which reciprocal interactions between individuals and their environment influence the developmental outcome. Some risk factors may be more significant (principal or primary cause of mental retardation), and others may be less significant (contributing or secondary cause), but the interaction between them is almost always important. For example, a child with phenylketonuria may be functioning at a much lower level because of both environmental deprivation and poor dietary compliance.

II. **Making the diagnosis**

A. **Signs and symptoms.** Mental retardation should be suspected in any child who is significantly below the normative developmental milestones for his or her age. Additionally, children with *established* risk (e.g., Down syndrome) are very likely to have mental retardation.

B. Evaluation of the etiology

1. An understanding of the etiology of mental retardation begins with a **complete medical and psychosocial history** and a **complete physical and neurologic examination.** This preliminary assessment results in a list of possible causes or differential diagnosis, which should include consideration of any and all potential risk factors.

2. The differential diagnosis should be thought of as a set of **hypotheses about the etiology,** so that the subsequent workup is designed to test the most reasonable hypotheses. Table 44-1 is designed to help the primary care clinician design an appropriate workup based on the most likely hypotheses in a particular case. This table lists a series of possible hypotheses based on whether the potential risk occurred prenatally, perinatally, or postnatally. A set of possible strategies for testing each of these hypotheses is then suggested.

3. **There is no single diagnostic workup that is appropriate to all cases.** In some cases the workup will be very simple (as in chromosomal analysis when Down syndrome is suspected). In most cases, however, the etiology will not be obvious, and a careful workup will be needed. Such an evaluation, however, will result in identification of the principal or primary cause of mental retardation in only about one-third of cases. Because new diagnostic measures for mental retardation are emerging rapidly, the etiologic evaluation of idiopathic mental retardation should be considered an ongoing process that can take advantage of the newest research.

    In ambiguous cases, the following tests are usually advisable:

    a. **High-resolution chromosomal analysis and fragile X studies** should be strongly considered because not all chromosomal abnormalities lead to obvious physical signs.

    b. **Radiologic imaging of the brain** (e.g., MRI or CT scan) often helps to detect inapparent CNS pathology.

    c. **Metabolic screens** for amino acids and organic acids may identify potentially treatable disorders, especially when a degenerative clinical course is suggested.

III. Management

A. Conveying the diagnosis and prognosis

1. **Diagnosis.** Primary care clinicians are often present when the diagnosis is first made. Unfortunately, parents often have unpleasant memories about how the diagnosis was first conveyed to them. To avoid this and to help ensure that the diagnosis is conveyed sensitively, clinicians can follow these guidelines:

    a. **Listen to what the parents say about the child.** This will give the clinician a sense of their level of sophistication, understanding, and emotional acceptance of the child's problems.

    b. **Ask the parents about which particular aspects of their child's problems bother them the most.** This will help to address the issues *most important to them.*

    c. **Review the results of the evaluation in a way that is easily understandable and unambiguous.** Avoid technical jargon and overly complex explanations. Assess parental understanding by asking them to rehearse how they will explain their child's problem to a family member.

    d. Parents will be all too eager to assume the responsibility and guilt for their child's problem. **Consistent and persistent reassurance that the condition was not their fault is always indicated.**

    e. **The clinician should respect the parents' preference for an alternative term to "mental retardation"** (such as "special needs" child). It is, however, important for them to understand that their child meets the diagnostic criteria for mental retardation and such a designation provides eligibility for important supports and services.

Table 44-1. Hypotheses and strategies for determining etiology of mental retardation

Hypothesis	Possible strategies
Prenatal onset	
Chromosomal disorder	Extended physical examination
	Referral to geneticist
	Chromosomal analysis, including fragile X study and high-resolution banding
Syndrome disorder	Extended family history and examination of relatives
	Extended physical examination
	Referral to clinical geneticist or neurologist
Inborn error of metabolism	Screening for amino acids and organic acids
	Quantitation of amino acids in blood, urine, and/or CSF
	Analysis of organic acids by GC-MS or other methods
	Blood levels of lactate, pyruvate, carnitine, and long-chain fatty acids
	Arterial ammonia and gases
	Assays of specific enzymes
	Biopsies of specific tissue for light and electron microscopic study and biochemical analysis
Developmental disorder of brain formation	CT or MRI scan of brain
	Detailed morphologic study of brain tissue (e.g., biopsy)
Environmental influences	Growth charts
	Placental pathology
	Maternal history and physical examination of mother
	Toxicologic screening of mother at prenatal visits and of child at birth
	Referral to clinical geneticist
Perinatal onset	Review maternal records (prenatal care, labor and delivery)
	Review birth and neonatal records
Postnatal onset	
Head injuries	Detailed medical history
	Skull x rays, CT or MRI scan (for evidence of sequelae)
Infections	Detailed medical history
Demyelinating disorders	CT or MRI scan
Degenerative disorders	CT or MRI scan
	Evoked potential studies
	Assays of specific enzymes
	Biopsy of specific tissue for light and electron microscopy and biochemical analysis
Seizure disorders	Electroencephalography
Toxic-metabolic disorders	See "Inborn error of metabolism"
	Toxicologic studies
	Heavy metal assays
Malnutrition	Body measurements
	Detailed nutritional history
	Family history of nutrition
Environmental	Detailed social history
	Psychological evaluation
	Observation in new environment

2. **Prognosis.** The primary care clinician should help the family to prepare for the future. This requires an understanding of the child's prognosis for functioning as an adult. In general, pediatric clinicians tend to *underestimate* the level at which adults with mental retardation can function in the community. The clinician must achieve the delicate balance of not giving overly optimistic predictions of the child's potential capabilities (thereby engendering intense disappointment over time) and not underestimating his or her long-term potential (thereby creating a negative self-fulfilling prophecy).

The clinician should ensure, over time, that the family accepts the prognosis, incorporates it into their family planning (e.g., for guardianship and financial trusts), and has realistic expectations for the child's future.

B. Clinical Issues

1. Primary care issues include **health supervision, immunizations, nutrition and growth, gynecologic care, and sex education.** Some children with mental retardation also have other problems that may require referral to a specialist (e.g., neurologist, psychiatrist, orthopedist, or physiatrist). The primary care clinician should work collaboratively with the family and with any specialists involved in the child's care.

2. The primary care clinician should closely monitor the **academic progress of the child** with mental retardation. A young child (less than age 3 years) should be referred for early intervention services as soon as a developmental problem is identified (often before the diagnosis of mental retardation is actually made). An older child should be referred to the public school system to ensure that a comprehensive evaluation is done and an appropriate educational plan is developed.

3. As the child gets older, the clinician will need to anticipate concerns about the **transition to adult living:** guardianship, living arrangements, work, sexuality, and family planning, among others.

Bibliography

For Parents

Arc (formerly called the Association for Retarded Citizens), (817) 261-6003.
The largest organization for parents of children with mental retardation. Many local Arc's have parent support groups as well as case advocacy and specific supports and services.

Every state has a government agency responsible for providing services to people with mental retardation.

For Professionals

Associations

American Association on Mental Retardation, (800) 424-3688.
Conducts workshops and publishes journals and books on mental retardation.

American Association of University Affiliated Programs for Developmental Disabilities, (301) 588-8252.
Coordinates a network of regional training and service programs.

Publications

Coulter DL. An ecology of prevention for the future. *Ment Retard* 30:363–369, 1992.

Luckasson R, et al. *Mental Retardation Definition, Classification and Systems of Supports.* Washington DC: American Association on Mental Retardation, 1992.

McLaren J, Bryson SE. Review of recent epidemiological studies of mental retardation: Prevalence, associated disorders and etiology. *Am J Ment Retard* 92:243–254, 1987.

Rubin IL, Crocker AC. *Developmental Disabilities: Delivery of Medical Care for Children and Adults.* Philadelphia: Lea and Febiger, 1989.

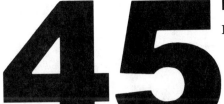

Motor Delays

Peter A. Blasco

I. Description of the problem. Motor development is the highest-ranking concern of most parents when their children are between ages 6–12 months. Parental concerns about neuromotor development are most often about delayed motor milestone achievement. Related complaints include vague references to tone abnormalities ("too stiff" or "too weak"), perceived structural abnormalities (most commonly the legs), or an awkward/clumsy gait in the ambulating child.

A. Epidemiology
- The prevalence of significant motor delays in the general pediatric population is not known. By statistical definition, 2–3% of infants will fall outside the range of normal motor milestone attainment. A minority of these milestone-delayed children (15–20%) will prove to have a significant neuromotor diagnosis, most commonly cerebral palsy or a birth defect, rarely some progressive nervous system or muscle disease.
- Early motor delays in the remainder of children often represent a marker for subtle neurologic dysfunction, which manifests itself more definitively in later childhood as troublesome awkwardness, attention deficit hyperactivity disorder, and/or specific learning disabilities.

II. Making the diagnosis

A. Evaluation. To make a meaningful statement about an infant's motor competence, the clinician should organize data gathered from the history, physical examination, and neurodevelopmental examination into three domains: motor developmental milestones, the classic neurologic examination, and markers of cerebral neuromotor maturation (primitive reflexes and postural reactions).

1. **Motor milestones** are extracted from the developmental history, as well as from observations during the neurodevelopmental examination (Tables 45-1 and 45-2). Milestone assessment is best summarized as a single (or narrow) motor age for the child. The motor age can be converted to a motor quotient (MQ) giving a simple expression of deviation from the norm:

$$MQ = \frac{\text{motor age}}{\text{chronologic age}} \times 100.$$

A motor quotient above 70 is considered within normal limits. Those falling in the 50–70 range are suspicious and deserve further evaluation (though most of these children will turn out to be normal). An MQ below 50 is abnormal.

2. **Neurologic examination.** Motor milestones do not take into account the *quality* of a child's movement. The motor portion of the **neurologic examination** includes assessments of tone (passive resistance), strength (active resistance), deep tendon reflexes, and coordination plus observations of station and gait. The best clues often come from observation, not handling.

a. **Tone.** Spontaneous postures (e.g., frog legs seen with hypotonia or scissoring with spasticity) provide visual clues to tone abnormalities.

b. **Strength.** Spontaneous or prompted motor activities (e.g., weight bearing in sitting or standing) require adequate strength. A classic example is the Gower's sign (arising from floor sitting to standing using the hands to "walk up" one's legs), which indicates pelvic girdle and quadriceps muscular weakness.

Table 45-1. Gross motor development timetable

Prone	
Head up	1 mo
Chest up	2 mo
Up on elbows	3 mo
Up on hands	4 mo
Rolling	
Front to back	3–5 mo
Back to front	3–5 mo
Sitting	
Sit with support ("tripod" sitting)	5 mo
Sit without support	7 mo
Get up to sit (unassisted)	8 mo
Walking	
Pull to stand	8–9 mo
Cruise	9–10 mo
Walk with 2 hands held	10 mo
Walk with 1 hand held	11 mo
Walk alone	12 mo
Run (stiff-legged)	15 mo
Walk up stairs (with rail)	21 mo
Jump in place	24 mo
Pedal tricycle	30 mo
Walk down stairs, alternating feet	3 yr

   c. Station refers to the posture assumed in sitting or standing and should be viewed from anterior, lateral, and posterior perspectives looking for body alignment.

   d. Gait refers to walking and is examined in progress. Initially, the toddler walks on a wide base, slightly crouched, with the arms abducted and elevated a bit. Forward progression is more staccato than smooth. Movements gradually become more fluid, the base narrows, and arm swing evolves, leading to an adult pattern of walking by age 3 years.

3. **Primitive reflexes** are movement patterns that develop during the last trimester of gestation and generally disappear between the third and sixth month after birth. Each requires a specific sensory stimulus to generate the stereotyped motor response.

   The Moro, tonic labyrinthine, asymmetric tonic neck, and positive support reactions are the most clinically useful (Figs. 45-1, 45-2, and 45-3). Normal babies and infants demonstrate these postures inconsistently and transiently, whereas those with neurologic dysfunction show stronger and more sustained primitive reflex posturing. Though primitive reflexes are somewhat tricky to gauge, even in expert hands, the clinician should keep attuned to four factors.

   a. Some form of primitive reflex response should be clearly elicitable in the newborn through ages 2–3 months.

   b. Symmetry of response is important, especially with the Moro.

   c. An obligatory primitive reflex is abnormal at any time. This is the situation where the child remains "stuck" in the primitive reflex posture as long as the stimulus is imposed and breaks free only when the stimulus is removed.

   d. Visible primitive reflexes **should no longer be present after ages 6–8** months.

4. **Postural reactions** consist of countermovements, which are much less stereotyped than the primitive reflexes and involve a complex interplay of cerebral and cerebellar cortical adjustments to a barrage of proprioceptive, visual, and vestibular sensory inputs. They are not present at birth but sequentially develop between ages 3–10 months. Postural reactions are

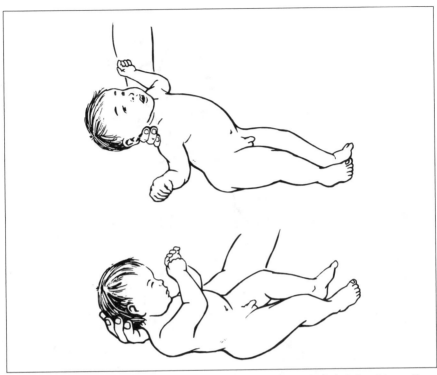

Figure 45-1. Tonic labyrinthine reflex. In the supine position, the baby's head is gently extended to about 45 degrees below horizontal. This produces relative shoulder retraction and leg extension, resulting in the "surrender posture." With head flexion to about +45 degrees, the arms come forward (shoulder protraction) and the legs flex. (Reprinted with permission from Blasco PA. *Pediatr Rounds* 1(2):1–6, 1992.)

Table 45-2. Fine motor development timetable

Retain ring (rattle)	1 mo
Hands unfisted	3 mo
Reach	3–4 mo
Hands to midline	3–4 mo
Transfer	5 mo
Take 1-in. cube	5–6 mo
Take pellet (crude grasp)	6–7 mo
Immature pincer	7–8 mo
Mature pincer	10 mo
Release	12 mo

sought in each of the three major categories: righting, protection, and equilibrium (Fig. 45-4). Though easy to elicit in the normal infant, they are markedly slower in their appearance in the baby with nervous system damage.

B. Classification of motor impairments

    1. Static central nervous system disorders indicate some type of nonprogressive brain damage. The insult may have arisen during early fetal development, resulting in a CNS anomaly. Alternatively, a brain developing in a normal fashion can be damaged before, during, or after birth by a wide variety of infectious, traumatic, and other insults. When a motor impairment

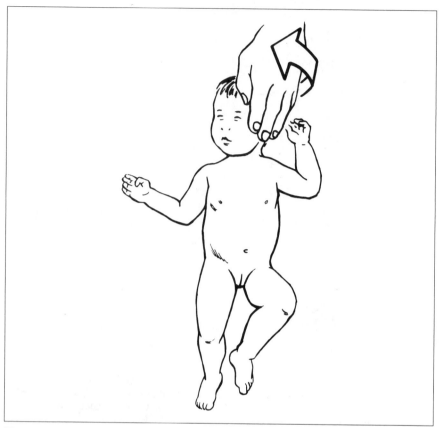

Figure 45-2. Asymmetric tonic neck reflex (ATNR). The sensory limb of the ATNR involves proprioceptors in the cervical vertebrae. With active or passive head rotation, the baby extends the arm and leg on the face side and flexes the extremities on the occiput side (the "fencer posture"). There is also some mild paraspinous muscle contraction on the occiput side producing subtle trunk curvature. (Reprinted with permission from Blasco PA. *Pediatr Rounds* 1(2):1–6, 1992.)

is due to a brain anomaly or to a static lesion that occurs before cerebral maturation is complete (roughly age 16 years), the disorder is referred to as cerebral palsy. This group represents the largest number of children with disabling motor problems (see Chapter 20).

2. **Progressive diseases** of the brain, the peripheral nerves, or the muscles produce motor impairment that worsens with time (e.g., Duchenne muscular dystrophy, Werdnig-Hoffman spinal muscular atrophy, nervous system tumors). Children with progressive conditions initially experience a period of normal or near-normal development. Evidence of a progressive disease is determined by careful history and/or by repeated examinations over time. The fraction of all motor-impaired children with progressive diseases is small. Uncovering the specific diagnosis helps one anticipate the rate of progression, provides other prognostic information, and forms the basis for accurate genetic counseling.

3. **Spinal cord and peripheral nerve disorders** are all static conditions except for the rare instances of an intrinsic spinal cord tumor or a progressive extrinsic compression syndrome. The largest single group in this category consists of children with myelodysplasia.

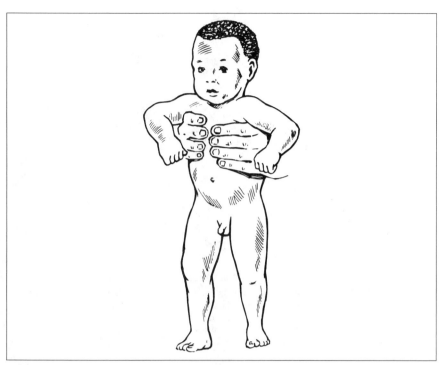

Figure 45-3. Positive support reflex. With support around the trunk, the infant is suspended and then lowered to pat the feet gently on a flat surface. This stimulus produces reflex extension at the hips, knees, and ankles so the subject stands up, completely or partially bearing weight. Children may go up on their toes initially but should come down onto flat feet within 20–30 secs before sagging back down toward a sitting position. (Reprinted with permission from Blasco PA. *Pediatr Rounds* 1(2):1–6, 1992.)

    4. Structural defects refer to conditions in which an anatomical structure is missing or deformed (e.g., a limb deficiency) or in which the support tissues for nerves and muscles are inadequate (e.g., connective tissue defects, abnormal bones). On the mildest end of the spectrum, there exist a wide variety of fairly common orthopedic deformities, which may or may not affect early motor milestones (club feet, developmental hip dysplasia, etc.). More severe disorders in this category include osteogenesis imperfecta and some varieties of childhood arthritis.

III. Management. Direct treatment for the child with a motor disability falls into five categories: (1) counseling and support for the child and family, (2) hands-on therapy, (3) assistive devices, (4) medication, and (5) surgery. A subspecialty team should be consulted to provide state-of-the-art evaluation, treatment services, and counseling in all needed disciplines. Professionals skilled in many different disciplines need to work together and *in concert with the parents*. The primary clinician's roles include seeing to the patient's general health, monitoring overall development, helping the child and family cope with many stresses (especially at anniversary and transition times), promoting the child's self-esteem and long-term adaptation to disability, and helping parents keep the multitude of subspecialty inputs in perspective.

Bibliography

For Parents
Swanson MJ, Harris SR. *Teaching the Young Child with Motor Delays.* Austin TX: Pro-Ed, 1986.

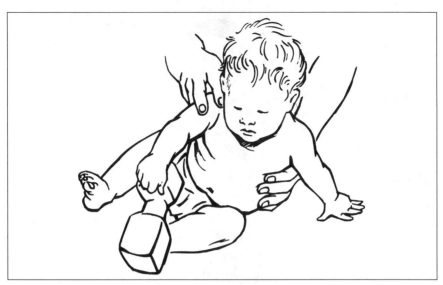

Figure 45-4. Postural reactions. The infant is comfortably seated, supported about the waist if necessary. The examiner gently tilts the child to one side noting righting of the head back toward the midline, protective extension of the arm toward the side, and equilibrium countermovements of the arm and leg on the opposite side. (Reprinted with permission from Blasco PA. *Pediatr Rounds* 1(2):1–6, 1992.)

For Professionals

Baird HW, Gordon EC. *Neurological Evaluation of Infants and Children.* London: Heinemann Medical Books, 1983.

Blasco PA. Normal and abnormal motor development. *Pediatr Rounds* 1(2):1–6, 1992.

Capute AJ et al. Normal gross motor development: The influence of race, sex, and socioeconomic status. *Dev Med Child Neurol* 27:635–643, 1985.

Shapiro BK. The pediatric neurodevelopmental assessment of infants and young children. In AJ Capute, PJ Accardo (eds), *Developmental Disabilities in Infancy and Childhood.* Baltimore: Brookes, 1991.

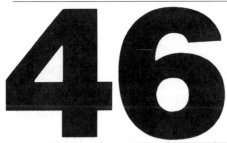

Night Terrors and Nightmares

Barry Zuckerman

I. Description of the problem

A. Night terrors. Children with night terrors bolt upright from their sleep and cry inconsolably for 5–20 minutes (in rare cases, even longer). Night terrors are associated with autonomic signs including a rapid pulse, increased respiratory rate, and sweating. The child has a glassy-eyed stare, which is due to the fact that the child is in rapid-eye-movement (REM) sleep and not actually awake. Following resolution, children easily return to sleep and have amnesia for the event in the morning.

   1. Pathophysiology. Night terrors are a *disorder of arousal*, occurring during an abrupt (rather than the usual slow) transition from stage 4 non-REM sleep to REM sleep.

   2. Epidemiology
   • Occurs in approximately 3% of children.

B. Nightmares. Nightmares are upsetting dreams that occur during REM sleep. Nightmares and night terrors are compared in Table 46-1. Nightmares are a universal occurrence in childhood and usually not due to a significant definable environmental problem.

II. Management

A. Night terrors. Because of the inconsolable crying and glassy-eyed stare, parents are usually terrified that something is wrong with their child. After the child returns to sleep, the parents may remain awake with their own terrors.

   1. The primary goal in management is to **reassure the parents** of the benign nature of these episodes. Management involves demystifying night terrors by explaining the physiologic basis of the behavior. Using an analogy like a myoclonic jerk during light sleep can help parents understand the physical nature of the night terrors. Most important, parents need to be assured that night terrors are not due to psychopathology or horrible life events. When parents know that there is nothing wrong with their child, they can usually tolerate periodic episodes.

   2. When the episodes are frequent and/or disrupt the sleep of others (especially siblings), **the child can be awakened prior to the time the episode usually occurs.** This is thought to alter the sleep cycling and prevent a night terror from occurring.

   3. Diazepam which should be used only rarely, will stop the attacks by suppressing REM sleep and provide the beleaguered family with temporary relief.

B. Nightmares. While night terrors are more frightening for parents to witness, nightmares are more distressing for the child. Although children may know that the nightmare is a dream, they remain frightened nevertheless.

   1. Parents need to **accept the child's fear** and not dismiss it as "just a bad dream."

   2. Parents should **comfort and stay with the child** until the child's distress has abated.

   3. Parents should **empathize with the child's fright** and tell him or her that

Table 46-1. Comparisons of nightmares and night terrors

	Night terrors	Nightmares
Stage of sleep	NREM	REM
Consolability	Poor	Good
Amnesia for event	Yes	No
Interest in returning to sleep	High	Low

while they cannot personally banish scary dreams, they will always come whenever the child is afraid.

4. **While dreams have magical properties, so do parents.** They should assure the child that nothing will harm him or her.

5. **Transitional objects** (e.g., a teddy bear, a favorite blanket) should be at the ready; a nightlight may be comforting. Ask the child what (besides a parent) is comforting after a nightmare.

6. In selected instances **parents may have to remain with the child** or even take the child to their own bed.

7. Parents should **discuss the nightmares and explain what nightmares are with the child** in the comforting light of day.

Bibliography

Schmitt BD. Dealing with night terrors and sleepwalking. *Contemp Pediatr* 6:119–120, 1989.

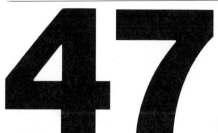

The Noncompliant Adolescent

Vaughn Rickert and
Susan Jay

I. **Description of the problem.** Compliance refers to the extent to which patients follow instructions related to taking medications, changing life-style behaviors, following diets, and maintaining preventive health practices.

A. **Epidemiology**
- Among selected subpopulations of adolescents, the rates of noncompliance are quite variable, in some cases as high as 80%.
- Compliance with preventive health measures is markedly lower than is compliance with treatment for acute illnesses.
- Generally, as with adults, full adherence to medical regimens has been estimated to be about 50%.

B. **Issues in noncompliance**

1. **Psychosocial development.** Encouraging compliance among adolescents requires the primary care provider to be aware of the cognitive changes and related developmental factors of adolescence. These include identity formation, self-esteem, and autonomy issues. For example, younger teenagers often resent being "lectured." They prefer to be treated with a shortened verbal message, supplemented with written instructions, because it is perceived to be more adultlike.

2. **Confidentiality.** Compliance is enhanced when the teenager's perception of the confidentiality of each visit is honored. Frequently adolescents present to the clinician with a hidden agenda. The patient may relate one concern to the parent or nurse, but it may be another issue entirely with which he or she wishes assistance. Unless the patient's real agenda is addressed, compliance will suffer. Equally important is for clinicians to know how to offer help without a direct request.

3. **Side effects of treatment.** Chronically ill adolescents may stop taking or outwardly refuse to take medication because of undesirable side effects. For example, the adolescent with Crohn's disease who is on high dosages of steroids is likely to become noncompliant if he or she is concerned with the weight gain and facial puffiness.

4. **Nature and duration of disease.** The type and length of the disease process can affect compliance. Generally, the length of the treatment regimen and the necessity of life-style changes are inversely related to compliance.

5. **Cost of care.** Health insurance (or lack thereof) for the medical visit and subsequent prescriptions remains a major obstacle in obtaining and using needed services.

6. **Family variables.** On occasion, compliance with a treatment protocol can become a battleground between teenager and parent. This scenario is often seen in the chronically ill adolescent who asserts autonomy and independence by not taking a particular medication. When these conflicts occur, the clinician is often expected to force the patient to comply with both the medical protocol and parental rules.

7. **Medical environment.** The time that the adolescents spend waiting to be seen by the provider affects their willingness to comply. Clinicians should not be surprised when their message and prescription are not enthusiastically received after the patient sat in the waiting room for 45 minutes.

Table 47-1. Patterns of noncompliance

Ambulatory attendance
  Delaying or failing to seek care
  Failing to keep scheduled appointments
  Terminating treatment prematurely
Behavioral aspects
  Not taking recommended preventive measures
  Incompletely following through with a prescribed regimen
  Sabotaging treatment regimens or not participating in prescribed health
    programs
  Improvising, creating, or substituting ready-made treatment regimen
Medication alterations
  Failing to fill the prescription
  Taking only a portion of a prescribed regimen or none at all despite filling the
    prescription
  Taking a medication that has not been prescribed (e.g., taking a friend's)
  Altering the prescription (e.g., changing dosage or frequency of medication)

Source: Jay MS, DuRant RH. Compliance. In ER McAnarney, RE Kriepe, DP Orr, GD Comerci (eds), *Textbook of Adolescent Medicine*. Philadelphia: Saunders, 1992, 207, with permission.

II. Making the diagnosis

A. Patterns of noncompliance are reported in Table 47-1. Accurate prediction of noncompliance during adolescence is difficult, if not impossible. The most direct approach, and usually the easiest, is to simply ask the teenager directly about his or her compliance behavior.

B. Patients often overestimate their compliance in order to "look good" to the clinician. However, adolescents who do admit "forgetting" to take their medicine are also the most likely to respond to treatment interventions.

C. Although noncompliance should be suspected when symptoms persist despite an effective regimen, clinicians must remember that **disease severity, life-style behaviors, and stress may also affect recovery.** Clinicians should not view adolescents as either wholly noncompliant or totally compliant. Rather, compliance and noncompliance are on a continuum which is affected by multiple factors.

D. Adolescents who are noncompliant with parental requests are similarly noncompliant around medical treatment.

III. Management

A. Avoid scare tactics and nagging. Education is the first step in promoting compliance. However, many clinicians use scare tactics when providing office-based education to adolescents, especially concerning substance abuse and motor vehicle injuries. These tactics may paradoxically challenge the adolescent to experiment with these substances or to engage in high-risk behaviors. Some health-related videotapes also rely on fear-arousal techniques instead of more effective strategies, such as minimizing peer influence. "Nagging," or using the same educational message at each visit, must be avoided because it leads to a decline in motivation and interest. It behooves the clinician to vary interventions across time and modify the features of these to the receptivity of the adolescent.

B. Relate an accessible message. Educational messages and information are often enhanced when visual aids are employed. It is also important to focus on the immediate concrete benefits of treatment (e.g., improved odor after quitting smoking). The primary provider should include the adolescent in the decision process whenever possible, for example, by providing the option to take a pill 4 times per day versus taking a different one 2 times per day.

C. Social inoculation. Social inoculation is a strategy in which the clinician provides verbal messages that the youth subsequently can use in specific situations to avoid peer pressures (Table 47-2). The use of social inoculation may deter the use of alcohol, smoking, and related health-compromising substances. In the confines of the examination room, behavioral rehearsal or practice sessions di-

Table 47-2. Management strategies to improve compliance by adolescents

Strategy	Use
Education	Regardless of specific health message, avoid scare tactics and use written/verbal instructions and/or videos.
	Simplify both verbal and written instructions of drug regimen.
	Computer-assisted instruction can be a useful vehicle for promoting healthy behaviors.
Environment	Waiting room decor needs to be sensitive to adolescents (e.g., no Sesame Street).
	Age-appropriate written materials that promote health and are attractively packaged contribute to a willingness to read this material.
	Interactive videodiscs on health-related topics are effective.
Provider behavior	Like adults, adolescents do not like to be kept waiting.
	Use a nonjudgmental approach.
	Be sensitive to developmental, psychosocial, and related cultural issues.
	Address confidentiality issue at first visit. If possible, allow teenager to make own subsequent appointment(s).
	Determine the best method by which to provide teenager with laboratory results or other patient follow-up information (e.g., telephone, mail, or teenager to call the provider).
	When calling, ask to speak to the adolescent patient by name.
	Link compliance with medication to a particular time during the day or to a specific behavior that the teenager already engages in.
	Provide options or choices whenever possible for treatment.
	Always delineate side effects, especially those that can be seen by others.
Self-monitoring	Determine a simple method for the adolescent to document symptom frequency or specific health-related behaviors (e.g., a golf wrist counter for the number of times the teenager experiences dizziness).
Behavioral rehearsal	Provide specific words to the teenager that can be used with peers. Teach verbal messages accompanied by assertive body language (e.g., hands on hips). This strategy is especially useful for younger teenagers who find it hard to express their opinions. For example, some messages that the physician can teach to promote nonuse of smokeless tobacco include, "It will stain my teeth," "My breath smells awful," "Did you know that it causes mouth cancer?" For alcohol use: "I can't have a drink because I am the designated driver," "I have to get up real early tomorrow."
Behavioral contracting	Draw up a written plan outlining the behavior(s) of concern and the goals that both patient and provider sign (e.g., a prom contract for no drinking and driving).
	Encourage the teenager to make a statement of intent such as, "I will not drink and drive, Doc," followed by a handshake.
Psychotherapy	Prescribe early in the treatment regimen when clinically significant noncompliance has been documented or a concomitant mental health disorder exists.
	For chronically ill adolescents, support groups may be helpful.

rected by the provider can be a way for the teenager to build "antibodies" to resist verbal challenges made by friends or peers that may compromise his or her health.

D. Behavioral modification. If noncompliance is suspected as the cause of a poor clinical response, have the adolescent keep a diary or record of his or her compliance behavior. Research suggests that behavior often changes in the desired direction when it is being monitored. Self-monitoring records are most effective when combined with a positive feedback system for compliance. Clinicians, however, must recognize that some cheating is likely among chronically ill adolescents. Education should include instructions on how to minimize the impact of occasional noncompliance on health.

E. Behavioral contract. A behavioral contract between patient and health care provider is another effective strategy to improve compliance. The contract is a written agreement between the primary care clinician and patient that stipulates behaviors that each party needs to complete in order to achieve a common goal. The consequences for failing to comply and rewards for meeting desired goals are articulated in this agreement. Verbal statements of intent to comply with treatment that are accompanied with a handshake or signature also may improve compliance.

F. Self-management of chronic illnesses. A self-management strategy is best suited for the compliant adolescent with chronic illnesses. These programs rely on a combination of self-monitoring, self-reinforcement, and problem-solving skills. For example, a young adolescent with Crohn's disease would be instructed to monitor daily caloric intake and provide himself or herself with rewards (e.g., extra time to play video games) for meeting desired goals. These types of programs are complicated and frequently require additional professionals because of the time necessary to teach elements of behavioral change, problem-solving skills, and coping mechanisms. Self-management programs should be time limited and require monitoring by a health provider.

IV. Clinical pearls and pitfalls
- Assume noncompliance is a product of poor education rather than a purposeful act.
- Make inquiries as to the positive exceptions (when the teenager remembers to take medication or minimizes alcohol intake).
- Ask the teenager how parents or other important adults can help.
- Explore prior strategies that have been unsuccessful.
- Provide opportunities for the teenager to be a part of the treatment decision.

Bibliography

For Parents

American Academy of Pediatrics. *Caring for Your Adolescent.* New York: Bantam Books, 1991.

Kolodny RC, Kolodny NJ, Bratter TE, Deep CA. *How to Survive Your Adolescent's Adolescence.* Boston: Little, Brown, 1984.

Powell DH. *Teenagers: When to Worry and What to Do.* Garden City, NY: Doubleday, 1986.

For Professionals

Cromer BA, Tarnowski KJ. Noncompliance in adolescents: A review. *J Dev Behav Pediatr* 10;207–215, 1989.

Friedman IM, Litt IF. Adolescents' compliance to therapeutic regimens. *J Adolesc Health Care* 8:955–973, 1987.

Jay MS, DuRant RH. Compliance. In ER McAnarney, RE Kriepe, DP Orr, GD Comerci (eds), *Textbook of Adolescent Medicine.* Philadelphia: Saunders, 1992.

Krasnegor NA, Epstein L, Johnson SB, Yaffe SJ (eds). *Developmental Aspects of Health Compliance Behavior.* Hillsdale NJ: Erlbaum, 1993.

Rickert VI, Jay MS. Adolescent wellness: Facilitating compliance in social morbidities. *Med Clin North Am* 74:1135–1148, 1990.

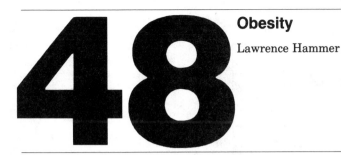

Obesity

Lawrence Hammer

I. **Description of the problem.** Commonly accepted definitions of obesity in childhood include weight in excess of 20% above "ideal" for age and sex and skinfold thickness in excess of the 85th percentile for age and sex. The clinical assessment of obesity must include consideration of the impact of the child's weight on his or her general well-being, relationships with peers, and family function.

A. **Epidemiology**
- 29% of boys and 25% of girls in the 6–11 age range and 18% of boys and 25% of girls in the 12–17 age range are obese.
- In childhood, obesity is more common among upper socioeconomic groups. This trend remains true in adult life, except among upper-income Caucasian women, who tend to be thinner than lower-income women.

B. **Familial transmission/genetics.** Obesity clearly "runs in" families, but familial transmission may involve both genetic and environmental influences. Adoption and twin studies point to a strong genetic component. Roughly 80% of children in families with two obese parents will become obese, while only 40% of children in families with one obese parent are likely to become obese.

C. **Etiology/contributing factors**

1. **Environmental.** Numerous studies have reported minimal differences in food intake and physical activity between obese and nonobese children. However, small differences in daily food intake or physical activity, when extended over long periods of time, may account for the excessive weight gain of some children. In clinical practice, the diet history of obese children almost always reveals either regular or periodic intake of excessive calories and high-fat foods. The intake may be excessive in portion size or due to high-caloric food selection.

2. **Organic.** Obese children do not have lower basal metabolic rates than their nonobese peers. However, studies of metabolic rate and energy expenditure following exercise or meals do reveal a lower rate in obese versus nonobese adults.

    A number of medical conditions may contribute to obesity, especially those causing restrictions in physical activity. Finally, there are children with abnormalities of appetite or satiety, due to CNS lesions, who may be predisposed to the development of obesity.

3. **Developmental.** There is a developmental pattern to the deposition of body fat through childhood and adolescence. During the first year of life, children tend to accumulate "baby fat," followed by a relative reduction in body fatness over the next several years as the child gains proportionally greater height than weight. Most children again begin to accumulate body fat at ages 5–6 years. This rebound in adiposity continues at a steady rate until puberty, after which there is a slower trend toward increasing fat deposition. Investigators have noted that children whose rebound in adiposity occurs earlier than age 5½ years tend to have a higher likelihood of obesity during adolescence.

II. **Making the diagnosis**

A. **Signs and symptoms.** The easiest clinical approach to making the diagnosis of childhood obesity is direct observation and examination. The child who appears

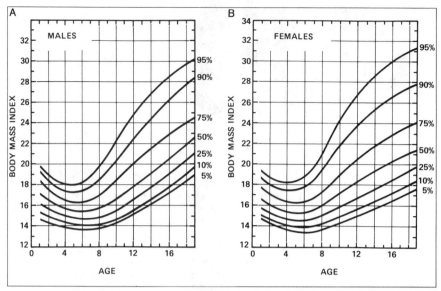

Figure 48-1. Body mass index curves for males (*A*) and females (*B*) through age 19 years. Derived from the First National Health and Nutrition Examination Survey, 1971–1974. (Reprinted with permission from Hammer LD, et al. Standardized percentile curves of body mass index for children and adolescents. *Am J Dis Children* 145:259–263, 1991. Copyright 1991, American Medical Association.)

to be obese probably is obese. In order to confirm the diagnosis, an assessment of the child's fatness must be performed. Weight alone is not a sufficient criterion for obesity in childhood, as weight varies with age and height. Weight greater than 20% above the "ideal" for height and age can be used as a criterion for diagnosis.

An alternative approach to the use of height and weight information in the diagnosis of obesity is to use a combination of the two as an index. The body mass index (BMI),

Weight (kg) ÷ height (ms)^2

can be plotted on a percentile curve (Fig. 48-1). A criterion of 90th percentile is useful for identifying overweight children. Serial measurements of BMI are useful in monitoring a child over time.

One of the problems with using weight and height as diagnostic criteria for obesity is their inability to distinguish between two children who have the same weight and height but differ in fatness or muscle mass. A skinfold thickness measurement may add additional valuable information to the diagnostic assessment of the child, although measurement of subcutaneous fat is not directly proportional to total body fat.

B. Differential diagnosis. Only about 5% of obese children have an underlying endocrinopathy or genetic syndrome. The endocrinopathies that are associated with child obesity include hypothyroidism, Cushing's syndrome, pseudohypoparathyroidism, and growth hormone deficiency. Syndromes associated with child obesity include Prader-Willi, Alström, Carpenter, Cohen, and Laurence-Moon-Bardet-Biedl.

Children with endocrinologic disorders or clinical syndromes manifest clinical histories and physical findings that distinguish them from children with idiopathic obesity. One key difference in such children is the presence of shorter-than-expected stature for the child's age and weight. In fact, a careful history and physical examination can successfully rule out these underlying disorders in the vast majority of children. Laboratory examination is rarely necessary except to confirm a clinically suspected diagnosis.

C. History: Key clinical questions

1. *What was the child's weight at birth and at subsequent points during childhood?* The clinician should plot the child's weights on a growth chart from birth to the present time. It is important to identify the child who has had an unusual pattern of weight gain, a sudden increase in weight, or a pattern that suggests an increase in the risk of long-term obesity, such as an early adiposity rebound.

2. *Are there any factors that may have influenced your child's weight gain at particular periods in his or her life?* The parents should contribute their thoughts regarding the child's excessive weight gain.

3. *Does your child's pattern of weight gain appear similar to that of others in the immediate or extended family?* The parents should describe other members of the family with weight problems and describe their own patterns of weight gain.

4. *What is it about your child's weight that concerns you?* This question provides an opportunity for parents to describe their concerns and motivation for seeking evaluation or treatment.

5. *How does your child's weight influence him or her directly or indirectly?* Does the child's weight seem to get in the way of physical activity, participation in school activities, performance in sports, interaction with peers, and other elements of social development and maturation?

6. *How does your child's weight influence the family?* Parents and child should discuss ways in which concern for the child's weight may influence family activities, such as vacations, outings, or physical activity, and describe the impact of the child's weight on their relationships with each other. For example, many parents shield their children from the impact of obesity by avoiding situations in which the child's obesity is more public. Parents may describe their conflicts over the importance of the child's weight problem, its severity, and their differing approaches to it.

7. *What might happen if your child's obesity becomes a life-long problem?* This question encourages parents to express their deepest fears about the impact of the child's obesity on his or her life and to discuss ways in which their own experiences with weight may have influenced their decision to seek help with this problem. Many parents seek to protect their children from the misery they themselves have experienced in relation to their weight.

8. *I would like to learn a little bit about your child's regular eating habits. Please try to recall each of the meals and snacks that your child has eaten over the last 24 hours and give me as much detail as possible about them. Please let me know if you would call this a typical eating day for your child or if there are any differences that I should be aware of. Are there any times when your child appears to "lose control," leading to a binge or overeating?* These questions introduce the notion that dietary intake is relevant and fulfills the parents' expectation that modification of dietary intake may be part of the approach to the problem. It is helpful to point out that although the child may not appear to have excessive dietary intake, there may still be an opportunity for dietary modification as part of the overall approach to the problem.

9. *Do you consider your child to be physically active on a regular basis? Please describe some of the vigorous physical activities that your child participates in. How often and for what period of time does your child participate in these activities? Is your child part of an organized sports program? Do you and your child ever exercise together? Please describe your own physical activity.* This question opens up discussion of the child's physical activity and gives the clinician insight into the parents' perception of their own physical activity and level of exercise. Opportunities for ways to increase regular physical activity may be discovered during the discussion.

10. *Does your child have any difficulties with sleep?* Children with severe obesity may have secondary sleep problems, such as daytime somnolence and

obstructive sleep apnea. These children should be evaluated by a sleep disorder specialist for central hypoventilation and obstructive sleep apnea.

D. **Behavioral observations.** During the process of evaluating the obese child and his or her family, it is useful to observe the interaction of family members and observe their expression of concern, criticism, or support of the child in dealing with this problem. It is also important to note parents' responses to the child's requests for food during the visit. Although overeating may not be the primary factor contributing to the child's obesity, interactions with food are often salient to the evaluation and treatment process.

E. **Physical examination.** A careful general physical examination is useful in the evaluation of the obese child. Such an examination yields identification of physical findings that may suggest an underlying endocrine syndrome or genetic disorder. The physical examination should include an overall assessment of the child's body habitus and notation of the pattern of fat distribution. Careful measurement of the height and weight of the child is important to rule out underlying short stature, which may indicate an associated endocrine or genetic abnormality. The presence of a buffalo hump, moon facies, short stature, and hypertension may suggest Cushing's syndrome (although many normal obese children have extra fat deposition over the upper back). Hypogonadism is present in a number of syndromes (Prader-Willi, Laurence-Moon-Bardet-Biedl, and Carpenter's). Short stature, short metacarpals and metatarsals, subcutaneous calcifications, and retardation are present in pseudohypoparathyroidism.

F. **Tests.** Laboratory tests should be used to confirm suspected underlying diagnoses rather than as routine screening. Obese children who are tall, of normal intelligence, and without stigmata of underlying syndromes do not require routine thyroid screening, for example.

III. **Management**

A. **Primary goals.** It is reasonable to establish a target weight for the child. This does not imply that the child must lose weight. Rather, taking into account appropriate rates of growth, the child's weight should fall into a healthy range for height and age, defined as 20% above or below the ideal weight for height and age, or at a BMI level below the 75th percentile. The process of establishing a goal weight or BMI goal for the child should be revised periodically, depending on the child's age and the family's ability to participate in the treatment program.

For many children, particularly those who are prepubertal, weight loss may be a less desirable goal than maintenance of weight at a particular level or reduction in the rate of weight gain. For children who are more than 40% overweight, such a goal may be difficult to achieve without periods of weight loss alternating with periods of weight maintenance. For children who are beyond puberty, it may be more appropriate to establish goals for weight loss. A reasonable rate of weight loss for children under age 12 years is ½–1 lb/week. Adolescents may safely lose 1–2 lb/week while still maintaining adequate nutritional status.

In addition to weight loss, it is important to emphasize associated goals of improved fitness, self-esteem, social interaction, and family harmony.

B. **Information for the family.** The family's involvement is critical to the evaluation and management of childhood obesity. A focus on the impact of the child's obesity on the family and on the child can lead to effective intervention. For example, rather than using the dietary history as a means of proving the presence of excessive dietary intake, the provider should use the dietary history as a means of identifying opportunities for dietary change. In discussing the child's regular physical activity, it should be possible to identify opportunities for increasing this activity. The clinician can approach intervention as a process of gradually modifying the child's eating behavior and physical activity over time, in the context of the whole family. It is critical that the family engage in this process in an active way and agree to initiate and maintain change in the whole family's food and exercise habits. Attempts to modify the child's diet in isolation rarely succeed and lead to an environment of blame.

Table 48-1. Behavioral strategies for weight loss

Establish goals for behavior change	Establish goals for small changes in the diet and physical activity on a weekly basis to increase the likelihood of success.
Self-monitor diet and physical activity	Self-monitoring provides the child with a heightened awareness of his or her efforts and successes.
Record review and parental reinforcement	One-on-one review of the record with the child provides an opportunity for parents to provide positive feedback for demonstrable change.
Establish a behavioral contract and use a simple reward system	By setting realistic goals each week, the parent and child can contract for a limited reward system.
	Expensive rewards, or those that can be achieved only after a significant period of time, are less effective than rewards that can be delivered immediately or soon after the demonstrated behavior change.
	A dual-level reward system may be useful in providing initial reinforcement for short-term change and greater levels of reinforcement for long-term success. This reward system can later be extended to the maintenance period so that reinforcement is delivered periodically for maintenance of behavior change. Simply rewarding weight loss alone should be discouraged.
Praise	Parents can use praise very effectively to reinforce and maintain desired behavior change.
	Criticism and punishment are ineffective and counterproductive.
Environmental control	Identify and eliminate factors within the environment that tend to promote overeating. For example, remove high fat, high-calorie foods from the household, increase the availability of cut-up vegetables rather than chips or pretzels for snack time, avoid television viewing during mealtimes, reduce the amount of time indoors during daylight hours, and increase the expectation for daily physical activity.
Cognitive restructuring	Identify and reject thoughts that may be demeaning, degrading, or pessimistic. Emphasis should be placed on successes, not failures.

Source: Reprinted with permission from Hammer LD, et al. Standardized percentile curves of body mass index for children and adolescents. *Am J Dis Children* 145:259–263, 1991. Copyright 1991, American Medical Association.

C. Treatment

1. **Initial strategies.** Intervention for child obesity begins during the evaluation process. Involving the family in the evaluation gives the message that they are part of the solution. In the course of evaluation, if the family appears to be dysfunctional, it is appropriate to delay the implementation of behavioral strategies until the family has had more extensive evaluation and entered into family counseling. Referral to a family therapist, particularly one familiar with many of the issues associated with obesity, can be extremely helpful.

For families who are capable of supporting the child's efforts, the initial strategies are focused on gradual alterations of the child's eating and physical activity. There are a number of behavioral strategies that are useful in the office-based approach to child obesity (Table 48-1).

Intervention does not require calorie counting or specific calorie intake. An alternative approach is to categorize foods as more or less desirable and to set goals for the reduction of less desirable foods and encouragement of more desirable foods. One such system of categorization is described in *The Stoplight Diet for Children,* which categorizes food as "red light," "yellow light," and "green light." By identifying foods in this way, parents can support the child's efforts to reduce intake of "red light" foods and increase intake of foods from the other categories. Gradual reduction in intake of "red light" foods can be rewarded and sustained in association with goals of weight loss or maintenance.

2. **Follow-up.** The primary care provider should provide regular follow-up for the child who is involved in either an office-based or a group treatment program. This follow-up can include periodic monitoring of the child's weight and height, review of the child's self-monitoring records for diet and physical activity, and encouragement to persevere.

D. **Criteria for referral.** Most obese children and their parents who are interested in participating in a treatment program can benefit from the peer support available through a group treatment program. The primary care clinician should investigate the options that are available in the community and provide that information to the family. The family that is too dysfunctional to participate in an office-based or group-based program should be referred for family evaluation and therapy. The family may benefit from such additional professional involvement as it struggles to help the child overcome the effects of obesity.

IV. **Clinical pearls and pitfalls**
- Obesity is a problem that develops over time and is not easily treated. Unless the patient is experiencing life-threatening complications due to severe morbid obesity, the problem should be approached in a nonemergent fashion.
- Obesity rarely occurs in isolation. There are commonly other family members who have struggled with weight and whose experience can be valuable in helping to develop a realistic set of goals for the child and family.
- The tendency for families to feel defeated by obesity comes from their unrealistic expectation of dramatic and continued change. In order to avoid the trap of setting unrealistic goals and expectations, the family should be encouraged to identify situations in which their attempts at change have been successful. Once these small victories are identified, they can be used to help identify other opportunities for change and to create an environment of positive expectation.
- Obesity is not the child's problem alone. The child lives within the family environment, and the family must be drawn into the process of evaluation and change.

Bibliography

For Parents
Epstein LH, Squires S. *The Stoplight Diet for Children: An Eight-Week Program for Parents and Children.* Boston: Little, Brown, 1988.

Mellin L. *Shapedown: Weight Management Program for Adolescents.* San Francisco: Balboa Publishing, 1983.

For Professionals
Burton BT et al. Health implications of obesity: An NIH consensus development conference. *Int J Obesity* 9:155–169, 1985.

Dietz WH. Childhood obesity: Susceptibility, cause, and management. *J Pediatr* 103:676, 1983.

Epstein LH, Wing RR, Valoski A. Childhood obesity. *Pediatr Clin North Am* 32:363, 1985.

Rosenbaum, M, Leibel RL. Pathophysiology of childhood obesity. *Adv Pediatr* 35:73–138, 1988.

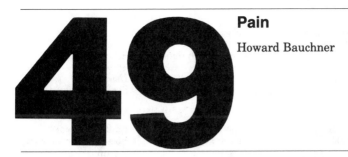

Pain

Howard Bauchner

I. **Description of the problem.** The International Association for the Study of Pain defines pain as "an unpleasant sensory and emotional experience associated with actual or potential tissue damage, or described in terms of such damage." Historically, neonates, infants, and children have not received adequate therapy for pain because health care providers assumed that neurologic immaturity rendered them incapable of fully experiencing painful stimuli. Recent research has demonstrated that even neonates have measurable biochemical and behavioral responses to painful stimuli. The goal of moving toward a "pain-free pediatrics" has become one of the most exciting new pediatric initiatives.

II. **Making the diagnosis.** There are a number of observational scales for the assessment of pain in children. These scales, however, are used principally for research purposes and are less helpful in the day-to-day management of children in pain. For most children, pain can be assessed by careful observation or by simply asking the child how much pain he or she is feeling. It is often helpful to phrase the question in such a way that a scale is implied: "On a scale of one (the least pain) to ten (the most), how much pain are you feeling?"

For neonates, infants, and preverbal children, pain must be assessed indirectly. For neonates, marked changes in facial expression, high-pitched crying, thrashing, the inability to be consoled, and changes in vital signs may indicate pain. Similar responses to pain may be seen in infants and toddlers, along with loud crying, the withdrawal of an exposed limb, the use of an arm or leg to resist, and a lack of cooperation.

III. **Management**

A. **Primary goals.** The primary goals are to reduce the pain and anxiety a child is experiencing and to help the child and parents develop coping strategies to deal with future painful experiences.

B. **Initial treatment strategies.** Both behavioral-cognitive and pharmacologic approaches are essential to the management of pain. Depending on the age of the child and the nature of the painful stimulus, one approach may be more important than the other. Most often, both are useful. For example, a child with a fracture should have the comforting presence of a parent while an intravenous catheter is placed for the administration of analgesics.

1. **Behavioral and cognitive approaches**

a. **Parental presence.** The presence of a comforting and soothing parent is usually invaluable. Many parents, however, are frightened of procedures. They need to be taught to talk, touch, and stay in sight of their child during the procedure in order to provide maximal comfort. Their presence allows the child to concentrate on the parents and listen to their instructions. For young children, parents can tell their children that they do not know if a particular procedure will hurt but that they can help by using "magic" (e.g., reading a book, blowing some bubbles, or helping the child pretend he or she is elsewhere). For older children, empathy with the pain and support in remaining cooperative during the procedure may suffice.

b. **Age-appropriate pain-reduction techniques.** Behavioral and cognitive techniques to reduce pain need to be appropriate to the child's age and developmental stage (Table 49-1). In general, sensory stimulation, dis-

Table 49-1. Age-specific approaches for pain reduction

Age	Pain reduction techniques	Specific strategies
Neonates and infants	Auditory, visual, tactile, proprioceptive stimulation	Use pacifier Stroke and swaddle, rock, or sing to child Visual distraction
Toddlers and preschoolers	Parental presence, distraction, alternate sensory stimulation	Educate parent Rock, rub, or blow on site of pain Focus visual attention (e.g., on jewelry) Read favorite book
School age	Parental presence, distraction, relaxation, hypnosis	Ask child what works best Incorporate child into story Have child blow pain away Use music or ice/heat
Adolescents	Relaxation, distraction, self-hypnosis	Ask what works best and individualize approach

Table 49-2. Commonly used drugs for office pain management in children

Drug	Pediatric dosage	Comments
Acetaminophen	PO, 10–15 mg/kg q4 h	Often underdosed
Aspirin	PO, 10–15 mg/kg q4 h	Do not use with febrile illness
Ibuprofen	PO, 4–10 mg/kg q6–8 h	
Naprosyn	PO, 5–7 mg/kg q12 h	
Opioids		
Codeine	PO, 1–2 mg/kg q3–4 h, max. 60 mg	
Methadone	PO, 0.1–0.2 mg/kg q4–12 h	Excellent, long-acting, oral analgesia
Morphine	PO, 0.3–0.6 mg/kg q12 h	Time released
Oxycodone	PO, 0.08–1.0 mg/kg q4–6 h	Tablets 4.5 mg, available with acetaminophen as Percocet-5 (5 mg oxycodone, 325 mg acetaminophen)
Sedatives		
Chloral hydrate	PO, 50–100 mg/kg single dose, max. 2 g	Useful in neurologically intact children for sedation
Diazepam	PO, 0.2–0.5 mg/kg single dose	Tablets 2, 5, 10 mg
Local Anesthetics		
Eutectic mixture of local anesthetics lidocaine and prilocaine	Topical, 2.5 g/application	Apply at least 1 h prior to procedure (IV, venipuncture)

traction, and the presence of a comforting parent are important for young children. School-aged children and adolescents can be taught helpful techniques, such as imagery, thought stopping (e.g., a school-aged child can say, "This won't hurt; I won't feel it") and self-hypnosis (see Chapter 13).

For most clinicians, the most common cause of pain in their patients is related to medical procedures. It is important for clinicians to have a number of strategies available to help children and adolescents cope with these procedures, including blowing bubbles, strategically placed mobiles, age-appropriate books, and a cassette player with an assortment of tapes.

    c. Engaging the child. Prior to employing any technique to reduce a child's pain, it is important to try to engage the child in a supportive relationship. Seeing the clinician as a powerful benign force is, in itself, a pain- and anxiety-relieving experience.

    It is important to ask older children what would be helpful with the pain. They may, for example, suggest listening to rock music, "just saying it won't hurt," "thinking of girls," and "knowing I can miss school." With a communicative child, the clinician should always ask, and not assume he or she knows, which technique would be best.

2. Pharmacologic approaches. The pharmacologic armamentaria available for pain management has increased significantly in the past decade. Table 49-2 lists commonly used, currently acceptable oral drugs for the outpatient treatment of pain in neonates, infants, children, and adolescents.

Bibliography

Acute Pain Management in Infants, Children, and Adolescents: Operative and Medical Procedures. Washington DC: US Department of Health and Human Services, Agency for Health Care Policy and Research, 1992.
Order by calling (800) 358-9295.

Bauchner H. Procedures, pain, and parents. *Pediatrics* 87:563–565, 1991.

McGrath PA. *Pain in Children—Nature, Assessment and Treatment.* New York: Guilford Press, 1990.

Schechter N, Berde C, Yaster M. *Pain in Infants, Children, and Adolescents.* Baltimore: Williams & Wilkins, 1993.

50

Physical Abuse

Eli Newberger

I. **Description of the problem.** Child abuse refers to physical and sexual assaults on children, child neglect, emotional abuse, and the deprivation of necessary physical and moral supports for a child's development.

A. **Epidemiology**
- Some form of child physical abuse occurs in as many as 10% of American families.

B. **Etiology/contributing factors.** A model for understanding child abuse must consider sociocultural factors and stresses in the family that may have originated in the child, the social situation, or the parent. These forces conspire to produce a triggering situation that culminates in the child's maltreatment (Fig. 50-1).

II. **Making the diagnosis**

A. **Signs and symptoms.** Abuse should be considered when a child presents with an unusual injury or symptom pattern, when illogical or changing explanations are offered by a parent to account for an injury, or when there is concomitant abuse of a child's mother.

A myriad of injuries have been reported in child abuse: fatal aspirations, intentional microwave oven burns, hypernatremic dehydration, toxic ingestions, pancreatic injuries, and "tin ear" syndrome (unilateral ear bruising, ipsilateral cerebral edema, and hemorrhagic retinopathy). A rare but noteworthy abuse syndrome is Munchausen's syndrome by proxy in which symptoms are created in children by their parents. In nearly all reported cases, the mother (who typically has a background in the medical field) misuses medications, withholds needed drugs, or exposes the child to toxic substances in an effort to provoke medical diagnostic explorations and medical treatments. Some cases have culminated in fatalities; others appear to be less egregious variants of parental neediness in which the child's symptoms offer a ticket into the health care system and all of its attendant attention and sympathy.

B. **Differential diagnosis.** The history and physical examination guides the approach to laboratory studies and excludes the many competing diagnostic possibilities that may masquerade as child abuse. Table 50-1 summarizes the principal diagnostic entities, clinical findings, and laboratory, radiographic, and specialized studies.

C. **History: Interviewing guidelines.** The clinician's interview creates an opportunity to gather the data that will guide the physical examination and inform the choice of subsequent laboratory study. It also serves the equally important function of establishing a therapeutic relationship with the parent and child that can enable the family to be open to services and interventions. Since many of these families do not have regular contact with people who can provide them with help in times of distress, the clinician's interview may be one of the first experiences a parent has had in which someone inquires thoughtfully and sympathetically about the child and their life situation.

1. **Interviewing the parents.** Each parent should be interviewed separately when possible to convey a sense of respect for the person as an individual and enable each parent to discuss sensitive issues (e.g., drug abuse or whether the mother is being victimized). The goal of the interview is to gather specific data and to assemble a historical sequence of important events that may be associated with a child's risk of victimization. It is *not* to establish who did

Sociocultural Factors

Values and norms concerning violence and force; acceptability of corporal punishment
Inegalitarian, hierarchical social structure; imbalanced interpersonal relationships
Value concerning competition versus cooperation
Exploitative, alienating economic system; acceptance and encouragement of permanent
  poor class
Devaluation of children and other dependents
Institutional manifestations of the above factors in areas such as law, health care, education,
  welfare system, sports, and entertainment

↓

FAMILY STRESSES

↓ Child-Produced Stresses	↓ Social-Situational Stresses	↓ Parent-Produced Stresses
Physical difference (e.g., handicapped)	Structural factors: poverty, unemployment, mobility, isolation, poor housing	Low self-esteem
Mental difference (e.g., retarded)		Abused as child
		Depression
Temperamental difference (e.g., difficult)		Substance abuse
	Parental relationship: patterns of discord-assault, domination-submission	Character disorder
Behavioral difference (e.g., hyperactive)		Ignorance of childrearing; unrealistic expectations
Foster child	Parent-child relationship: attachment problems, perinatal stress, punitive childrearing style, scapegoating, role reversal, excess or unwanted children	

↓

Triggering Situation

Discipline
Argument; family conflict
Substance abuse
Acute environmental
  problem

↓

Maltreatment

Injury
Inability to provide care
Poisoning
Psychological maltreatment

Figure 50-1. Model for understanding child abuse. (Adapted with permission from Bittner S, Newberger EH. Pediatric understanding of child abuse and neglect. *Pediatr Rev* 2:197–208, 1981.)

what, to whom, and with what. Such a detailed level of disclosure should not be sought in a medical interview, lest it be confused with a criminal investigation and inhibit the potential of providing therapeutic care in the future.

a. The interview can start with a short discussion of the reason the child and parents are in the office. This is best done with sympathetic, open-ended questions (e.g., *What is your understanding of why you are here today?*). The initial questions should be nonthreatening ones with easy answers (e.g., *How much did James weigh when he was born?*). Such neutral questions about the early perinatal course naturally flow into more significant questions, such as *How was the pregnancy?* This question often prompts the mother to reflect on her relationship with the

Table 50-1. The differential diagnosis of child abuse

Clinical findings	Differential diagnosis	Differential tests
Cutaneous lesions		
Bruising	Trauma	
	Hemophilia	Prothrombin time, partial thromboplastin time
	Von Willebrand's disease	Bleeding time
	Anaphylactoid purpura	Rule out sepsis
	Purpura fulminans	Rule out sepsis
	Ehlers-Danlos syndrome	Hyperextensibility
Local erythema of bullae	Burn	
	Staphylococcal impetigo	Culture, Gram's stain
	Bacterial cellulitis	Culture, Gram's stain
	Pyoderma gangrenosum	Culture, Gram's stain
	Photosensitivity and phototoxicity reactions	History of sensitizing agent, oral or topical
	Frostbite	Clinical history and characteristics
	Herpes, zoster or simplex	Scraping
	Epidermolysis bullosa	Skin biopsy
	Contact dermatitis, allergic or irritant	Clinical characteristics
Ocular findings		
Retinal hemorrhage	Shaking or other trauma	
	Bleeding disorder	Coagulation studies
	Neoplasm	
	Resuscitation	History
Conjunctival hemorrhage	Trauma	
	Bacterial or viral conjunctivitis	Culture, Gram's stain
	Severe coughing	History
Orbital swelling	Trauma	
	Orbital or periorbital cellulitis	Complete blood count, culture, sinus radiographs
	Metastatic disease	Radiograph, CT scan; CNS examination
	Epidural hematoma	Radiograph, CT scan; CNS examination
Hematuria	Trauma	Culture
	Urinary tract infection	Renal function tests, biopsy
	Acute or chronic forms of glomerular injury (e.g., glomerulonephritis)	
	Hereditary or familial renal disorders (e.g., familial benign recurrent hematuria)	History
	Other (e.g., vasculitis, thrombosis, neoplasm, anomalies, stones, bacteremia, exercise)	History, cultures, intravenous pyelogram
Acute abdomen	Trauma	Rule out other disease
	Intrinsic gastrointestinal disease (e.g., peritonitis, obstruction, inflammatory bowel disease, Meckel's diverticulum)	Radiographs, stool tests, and others

Table 50-1. (continued)

Clinical findings	Differential diagnosis	Differential tests
	Intrinsic urinary tract disease (infection, stone)	Culture, intravenous pyelogram
	Genital problem (e.g., torsion of spermatic cord, ovarian cyst)	History, physical examination, radiograph
	Vascular accident, as in sickle cell crisis	Angiography, sickle preparation
	Other (e.g., mesenteric adenitis, strangulated hernia, anaphylactoid purpura, pulmonary disease, pancreatitis, lead poisoning, diabetes)	As appropriate
Osseous lesions Fractures (multiple or in various stages of healing)	Trauma	
	Osteogenesis imperfecta	Radiograph and blue sclerae
	Rickets	Nutritional history
	Birth trauma	Birth history
	Hypophosphatasia	Decreased alkaline phosphatase
	Leukemia	Complete blood count, bone marrow
	Neuroblastoma	Bone marrow, biopsy
	Status after osteomyelitis or septic arthritis	History
	Neurogenic sensory deficit	Physical examination
Metaphyseal lesions	Trauma	Radiograph and nutritional history
	Scurvy	History
	Menkes syndrome	Decreased copper, decreased ceruloplasmin
	Syphilis	Serology
	"Little League" elbow	History
	Birth trauma	History
Subperiosteal ossification	Trauma	
	Osteogenic malignancy	Radiograph and biopsy
	Syphilis	Serology tests
	Infantile cortical hyperostosis	No metaphyseal irregularity
	Osteoid osteoma	Response to aspirin
	Scurvy	Nutritional history
Sudden infant death syndrome	Unexplained	Autopsy
	Trauma	Autopsy
	Asphyxia (aspiration, nasal obstruction, laryngospasm, sleep apnea)	"Near-miss" history
	Infection (botulism?)	Cultures, bacterial and viral
	Immunodeficiency?	Immunoglobulins
	Cardiac arrhythmia?	Autopsy
	Hypoadrenalism?	Electrolytes
	Metabolic abnormality (calcium? magnesium?)	$CA++$, $Mg++$

Source: Reproduced with permission from Bittner S, Newberger EH. Pediatric understanding of child abuse and neglect. *Pediatr Rev* 2:197–208, 1981.

child's father, points of distress and discomfort in personal relationships, and her hopes and expectations for the baby. Asking *What was this time like for you?* or *Was this a happy time for you?* in a sympathetic, caring way, and listening thoughtfully and attentively to the responses often elicit the precursors and harbingers of the troubles to come.

b. A general pediatric history should follow, including information about the perinatal, early infancy, and toddler periods. During the interview, it is of value to affirm the parent's emotional reactions with comments like, *That must have been difficult for you* or *I can see it makes you sad to talk about that.* This prelude affords a chance to lay the groundwork for the more sensitive discussions to come that address the possible victimization of the child.

c. Mothers should be asked about their relationships with their partners, because 50% of partners who have abused the child have also abused the other parent. Additional questions about the child's behavior and temperament can be revealing. Persistently negative characterizations about the child and conflicts between adults about how best to care for the child should be of concern. Finally, sensitive questions about the parent's own childhood (e.g., *How were you punished as a child? Where you ever injured by an adult?*) can uncover an intergenerational perpetuation of abuse.

d. The approach to the possibility of abuse or neglect should be framed with sympathetic, open-ended questions such as, *What happened then?* and *What did she say to you?* Leading questions (e.g., *Tell me how you hit him with the belt.*) and telegraphing of a specific anticipated response (e.g., *His father didn't abuse you, did he?*) should be avoided. An interviewer alert to the parent's emotional responses who indicates a capacity to listen and to support their expression will have a better chance of hearing specifics with regard to what actually happened to the child.

e. Often it is at the end of the interview, sometimes in response to, *Do you have any questions for me?* that the most important information emerges. Therefore, the clinician should always leave time for questions and listen for the information contained in a parent's queries. He or she should let parents know at this time that he or she will be available to them no matter what happens and that not everything has to be decided at the initial interview.

2. **Interviewing the child.** A child old enough to report her or his experience should be interviewed privately. The child should be asked who gives child care, whether anyone has been hurting him or her, and how he or she feels about being at the doctor's for this visit. It is important to be sensitive to the child's own sense of vulnerability or shame, to be gentle and caring in approach, and to respect the child's confidences.

The provider should always talk with a child at his or her eye level and use age-appropriate language and toys. Nonloaded hypothetical questions should be asked (e.g., *Sometimes kids are really sad about what goes on in their homes. Is something making you sad?*) but never leading questions (e.g., *You're being abused, aren't you?*). The provider should always affirm children's statements of feeling (e.g., *It sounds like you're pretty angry about that*) and try not to challenge their desire to protect their parents.

D. **Physical examination.** The physical examination of a suspected victim of child physical abuse should be conducted in an unhurried way, with efforts made to make the child feel at ease. Prior to the examination, the child should be protected from hearing conversations (including medical history) in which the origins of injuries and conflicting stories are discussed. Particularly if there has been a seeming incongruity between the offered explanation for the child's injuries and the anticipated findings, the child may feel awkward and want to avoid frustrating or enraging his or her parents.

The room should be well lighted. Natural light is especially helpful in discerning nuances of skin color and texture and to ensure that one is not perceiving artifacts of shadow or lighting. The examination is conducted in the usual way, generally beginning with the head, eyes, ears, nose, and throat. One should *not* simply focus on areas of obvious injury.

Palpation of the head to identify subcutaneous hematomas and examination of the skin behind each ear are frequently useful maneuvers to identify abusive injuries. The neck should be examined with care as well. Especially in infants, the frenulum and oropharynx are vulnerable to bottles and spoons being jammed into the mouth; older children may suffer direct dental impact from blunt trauma to the face.

Facial injuries should be noted and simple drawings made of the distribution, shape, and color of each observed lesion. Retinal examinations should be conducted with care. Because the clinician using the indirect ophthalmoscope may not obtain a full impression of the eye grounds, ophthalmologic consultation may be sought to identify retinal hemorrhages.

As one proceeds to examine the chest, abdomen, and genitals, it is important to disrobe each portion of the body fully. Injuries of particular concern are often found on the upper, middle, and lower back and across the buttocks. These should be documented in writing and by drawing, taking care to identify all nuances of color of bruises and distinct shapes of any identified lesions. The absence of abdominal bruises should not be taken to signify an absence of underlying organ injury because the skin of the abdomen is so distensible that substantial traumatic force can be sustained without the development of bruising. Palpation must be done with care and an abdominal ultrasound examination and surgical consultation considered if history and presenting symptoms suggest intraabdominal injury.

E. Tests. Radiological tests, such as a skeletal series, are indicated when there are clear diagnostic clues, from history or physical examination, that suggest a likelihood of osseous trauma.

III. Management

A. Primary goals. The goal for the clinician in addressing possible child abuse is to give needed treatment, to ensure the child is protected, and to provide a bridge to services designed to prevent whatever may have happened from happening again.

B. Initial treatment strategies. The primary care clinician's main responsibility in child abuse management is diagnostic. In some cases, however, the clinician may play a continued intervention role, which should be tailored to the available resources.

There are a number of vital interventions following child abuse.

1. **Social casework** is the core service offered in child protection agencies. Social workers assess the needs of the child and family with a focus on the protection of the child. They may offer and coordinate counseling and other services designed to improve parental functioning and parent-child relationships.

2. **Psychotherapy** is often provided to individuals, couples, and families. It should be considered for children in all cases of abuse. This recommendation is made with a view to addressing the important child developmental and psychiatric burdens associated with the victimization experience.

3. **Health services** include continuing pediatric care and sometimes backup of public health nursing. Victims of child abuse appear to suffer more acute and chronic illnesses, yet their medical needs are often neglected (by both parents and social welfare agencies).

4. **Family-focused interventions** include homemaker services, parent aide programs, advocacy and social support. These are key ingredients of family preservation services, which are offered to prevent the breakup of the family. Other interventions of value are child care services and alcohol and substance abuse treatment for the families who need them.

5. **Substitute care,** which includes foster home and institutional care, may be given on a voluntary or court-mandated basis. It should be considered as a service, although too often it is proposed as a punishment.

6. **Battered women's services** are often essential in providing protection to children and parents.

7. **The criminal justice system** can be of value in protecting children, especially in the face of criminally deviant behavior by caregivers whose actions cry out for stringent social controls.

Bibliography

For Parents
Parents Anonymous (check local telephone directory).
A voluntary self-help movement with chapters and hot lines throughout the United States. It offers opportunities for parents who can benefit from talking through their problems with others.

For Professionals

Kleinman PK. *Diagnostic Imaging of Child Abuse*. Baltimore: Williams and Wilkins, 1987.

Ludwig S, Kornberg AE (eds). *Child Abuse: A Medical Reference*. New York: Churchill Livingstone, 1992.

Newberger EH (ed). *Child Abuse*. Boston: Little, Brown, 1982.

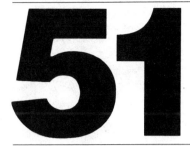

Prematurity: Follow-Up

James A. Blackman and
Robert J. Boyle

I. Description of the problem. Infants born before the thirty-seventh week of gestation are at risk for chronic medical, neurodevelopmental, and behavioral problems. The shorter the gestation and greater the number of associated medical and psychosocial complications, the higher the risk and need for close primary care surveillance.

A. Epidemiology
- Approximately 9% of all births are premature, with 2% having gestational age less than 32 weeks.
- While the incidence of prematurity has not declined over the past decade, mortality and morbidity risk for this group has declined dramatically (Table 51-1).

B. Risk factors for developmental and behavioral problems. Risk factors mandating especially close developmental surveillance include:
- Very low birth weight (< 1500 g)
- Intrauterine growth retardation
- Neonatal seizures
- Persistent head ultrasound/CT abnormalities, including ventricular dilatation or asymmetry, periventricular leukomalacia, or porencephalic cysts
- Chronic lung disease
- Persistent feeding problems (e.g., need to gavage feed beyond 34 weeks postconceptual age)

Biological risk alone does not determine outcome. Rather, it is the interaction of those risks with social and environmental factors that best predicts long-term functioning. Figure 51-1 is a clear illustration of this interaction. In the first 2 years, biological factors are strong predictors of developmental function, especially in the motor domain. However, after age 2 years, socioenvironmental factors assume a far more prominent role in determining cognitive outcome and school success. The primary care clinician is not able to change the preexisting organic insults but can alter and improve a child's developmental and behavioral functioning by supporting the social environment.

II. Evaluation

A. Common health problems of the premature infant. Since chronic medical problems and developmental and behavioral difficulties are inextricably linked, meticulous management of these problems will enhance the likelihood of good outcomes.

    1. Neurologic. Maintain good seizure control through judicious use of anticonvulsant medications.

    2. Ophthalmologic. Ensure that vision has been tested by an ophthalmologist.

    3. Audiologic. Be certain that hearing has been tested.

    4. Respiratory. Pulmonary symptoms can impede developmental progress. In concert with specialists in chronic lung disease, optimize pulmonary function.

B. Growth and feeding. High-risk infants often come home from the hospital with continuing feeding problems: tube dependency, inadequate caloric intake, or volume intolerance due to cardiopulmonary disease. Good nutrition provides the

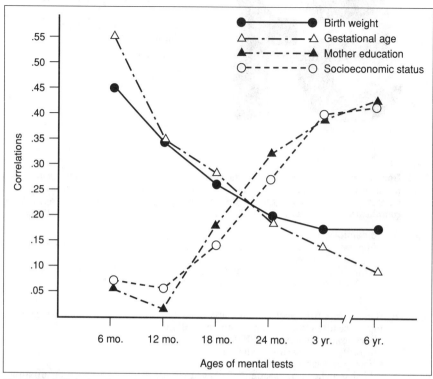

Figure 51-1. Relationship of biological and demographic variables with mental development. Prematurity exerts a potent but short-lived influence on mental development; heritage and home environment have a more lasting effect beyond age 2 years. (Reprinted with permission from Wilson RS. Risk and resilience in early mental development. *Dev Psychol* 21:792, 1985. Copyright 1985 by the American Psychological Association.)

necessary substrate for optimal developmental gain. Key questions to ask include the following:
• Is weight gain appropriate?
• What is the caloric density of the formula?
• What is the daily caloric intake?
• How long does it take to feed the child?
• Does the child have difficulty sucking or swallowing?
• Are the feeding techniques appropriate, given the child's development and capabilities?

Growth patterns should be interpreted from a longitudinal perspective using standard growth charts. For premature infants, measurements can be plotted on special growth charts for premature infants, or, after age adjustment (chronological age in weeks minus number of weeks premature), they can be plotted on a regular growth chart. Beyond ages 18–24 months, continued age adjustment is unnecessary.

1. Growth trends

   a. Dropping growth percentiles or moving further below the fifth percentile. This may be secondary to medical, nutritional, environmental, or neurologic factors. Further investigation is warranted.

   b. Catch-up growth or forward movement across percentiles. Catch-up growth may begin slowly and continue over the first 2 years of life.

Table 51-1. Risk by birth weight

Birth weight	Mortality	Major morbidity of survivors[a]	Minor morbidity of survivors[b]
< 800 g	50–60%	20–30%	20–30%
800–1000 g	30–40%	15–20%	15–20%
1000–1500 g	5–10%	10–15%	10–15%

[a] Includes developmental quotient below 70, cerebral palsy, epilepsy, and blindness
[b] Includes learning disabilities, borderline cognitive function, attention deficits, and poor school achievement (5–10% in the general population) among children without major morbidity.

    c. Growth parallel to fifth percentile. The child may continue to be small or catch up in future years. This pattern is often seen following extreme low birth weight and/or intrauterine growth retardation.

    d. Rapid head growth. Catch-up head growth is a good sign. However, when head circumference crosses percentiles more rapidly than length or weight, head ultrasound evaluation for hydrocephalus should be considered.

    e. Head growth lagging behind other parameters. This is an ominous sign, often associated with mental retardation.

C. Behavior and development

  1. History: Key clinical questions

    a. *Are you concerned that your baby is too passive or overly irritable?* Premature babies may be especially passive or irritable due to CNS injury or the prolonged hospital experience. Infants with CNS injury manifest the same problems as all other infants (e.g., colic, night wakening, temper tantrums), but they tend to be more intense or prolonged.

    b. *Do you see your child as especially fragile or vulnerable?* It is sometimes difficult for parents to modify their perception of the child from "fragile" to "healthy." Although it may take months (or years) for the child to achieve medical stability, it may take parents even longer to accept this reality. Common pediatric illnesses may be overinterpreted as evidence of continuing vulnerability. (See Chapter 89.)

    c. *Does your child seem either stiff or floppy?* Although hypertonia is readily associated with cerebral palsy, the first sign in infants may be persistent hypotonia. Frequently low tone evolves into high tone or spasticity over the first year of life.

    d. *Does your child have any unusual movement patterns?* Dragging the legs along in crawling, body rolling (instead of crawling), or seat scooting may be manifestations of neuromotor abnormalities.

  2. Assessment. Although developmental surveillance is recommended for all children, careful and regular assessment is even more important for premature children. (See Chapter 7.)
    There is much debate about whether and how much to "correct" for prematurity in interpreting developmental performance. As with growth, premature infants tend to catch-up to their like-aged peers over the first years of life. Furthermore, the older the child gets, the less relevance 2–3 months correction has. A practical compromise is to use a half-correction approach: subtract one-half the weeks premature from the child's chronological age and use this result as the expected level of developmental attainment. Some developmental screening tests recommend full correction until age 2–3 years. If the child is not achieving age-appropriate skills, an in-depth assessment by a developmental specialist or early intervention program is warranted.

D. Psychosocial issues

1. **Family dynamics and stress.** Shortened gestation interrupts the normal psychological preparation for life with a newborn. The long, uncertain intensive care experience can drain the family's physical and emotional stamina. Parents take home a normal but fragile, slow-starting, or clearly abnormal infant. The clinician should schedule an early "decompression visit" for the parents to discuss the neonatal intensive care unit experience and to give vent to their frustrations and fears. Counseling or family support groups may be helpful.

2. **Day care issues.** Due to the increased morbidity from respiratory infection in premature infants with a history of chronic lung disease, day care settings with extensive exposure to other children with respiratory illnesses should be avoided. Families may need assistance and guidance with appropriate day care arrangements.

III. Management. Each infant should have an identified medical home where primary care and regular developmental screening occur; the clinician must be aware of the infant's and family's needs and assist the family in obtaining and coordinating other necessary services. Follow-up should be seen as a multidisciplinary team function, with the primary care clinician, other medical specialists, early intervention services, and other therapies (occupational or physical) participating as needed.

IV. Clinical pearls and pitfalls
- Beware of overwhelming the family with services or appointments. Simplification and coordination of services as well as family involvement in the process will decrease family stress and ensure better overall compliance and satisfaction.
- Do not assume that the child will outgrow the problem. Appropriate evaluation and correction for the degree of prematurity should allow the clinician to make an informed judgment about the infant's status.

Bibliography

For Parents

Organizations

Parent Care, 101½ South Union Street, Alexandria VA 22314-3323.

Parents of Premature and High Risk Infants International, c/o CASE, 33 West 42d St., New York NY 10036.

Publications

Harrison H. *The Premature Baby Book*. New York: St. Martin's Press, 1983.

VandenBerg KA, Hanson MJ. *Homecoming for Babies after the Neonatal Intensive Care Nursery*. Austin: Pro-ed, 1993

For Professionals

Ballard RA. *Pediatric Care of the ICN Graduate*. Philadelphia: Saunders, 1988.

Bernbaum JC, Hofman-Williamson M. *Primary Care of the Preterm Infant*. St. Louis: Mosby Yearbook, 1991.

Sammons W, Lewis JM. *Premature Babies: A Different Beginning*. St. Louis: Mosby, 1985.

52

Psychosomatic Illness

Gordon Harper

I. **Description of the problem.** Psychosomatic illness refers to symptomatology in which both psychological and physiologic processes play prominent roles. Often the symptoms extend across disease categories, ranging from fatigue to shortness of breath to pain to weight loss. This multifactorial definition differs from the one-factor use of *psychosomatic* to mean "psychogenic." It also differs from the use of *psychosomatic* in popular culture as a term of disparagement, meaning "fake," "insignificant," or "unworthy." This chapter outlines two conditions in which psychosomatic interactions figure prominently: unexplained disability and insistent somaticism.

A. **Epidemiology**
   - Between 50 and 75% of office visits are occasioned not by organic pathology alone but by unexplained symptoms, reactions to symptoms, and fear of symptoms.
   - Psychosomatic interactions occur at all ages, from rumination and "nonorganic" failure to thrive in infants and toddlers, to conversion symptoms and eating disorders in older children and adolescents.

B. **Pathogenesis.** These disorders must be considered in terms of diseased organs and in terms of the meanings people make of the body and its symptoms. When child and family lack nonsomatic channels for communication, the body and its symptoms may be recruited for the purpose of expressing the child's distress—a distress often not even known to the child.

II. **Unexplained disability.** Unexplained disability implies dysfunction out of proportion to any demonstrable disease process.

A. **Features**

1. The **symptoms,** either nonspecific (e.g., malaise/fatigue) or specific (e.g., localized pain, limb disuse, vomiting), are associated with disability lasting for weeks or months.

2. There is a **pronounced family reaction** to illness: either overreaction (with frequent calls to clinicians and pressure for a quick diagnosis) or underreaction (with surprise that others are concerned).

3. There are often **many symptoms.**

4. There is an **apparent disease/illness discrepancy** in which the symptoms do not add up.

5. There may be a **lack of experience, in child or family, with acknowledging feelings** (especially anxiety, anger, or sadness), disbelief in the value of sharing pain or of being understood, and a disinclination to "talk about what can't be helped."

B. **Making the diagnosis**

1. **Remember the basics.** Specialized evaluations are unlikely to contribute to a diagnosis unless indicated by specific findings.

2. **Obtain data from both child and parent, separately.** Pooled data from separate interviews are more likely to yield relevant information. Key clinical questions include:

a. *What do you think is going on? I know you've come to me for my opinion, but I'm still interested in your ideas. You've been living with this for a long time.*

b. *Apart from these symptoms, how are things going?* This question applies to school, friends, family, sleep, appetite, future plans, managing conflict, and managing feelings.

c. *Who understands how it's been for you?*

3. **Take your time.** Despite pressure to reach diagnostic closure, let the disorder declare itself over time.

4. **Weigh the finding.** Parents who are overimpressed with technical findings need a clinician's help in interpreting irrelevant findings (e.g., a clinically insignificant, mildly abnormal EEG).

C. Management

1. **Seek a middle ground.** Despite pressure to say "It's medical" or "It's emotional," the clinician should not be afraid to equivocate. Temporizing is not a waste of time; it allows trust to develop and fear to subside, and a broader view of the situation to emerge.

2. **Stay involved as a primary care clinician.** These children need follow-up for serial assessments and health supervision. "Referred to" mental health services should not mean "referred out" of pediatric care.

3. **Acknowledge to the family how hard the evaluation has been.** Sympathetic validation soothes and heals—for example, "Bethany's pain is interfering with her life as a teenager, but she is fighting hard to manage it. We will help her in that fight. And I know that you as parents are worried sick, too."

4. **Support family stabilization.** Without labeling such problems as the "cause" of the child's symptoms, the clinician can sympathetically help parents attend to family business and their own lives as a couple, which may have been neglected while the patient has been ill.

5. **Help the child normalize his or her life.** The child may need medical permission and encouragement to get back to peers, school, and activity, even while symptoms continue.

6. **Do not put off referral to mental health colleagues** until "We are sure there's nothing physical." Such a reason for waiting reinforces mind-versus-body thinking and the feeling that acknowledging emotional stress is shameful and dangerous. It is preferable to suggest to the family a collaborative approach for a difficult problem.

7. **Hospital admission can help** by interrupting the ways in which the child has been managing distress and the family has been dealing with conflict. New ways of coping can then develop. Early in the course of the child's illness, it is useful to mention the possibility of admitting the child to a mental health or psychosomatic unit, not as "a psychiatric case" but as a case of "serious unexplained disability." Parents, child, and clinician may need to agree at that time on hospitalization at a future date if significant improvement has not occurred.

8. **Clinical pearls and pitfalls**
   • Do not use polarizing, stigmatizing language: "All the tests are normal"; "There is nothing wrong."
   • Avoid "over-and-out" referral: "I guess you have to see the psychiatrist" (said with regret and foreboding).

III. **Insistent somaticism.** Insistent somaticism is a more serious form of unexplained disability in which parents insist that psychological factors have no role in their child's disorder (even when no one has made such a suggestion). An "-ism" has here been made of the word *somatic* in order to capture an intensely held commitment to a particular way of thinking about their child's problems shown by these parents (and sometimes by the child as well).

A. **Features**

1. **Parents are terrified of psychological disorders:** "Better she should have cancer than an emotional problem." These parents are frightened not just of psychological distress in general but of the possibility that their child is unhappy or angry. To them, a hurting child who does not have a medical diagnosis is an unhappy child, and an unhappy child activates an unbearable self-reproach: "We must be bad parents." Behind the parents' argumentativeness lies a fear of frightening feelings, and behind that fear lies an equation of parent-child distress with separation and death.

2. **The family will shop for new doctors in a desperate hope of discovering a physical disorder.** In the process, the child may be subjected to dubiously indicated and potentially dangerous diagnostic and therapeutic procedures. The parents' terror over the possibility of psychological inquiry contrasts with the alacrity with which they accept medical procedures, even invasive or painful ones.

3. **The parents disparage mental health clinicians** and primary care clinicians who are open to considering the child's emotional state.

4. **At the extremes, these cases overlap with serious undiagnosed psychiatric disorder in a parent** (mood disorder, anxiety disorder, or personality disorder) or with frank factitious illness (Munchausen syndrome by proxy).

B. **Making the diagnosis: Key clinical questions**

1. *Has anybody understood what a time you've had?*

2. *In your heart of hearts, what do you worry might be going on?*

3. *Can we work together, with your bringing me all your questions and concerns, including your misgivings about how I am taking care of your child?*

4. *Can you imagine your child/yourself well and without these symptoms?*

C. **Management**

1. Remember that **the parents are terrified and feel shame and guilt** about their child's illness. Express appreciation for their efforts and commitment. The parents will hear everything said of the child to refer to themselves. Emphasize the child's strengths, including his or her courage and the parents' supportiveness.

2. **Centralize medical care.** One primary care clinician should coordinate the multiple consultants, approve any proposed tests, and meticulously present findings and recommendations to the parents. Tell the parents, "To be helpful, I have to know what's going on, what tests you're considering, what results you're trying to make sense of."

3. **Try to help the parents shift their focus from the question of etiology to the work of adaptation** and living with unwanted symptoms. "We want to help Billy get on with life, including school and friends, and we can help him with that even if we can't say for sure what causes all this." Avoid statements like, "There's no medical problem," or, "The tests were negative," which means to the parents, "There's an emotional problem [and you're a bad parent]." Avoid phrases like "medically clear" or "okay from the medical point of view." Instead, try something like, "Our evaluation indicates a serious problem with pain [or, with walking, or, with headache]." Don't try to talk the parents out of the belief that the child is medically sick.

4. **Stay involved.** Don't try to "just tell them it's a psychological problem" and refer "over and out" to mental health colleagues.

5. Be aware of these parents' intense self-blame and **look for ways to acknowledge medical limitations:** "You're right, medicine doesn't know enough as it should about this kind of problem."

D. **Clinical pearls and pitfalls**

• In contrast to patients with simple unexplained disability, for whom early participation of mental health colleagues is advisable, be careful about referring these families. Do not refer to mental health colleagues when the parents'

attitudes make them see any such referral as confirmation of their "badness" and as abandonment by the medical clinician when they are terrified of an undiagnosed disease.
- Avoid loose talk about "feelings" or depression.
- Do not act on the frustration and annoyance easily felt in these cases.
- Stay involved. Let parents know you appreciate their efforts.

Bibliography

DB Herzog, G Harper, Unexplained disability. *Clin Pediatr* 20:761–767, 1981.

EH Channing, SB Hauser, KA Shade, WT Boyce. Mental disorders in chronically ill children: Parent-child discrepancy and physician identification. *Pediatrics* 90:692–96, 1992.

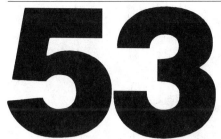

Recurrent Abdominal Pain

Leonard Rappaport

I. Description of the problem. Recurrent abdominal pain (RAP) is defined as repeated paroxysms of abdominal pain occurring at least once a month, lasting for at least 3 months, with intervening asymptomatic periods. Each episode is severe enough to interfere with normal activities.

A. Epidemiology
- Recurrent abdominal pain occurs in approximately one in seven children aged 5–12 years. It is one of the most prevalent of childhood symptoms brought to the attention of primary care clinicians.
- There is a slight female predominance.
- Prevalence is unrelated to social class, birth, or family size.

B. Etiology. Three factors, in varying combinations, have been implicated in RAP. For all factors, a family that is overinvolved with the pain symptoms may exacerbate the pain complaint.

1. Clear-cut organic pathology. While the list of possible etiologies is legion, only 10% of children presenting with recurrent abdominal pain have an identifiable organic etiology.

2. Psychogenic pain. This is often secondary to a combination of temperament, stress, family, and adjustment factors.

3. Physiological pain. This pain is generated intraabdominally as a result of normal physiologic processes (termed "dysfunctional RAP"). This category is subdivided into those with recognizable causes (e.g., imbalance between a stressor and a normal physiologic variant such as lactose intolerance) and those with nonspecific RAP (no organic etiology can be identified).

II. Making the diagnosis

A. Signs and symptoms. In RAP, the abdominal pain is typically periumbilical, lasts 30–60 minutes, and occurs during the day (rarely awakening the child from sleep). The child will often appear pale and diaphoretic. Alterations from this pattern have been associated with a higher incidence of organic pathology and have been termed "red flags" (Table 53-1).

B. Differential diagnosis. While recurrent abdominal pain can be caused by almost any pediatric disease process, most studies have shown that one-third to one-half of the identified pathology can be found in the genitourinary tract.

C. History: Key clinical questions

1. *When did the abdominal pain begin? How often does it occur? Where does it hurt?* Have the child locate the area by pointing with one finger.

2. *Are there associated symptoms when the pain occurs?* For example, is there fever, vomiting, dizziness, or other pain locations?

3. *Does the child have regular bowel movements?* A major cause of recurrent abdominal pain is constipation, and it is essential to know the child's stooling pattern.

4. *Has there been weight loss?*

Table 53-1. "Red flags": signs and symptoms

Pain farther away from the umbilicus
Fever
Weight loss
Blood in stools (guaiac positive)
Pain awakening the child at night
Anemia
Dysuria
Elevated ESR

Table 53-2. Initial work-up

Complete physical examination including:
    Rectal examination (including stool guaiac)
    Examination of spine
    Neurologic examination
Initial laboratory examination
    Urinalysis (culture in females)
    CBC and erythrocyte sedimentation rate
    Stool for ova and parasites (or *Giardia* antigen in geographic areas where
        Giardia is common)
    Lactose breath test (if suggested by history and physical)
    Abdominal ultrasound (if suggested by history and physical)

    5. [To both parent and child] *What do you think causes the pain? How upset does your child become and how much does it interfere with his or her activity? What is your response?* It is important to know how the family views this problem. Does it remind them of some bad occurrence in their family, such as a child with unrecognized appendicitis or a tumor? Has the family focused a great deal of energy on the abdominal pain? Is the family rewarding the child for having the pain, and has it become "the currency" of interaction in the family?

    6. *How is this pain interfering with your child's life?* It is important to establish whether the pain has been associated with a global withdrawal from school, family, and social interaction. This behavior has been termed the "extended syndrome" of RAP, in which the pain becomes the focus of the child's life.

    7. *What do you think causes the pain? Is there anything you can do to get rid of the pain?* It is essential to know just how important the pain is to the child. Often, for example, a child can say that the pain is mild but that everyone is worried about it.

  D. Behavioral observations. The clinician should observe the parents' interactions with the child. How upset do they appear over the pain symptom, and is the child acting at an age-appropriate developmental level? Do the parents allow the child to answer the questions?

  E. Physical examination. A complete physical examination, including a neurologic and rectal examination, is essential. Any area not examined at this time should be noted clearly so it can be examined in the future.

  F. Laboratory evaluation. If the history and physical examination suggest a specific etiology, appropriate tests should be ordered. Otherwise, the initial laboratory evaluation should be quite limited (Table 53-2).

III. Management

A. Primary goals. The primary goals in managing RAP are to identify and treat organic disease appropriately, lessen pain whenever possible, and decrease the impact of the abdominal pain symptom in the child's life. These goals are accomplished by a thorough initial examination and the institution of an explicit management and treatment plan with the family at the initial visit.

B. Initial treatment strategies

1. **Explanation.** On the day of the initial evaluation, the clinician should explain that only 10% of children will have an identifiable organic etiology for their pain and that some children will continue to have abdominal pain several years after the initial presentation. The clinician should explain that the objective of the initial visits is to find organic disease, if present, and to manage the symptoms with available interventions.

2. **Trial of fiber.** The initial history, physical examination, and laboratory screening are usually negative in recurrent abdominal pain. In most cases, management of the pain complex becomes the major issue. While there have been many suggested treatments for RAP, only one placebo-controlled trial has yielded positive results. This trial utilized fiber in a dosage of 5 g/day (in a fiber cookie). The group receiving this intervention had a significant decrease in abdominal pain during the study period. Therefore a trial of fiber would seem appropriate for most children with RAP.

3. **Parents' role.** It is important to outline the "red-flag" symptoms for parents—those the clinician should hear about immediately, should they occur (Table 53-1). This should include an explanation of the "extended syndrome" of recurrent abdominal pain, which includes social withdrawal.

C. Back-up strategies. Since the pain of RAP often persists even after a fiber intervention, it is essential for the clinician to remain vigilant for an etiologic cause and not to be discouraged. Care, rather than cure, is often the approach that must be taken at this time. Failure to find a cause or rid the child of the pain is disappointing to all parties, but the clinician should continue to focus energy on limiting the impact of the pain just as he or she does when coping with other chronic conditions for which there is no cure.

IV. Clinical pearls and pitfalls

- There is no substitute for a complete and thorough initial history and physical examination. Unnecessary laboratory and radiologic tests often lead parents to believe that there is an organic etiology for the abdominal pain. Under such circumstances, a negative work-up can lead to unnecessary repeat evaluations, which can be quite traumatic for the child.
- Stay in touch. It is helpful to see a child with RAP on a monthly or bimonthly visit to monitor the pain symptom. Show the parents that you are not ignoring the pain, and reassure the child that you will be monitoring the pain.
- Rectal examinations are more easily done with the child lying on the back facing you in a modified lithotomy position. You then tell the child to bear down as though they are going to have a bowel movement while the rectal examination is completed. In this way the child can look at you while you talk and can be distracted from whatever discomfort may be caused by the examination. Additionally, you can clearly see any discomfort the child is experiencing. Having the child face away from you on the examining table, as is often done, can be frightening to the child and provides no additional data.
- Explain to the child that abdominal pain is common in children their age and that the pain does not mean that there is something wrong. Often children are secretly afraid that something truly bad is occurring to them.
- If a family is uncomfortable with your evaluation of their child's abdominal pain, do not discourage a second opinion. It is often helpful to have a specialist in mind whom you feel has a reasonable approach to the care of children with RAP.
- When you note the onset of the extended syndrome, it is time to refer the child to a mental health professional who has an expertise in the management of chronic disease and pain symptoms.

Bibliography

Apley J. *The Child with Abdominal Pains*. London: Blackwell, 1975.

Barr RG. Recurrent abdominal pain. In MD Levine et al. (eds), *Developmental Behavioral Pediatrics*. Philadelphia: Saunders, 1983.

Feldman W et al. The use of dietary fibre in the management of simple childhood idiopathic recurrent abdominal pain: Results of a prospective double blind randomized controlled trial. *Am J Dis Child* 139:1216–1218, 1985.

Rappaport L, Leichtner A. Recurrent abdominal pain. In N Schechter et al. (eds), *Pain in Infants, Children, and Adolescents*. Baltimore: Williams & Wilkins, 1993.

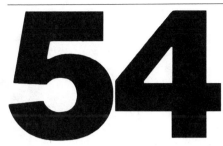

School Avoidance

Barton D. Schmitt

I. **Description of the problem.** Children with school avoidance repeatedly stay home from school or are sent home from school for physical symptoms of emotional origin. In the classic case, the child awakens with a stomachache on Monday morning, is allowed to stay home, and feels fine by midmorning. The terms *school refusal, school avoidance,* and *school phobia* are often used interchangeably.

A. **Epidemiology**
- School avoidance is the most common cause of vague physical symptoms in school-aged children.
- Approximately 5% of elementary school children and 2% of junior high school children have this disorder.
- The incidence of school refusal may be decreasing because of the increasing numbers of working mothers, which requires most children to master their separation fears long before entering kindergarten.

B. **Etiology.** There are two basic types of school avoidance syndrome.

1. **Anxiety-related school avoidance.** These children are excessively worried (e.g., about grades, being liked by other people, marital discord). Most of these children also have persistent separation anxiety, which normal children have mastered by ages 3–4 years. Many have a shy and sensitive temperament. Frequently there is an overprotective parent who worries too much about the child's experiencing stress in the neighborhood and school. These children are good to excellent students and cause no behavioral problems in the classroom. Girls outnumber boys, and the onset usually occurs in kindergarten. Approximately 20% of this group also have an acute precipitating event (e.g., being teased by someone at school).

2. **Secondary-gain school avoidance.** These children do not manifest any symptoms of anxiety. Their poor school attendance often follows an acute illness that seems to stretch on and on as they get further behind in their schoolwork. The desire to stay at home is also perpetuated by the sympathy they receive and the amount of television they are allowed to watch. They often have a lenient parent who does not place much value on education. Boys outnumber girls in this group, and often they are poor students.

II. **Making the diagnosis**

A. **Signs and symptoms.** Table 54-1 reviews common presenting symptoms. Most children with school avoidance complain of physical symptoms at the time of departure for school. The children with the anxiety-related type usually have physiologic manifestations of anxiety (e.g., headache, recurrent abdominal pain). The children with the secondary-gain type of school refusal usually fabricate or exaggerate symptoms (e.g., sore throat, leg pain).

B. **Confirming the diagnosis.** School avoidance is a diagnosis of inclusion that can be confirmed by documenting four diagnostic criteria.

1. **The child complains of recurrent vague, mysterious physical symptoms.**

2. **No physical cause is found on careful evaluation,** including a physical examination and appropriate laboratory tests. The discrepancy between how sick the child sounds and how well the child looks is one of the hallmarks of this disorder.

Table 54-1. Presenting symptoms for school refusal

General
Insomnia
Excessive sleeping
Fatigue
"Always tired"
"Fever"
"Always sick"
Skin
Pallor
Ear, nose, and throat
Recurrent sore throats
Recurrent sinus problems
"Constant" colds
Respiratory
Hyperventilation
Coughing tics
Cardiovascular
Palpitations
Chest pains
Gastrointestinal
Recurrent abdominal pains
Anorexia
Nausea
Recurrent vomiting
Diarrhea
Skeletal
Bone pain
Joint pain
Back pain
Neuromuscular
Headaches
Dizziness
Syncope
"Weakness"

Note: Symptoms in **boldface type** can be physiologic manifestations of anxiety. The other symptoms may be fabricated or exaggerated.

3. **Physical symptoms predominate in the morning** and are accentuated when the family tries to send the child to school. Often the symptoms clear by 10:00 A.M.

4. **The child has missed 5 or more days of school because of these physical symptoms.** By comparison, children with chronic physical diseases often have excellent school attendance records.

C. **Differential diagnosis.** Each physical symptom listed in Table 54-1 has a specific and lengthy differential diagnosis. The primary care clinician is obligated to rule out any physical disease as a cause of the school refuser's symptoms. Excessive or chronic school absence also can have other causes (Table 54-2). Some parents keep a child at home for a prolonged period of time because of mistaken beliefs regarding the need for bed rest or isolation (e.g., keeping a child home 10 days for streptococcal pharyngitis). Children with chronic physical disease or learning disabilities may become reluctant to attend school because they are unable to adapt well to the academic environment or to the other children. A *truant* is a youngster who is neither at home nor at school during school hours. These children are at risk for becoming school dropouts. The acute onset of school avoidance may relate to a precipitating event, such as a change of schools or the loss of a school chum. Other precipitants include family stresses (e.g., acute marital strife, the father's loss of a job, a sick mother, the birth of a sibling),

Table 54-2. Chronic school absence: A differential diagnosis

School refusal
  Anxiety-related type (school phobia)
  Secondary-gain type (school avoidance)
Overresponse to minor illnesses
Chronic physical disease with poor adaptation
Learning disability with poor adaptation
Truancy
Substance abuse
Depression
Psychosis
Teenage pregnancy
Family dysfunction

stresses that occur en route to school (e.g., a bully at the bus stop), academic stresses (e.g., an impending test, a requirement to recite in class, a poor report card), and school-based stresses (e.g., bathroom restrictions for children with small bladders, physical fitness requirements for overweight or clumsy children, teasing on the school grounds).

D. History: Key clinical questions

1. *How much school has your child missed because of these symptoms?* It is a mistake to assume that the parents will bring up poor school attendance to the clinician. They often believe that everyone keeps "sick" children at home and in bed.

2. *How many days of school did your child miss last year?* This information is needed when parents blame the problem on some illness or stress that began during the current school year.

3. *When are the symptoms worse?* In school avoidance, the symptoms are usually worse on Sunday nights, early mornings, Mondays, during September, and following holidays. Often the onset of symptoms dates to entering kindergarten or first grade.

4. *What do you think is causing the symptoms?* or *What is the worst diagnosis your child could have?* The parents may fear a specific disease that the child does not harbor.

5. *Have any major changes occurred in your family?* This question may help the family acknowledge stressors they had initially overlooked or denied.

6. *Does your child ever stay overnight with friends at their homes?* An inability to be away from parents at night supports separation issues.

7. *What is the worst possible thing that could happen if you sent your child to school with these symptoms?* The parents may fear that the child will emotionally decompensate at school, have embarrassing symptoms, or be teased.

E. Physical examination. The physical examination of these children should be completely normal. The performance of a meticulous examination is reassuring to the parents, as parents place an inordinate amount of faith in the ability of the examination to uncover hidden disease. During the examination, the clinician should discuss normal findings rather than proceed in silence. He or she can provide double reassurance for more skeptical parents by asking a partner to confirm the findings and comment briefly.

F. Tests. Each specific physical symptom will determine which laboratory studies (if any) are appropriate.

III. Management

A. Primary goals

1. **Convince the parents that their child is in excellent physical health.**

2. **Convince the parents that their child has school avoidance.**

3. **Return the child to full-time school attendance.**

B. **Information for the family.** The main barrier to successful treatment is changing the family's focus from organic to nonorganic. The following steps are usually helpful to this process.

1. **Explain what school avoidance is and that stress can cause real physical symptoms.** Explain the difference between physical symptoms and physical disease. Explain that pain is real, even when it has an emotional origin. Point out that everyone's body has a certain physical way of responding to emotional stress.

2. **Clarify for parents that school avoidance occurs in normal children and normal homes.** Mention that it is a "stress-related," not a "psychiatric," problem. Support the parents as being good caregivers.

3. **Clarify that the child is in excellent physical health.** Pronounce the child *unequivocally* physically well. Do not leave the parents hanging with statements such as, "He probably has school avoidance, but we can't be certain." If a clinician is unwilling to call the cause stress related, he or she can at least attribute the symptoms to some benign physiologic process, such as gas pains, a sensitive stomach, growing pains, or tension headaches.

4. **Tell parents why the symptom is not the result of physical disease.** Justify the nonorganic diagnosis by pointing to the timing of the symptoms, the age of onset that coincides with school entry, the presence of the symptoms during previous school years, the normal physical examination, and normal laboratory tests.

5. **Reassure parents that you can effectively treat this condition.** The primary care clinician can promise to provide a treatment plan that will reduce the symptoms in the majority of cases. The minimal goal of this discussion should be to get the parents to agree to regular school attendance pending additional observations, even if they cling to the idea that their child may have some rare disease.

C. **Initial treatment strategies**

1. **The mainstay of treatment is returning the child to regular school attendance.**

2. **Talk with the parents.** Once the primary care clinician has convinced the family that the youngster is physically well, he or she must insist on an immediate return to school. Being in school is intrinsically therapeutic and breaks the vicious cycle that occurs when a child gets out of step with schoolwork and friendships. Parents will need to be firm in the morning for several weeks. On any morning that the "child has to stay home for illness," the clinician is needed to reassess the child and send him or her to school if the condition is minor or a psychosomatic symptom.

3. **Talk with the child.** The clinician should reassure the youngster that she or he is in good physical health and in no physical danger. The symptoms can be blamed on worrying too much about competition, grades, bad things happening, or catching up with schoolwork. The clinician can offer a face-saving way to accept the diagnosis (e.g., headache from worrying too much) and emphasize that daily school attendance, a nonnegotiable requirement, will help the child feel better.

   a. **Secondary-gain school refusal.** Simply state, "You can't miss any further school because it is illegal to do so." This type of refusal responds quickly to this warning and limit setting.

   b. **Anxiety-related school refusal.** More sympathy is in order. If the child has severe symptoms at school, promise the availability of lying down in the nurse's office for 5–10 minutes. Clarify, however, that she or he cannot go home because of these symptoms.

4. **Contact the school staff.** Communication between the primary care clinician and the school nurse is essential. The clinician should be called if the child's

attendance remains poor or if the child is in the nursing station and wants to go home. The clinician and school nurse can then work together to decide whether the child should stay in school. School staff can also help to make the return to school as nontraumatic as possible, (e.g., cancelling some of the make-up work).

5. **Treat contributory stress factors.** Most school stresses can be dealt with by the parent, school principal, special education teacher, or the primary care clinician. Correction of most of these factors alone may produce little improvement in school attendance, because they only partially account for the child's preference for staying home. Changing to a different class or a different school generally is of no benefit except in those rare situations in which an unstable teacher is mistreating one or more children.

6. **Providing follow-up visits.** Follow-up visits are essential for monitoring attendance. Children with school avoidance should have return visits in approximately 1 week, 1 month, and again approximately 2 weeks into the following school year. These parents also need to call their clinician on the first day of acute illnesses to help decide whether the child needs to stay home.

D. **Criteria for referral.** The primary care clinician needs to refer the child with more severe, intractable emotional problems to a child psychiatrist, psychologist, or social worker. Most children who have been on prolonged bed rest should also be referred. Most of all, patients who are unresponsive to pediatric counseling also need referral.

IV. **Clinical pearls and pitfalls**
- Ask about school attendance whenever you evaluate a child for recurrent or persistent symptoms.
- Suspect school avoidance when no organic disease has this profile or keeps this timetable.
- Don't be misled because the child "likes school," is a good student, or "wants to go back."
- If in doubt about the diagnosis, request a 7-day symptom diary. It will be more helpful than any imaging study.
- Protect these children from unwarranted laboratory tests, procedures, prescriptions, hospitalization, and surgery.
- Request that children return to school, even while the evaluation is in process. Returning will be either diagnostic or therapeutic.

Bibliography

For Parents
Schmitt BD. When your child has school phobia (a parent information sheet). *Contemp Pediatr* 7(8):41–42, 1990.

For Professionals
Krugman RD, Krugman MK. Emotional abuse in the classroom. *Am J Dis Child* 138:284–286, 1984.

Schmitt BD. School refusal. *Pediatr Rev* 8:99–105, 1986.

Weitzman M et al. School absence: A problem for the pediatrician. *Pediatrics* 69:739–746, 1982.

55

School Failure

Paul H. Dworkin

I. **Description of the problem.** Over 10% of schoolchildren in the United States are receiving special education and other services because of difficulties with school performance. School failure is a complex issue that defies traditional methods of pediatric evaluation and management. While learning problems are of obvious multidisciplinary concern, the primary care clinician plays a vital role in clarifying the reasons for school failure and facilitating appropriate evaluation and intervention.

A. **Reasons for school failure.** A wide variety of causes may contribute to a child's failure in school. A simple classification scheme identifies **intrinsic** or child-related causes (e.g., specific learning disabilities, attention deficits) and **extrinsic** or environmental-related causes relating to either the home (e.g., parental separation or divorce) or the school setting (e.g., poor instruction). In most cases, school failure is not due to a single factor but rather the result of a complex interaction of child-, family-, and school-related variables.

B. **Specific causes**

1. **Learning disabilities.** As defined by federal legislation, *learning disabilities* "is a generic term that refers to a heterogeneous group of disorders manifested by significant difficulties in the acquisition and use of listening, speaking, reading, writing, reasoning, or mathematical abilities. These disorders are intrinsic to the individual and presumed to be due to central nervous system dysfunction. Even though a learning disability may occur concomitantly with other handicapping conditions or environmental influences, it is not the direct result of these conditions or influences."

Learning disabilities are characterized by a discrepancy between ability (as measured by intelligence tests) and actual academic achievement. Their prevalance is estimated at 3–15% of schoolchildren. While most learning disabled children have underlying weaknesses in language function, weaknesses in other higher-order cognitive functions (so-called metacognitive skills) have been increasingly recognized. Such children may have difficulties with reasoning, memory, or focusing their attention and have been described as "passive learners" because of their difficulties with selecting strategies for problem solving.

2. **Attention deficits** (see Chapter 40). There exists significant overlap between children with learning disabilities and attention deficit hyperactivity disorder (ADHD). From a clinical standpoint, distinguishing between children with an intrinsic deficit of attention (ADHD) and those with attention deficits secondary to other developmental-behavioral dysfunctions (e.g., language impairment, depression) is often difficult.

3. **Mental retardation** (see Chapters 43 and 44). Mild mental retardation is often not identified until children are confronted with the cognitive demands of school. At that time, a slow learning rate and ultimate acquisition of academic skills up to the fifth- or sixth-grade level is typically seen.

4. **Sensory impairment.** Hearing loss results in a significant educational handicap because language acquisition and communication skills are impaired. Such students typically experience difficulties in reading, arithmetic reasoning, and problem solving. They may exhibit classroom maladjustment, behavioral problems, and social immaturity. The prognosis directly relates to the age at which identification occurs. In comparison, blind children usually

fare better within the classroom. Visually impaired children who experience school failure tend to have multiple additional handicaps.

5. **Emotional illness.** From 30% to 80% of emotionally disturbed students have problems with academic achievement and classroom behavior. Emotional problems such as low self-esteem and poor self-image often exacerbate school failure brought on by other causes, such as learning disabilities.

6. **Chronic illness.** From one-quarter to two-thirds of chronically ill students have problems with academic achievement (see Chapter 21). Possible adverse influences on school performance include limited alertness or stamina, chronic pain, medication side effects, absenteeism, emotional maladjustment, low intelligence (primarily children with certain neurologic disorders), the inferior quality of alternative classroom placement, and inappropriate or unrealistic expectations by teachers and parents. Additionally, certain chronic diseases (e.g., epilepsy, cerebral palsy, myelomeningocele) are associated with an increased incidence of learning disabilities.

7. **Temperamental dysfunction** (see Chapter 66). The temperamentally "difficult" student may become easily frustrated and angry when confronted with material not easily mastered. The initial reluctance to participate and tendency to withdraw of the "slow-to-warm-up" child may be misinterpreted as anxiety or as a limited capacity for learning. Although the temperamentally "easy" student usually fares well, problems may arise when expectations for behavior markedly differ between home and school. For example, a student's mild intensity of reaction to situations or stimuli may be misinterpreted within the classroom as a lack of interest or motivation.

8. **Family dysfunction and social problems.** Family issues that contribute to school failure include parental separation and divorce, child abuse and neglect, the illness or death of an immediate family member, parental psychopathology, early parenthood, substance abuse, and poverty.

9. **Ineffective schooling.** School *processes* are more important determinants of students' performance than such features as whether schools are public or private, class size, the age and spaciousness of school buildings, and student-teacher ratio. Rather, the school's academic emphasis, expectations for attainment, amount of homework, teachers' actions during lessons, use of group instruction, and the use of rewards and praise are major influences on students' performance. Aspects of the school's social environment (such as the amount of praise offered to children) may be particularly important for children from disadvantaged homes in which less emphasis is placed on academic attainment and standards for classroom behavior.

II. **Making the diagnosis.** If psychoeducational evaluation has already identified the reasons for a student's school failure (e.g., learning disabilities, mild mental retardation), the goal of pediatric evaluation is to exclude medical problems as contributors to poor classroom performance. Additionally, the primary care clinician's familiarity with the child and family may be helpful in identifying social or emotional factors that further impair school performance. For the child with newly recognized school failure, the pediatric clinician must identify such conditions as sensory impairment or chronic illness, while searching for medical, neurophysiologic, and psychologic correlates of such other conditions as learning disabilities, mental retardation, and emotional illness.

Possible components of the evaluation of children with school failure include:

A. **History.** Important historic information should be sought from parents, teachers, and the child. Review of the student's perinatal and past medical history, developmental milestones, past and present behavior, and family and social history may yield findings with possible implications for school failure (Table 55-1).

B. **Key clinical questions**

1. *Which subjects are particularly difficult for the child?* The pattern of delays may suggest a specific etiology; for example, learning disabled children typically have discrete difficulties in select subjects, while mildly retarded students have more pervasive academic delays.

Table 55-1. The role of history in the evaluation of school learning problems

Aspect	Findings of specific learning disabilities
School functioning	
Academic achievement	Discrete delays in select subject (e.g., language)
	Adequate early performance, with difficulties emerging later (e.g., mathematics, writing)
Classroom behavior	Long-standing, pervasive problems with inattention, impulsivity, overactivity
	Disorganization and poor strategy formation
	Depression, moodiness
Attendance	Excessive absenteeism
	School avoidance
Past psychoeducational testing	Discrepancy between cognitive abilities and academic achievement
Special required school services	Response to "diagnostic teaching"
Perinatal history	Clusters of adverse events
	Maternal alcohol or drug intake
Medical history	Recurrent and/or persistent otitis media
	Iron deficiency anemia
	Lead poisoning
	Seizures
	Frequent accidents
	Chronic medication use
Development	Delayed or disordered language acquisition and communication skills
	Subtle delays in select milestones
	Uneven pattern of skills and interests
Behavioral history	Long-standing, pervasive problems with attention span, impulsivity, acting out, overactivity
	Sadness
	Poor self-esteem
Family history	Learning problems
	School failure among first-degree relatives
Social history	Child abuse or neglect
	Other stressors

Source: Reproduced with permission from Dworkin PH: School learning problems. In Hoekelman RA, et al. (eds): *Pediatric Primary Care.* St. Louis: Mosby-Year Book 1991, p. 648.

2. *How does the child behave in the classroom?* Classroom behavior may suggest attention deficits, poor self-image, or conduct disorder.

3. *How many days has the child missed school?* Poor school attendance may be due to chronic illness, school phobia, or poor motivation due to learning disabilities.

4. *Has past testing been performed?* Past educational or psychological testing may have identified causes of a child's school failure.

5. *What special services has the child received?* Responses to different instructional techniques ("diagnostic teaching") may suggest reasons for school failure.

C. **Physical examination.** The physical examination has a limited, but important, role in the evaluation of children with school failure. Certain specific aspects deserve special emphasis (Table 55-2).

Table 55-2. The physical examination and evaluation of school learning problems

Aspect	Findings suggestive of specific learning disabilities
General observations	Sadness, anxiety Short attention span, impulsivity, overactivity Tics
Phenotypic features	Stigmata of genetic syndromes (e.g., sex chromosome abnormalities, fetal alcohol syndrome) Minor congenital anomalies
Skin	Multiple café au lait spots "Ash-leaf" spots, adenoma sebaceum
Tympanic membranes	Signs of recurrent or chronic otitis media
Genitalia	Delayed sexual maturation in boys
Growth measurements	Short stature Microcephaly and macrocephaly
Sensory screening	Poor hearing or vision

Source: Reproduced with permission from Dworkin PH: School learning problems. In Hoekelman RA, et al. (eds.): *Pediatric Primary Care.* St. Louis: Mosby-Year Book, 1991, p. 649.

- **D. Mental status examination.** Simple projective techniques may suggest emotional issues such as depression, anxiety, or poor self-image as the cause or, even more likely, the consequence of school failure. Examples include:

    1. **"If you had three wishes, what would they be?"**

    2. **"If you could make three changes in your life, what would they be?"** The sad or anxious child may be unwilling to offer wishes or hope for changes in family or school circumstances.

    3. **"Draw a picture of your family"** may suggest concerns with family composition or reveal anxiety or uncertainty regarding the child's status within the family.

- **E. Neurodevelopmental assessment.** Surveying the child's abilities in different areas of development may help to identify weaknesses contributing to school failure. For example, the developmental profile of learning disabled children is typically characterized by an uneven pattern, with discrete areas of relative strength and weakness. The significance of minor neurologic indicators ("soft neurologic signs") is controversial; such findings should not serve as a basis for diagnosing learning disorders.

- **F. Laboratory studies.** No laboratory studies are routinely indicated in the assessment of school failure. Rather, tests should be performed based on specific indications. One possible exception is screening for lead poisoning.

- **G. Further investigations and referrals.** Psychoeducational evaluation is critically important in the evaluation of childen with school failure.

    1. **Goals.** The goals of such evaluations include:

        a. **To examine the student's academic strengths and weaknesses.**

        b. **To determine the child's cognitive ability,** including such higher-order functions as abstract reasoning, problem solving, and learning style.

        c. **To assess perceptual strengths and weaknesses.**

        d. **To examine communicative ability.**

        e. **To assess social and emotional adaptation.**

    2. **Performance.** Ideally, such evaluations are performed by the child's school system, in accordance with state and federal mandates. There is no one standardized evaluation appropriate for all children, and the specific tests used depend on the preference and expertise of the examiner and the child's needs. Examples include intelligence tests; tests of general learning abilities;

academic achievement tests; diagnostic reading, math, and writing tests; tests of perceptual and motor function; and such informal techniques as diagnostic teaching. School personnel performing such evaluations may include psychologists, special educators, learning disability specialists, speech-language pathologists, and social workers.

III. **Management.** For learning disabilties, mild mental retardation, and other common causes of school failure, educational intervention is the most crucial. Nonetheless, a variety of important primary care roles are both feasible and important in the management of school failure.

A. **Specific medical intervention** is the most traditional of pediatric roles. Examples include:

1. **The treatment of underlying medical conditions,** such as asthma or a seizure disorder, that influence school performance.

2. **Pharmacologic management** of attention deficits.

B. **Counseling** is a traditional mode of pediatric intervention. Aspects may include:

1. **Clarification of a student's strengths and weaknesses.**

2. **Anticipatory guidance regarding commonly encountered school difficulties** and the consequences of school failure (e.g., low self-esteem).

3. **Alleviation of guilt and anxiety.**

4. **Explaining the legal rights of students and families.**

5. **Guidance regarding the lack of effectiveness of nontraditional treatment strategies** (e.g., dietary manipulation, optometric training).

6. **Offering advice regarding specific behavior management strategies,** such as time-out and positive reinforcement.

C. The primary care clinician can assume an active role in monitoring the progress of children with learning problems. Office visits provide important opportunities to monitor self-esteem, search for signs of depression, and offer encouragement and praise for progress.

Bibliography

For Parents

Publications

Learning Disabilities and Children: What Parents Need to Know. Elk Grove Village Il: American Academy of Pediatrics, 1989.

Silver LB. *Attention Deficit-Hyperactivity Disorder and Learning Disabilities—Booklet for Parents.* Summit NJ: CIBA-GEIGY, 1990.

Silver LB. *The Misunderstood Child: A Guide for Parents of Learning Disabled Children.* New York: McGraw-Hill, 1984.

Organizations

Association for Children and Adults with Learning Disabilities, 4156 Library Road, Pittsburgh, Pennsylvania 15234; (412) 341-8077.

Council for Exceptional Children, 1920 Association Drive, Preston, Virginia 22091; (703) 620-3660.

Foundation for Children with Learning Disabilities, 99 Park Avenue, 6th Floor, New York, New York 10016; (212) 687-7211.

For Professionals

Dworkin PH. *Learning and Behavior Problems of Schoolchildren.* Philadelphia: Saunders, 1985.

Dworkin PH. School failure. *Pediatr Rev* 10:301–312, 1989.

Levine MD. Neurodevelopmental variation and dysfunction among school-aged children. In MD Levine, WB Carey, AC Crocker (eds), *Developmental-Behavioral Pediatrics* (2nd ed). Philadelphia: Saunders, 1992.

School Readiness

Judith S. Palfrey

I. **Description of the problem.** "School readiness" implies preordained criteria for school entry. Table 56-1 lists the skills typically considered prerequisites for entrance into kindergarten and first grade. The child who is not ready for school may not have attained the majority of these skills. There are a number of factors to consider when assessing academic readiness.

   A. **Lack of experience/stimulation/opportunity.** Children whose families are over-burdened by poverty, violence, and stress may not have been provided with the experiences that promote early academic skills. Children who do not have access to books, writing materials, and educational games in their homes and day care centers, for example, will not acquire the preacademic basics. Moreover, children whose parents have low expectations for their learning capacities will not be encouraged to explore such materials, even if they are available.

   B. **Specific cognitive disabilities.** Some children will not meet the expected pre-academic milestones because they have specific cognitive and learning deficits. Children may have expressive and/or receptive language delays, visual-motor integration problems, memory difficulties, or attentional concerns that keep them from mastering early material. Oromotor, fine, and gross motor problems may hinder children from expressing what they actually know.

   C. **Socioemotional problems.** Some youngsters are not ready for a traditional school because of emotional problems. For them, the regimentation of a school day—standing in line, sitting at a little table, listening to the teacher, sharing with other children, taking turns—proves to be intolerable. Their inability to master such tasks may be rooted in family problems, posttraumatic stress, or other environmental risks.

   D. **Immaturity.** A common presentation to pediatric clinicians at the time of school entrance is the issue of "immaturity." The school or family may be worried that the child acts younger than his or her chronological age and is not ready for a group setting. This question is often raised, but few children fall into this category. It is critical that the primary care clinician rule out specific developmental and emotional difficulties before assigning the child to the "immature" category.

   When a child does manifest immature behavior (such as thumb sucking, dependence on a "blanky" or special stuffed animal, clinging to parents), it is helpful to consider the reasons the child is persisting in these behaviors. First-born children may take on these babyish behaviors in order to stay close to home. This is especially relevant when there is a younger sibling who is vying for parental attention. The last-born children may be "babied" by parents who are trying to avoid the empty-nest syndrome. In such cases, the child should enter school to validate the desire to mature rather than the desire to remain a baby.

   E. **Shyness.** Children who are shy may also be considered "immature." While these children do need minor interventions to ensure a smooth transition into school, a call to the school to alert the teacher of the child's temperament and the importance of a supportive transition team is often all that is needed.

II. **Making the diagnosis.** In thinking about school readiness, the clinician should consider the following questions:
   • Does the child have a previously unrecognized developmental or behavioral problem?
   • Is the child delayed in all areas of functioning?

Table 56-1. School readiness skills

Kindergarten
Knows color names
Identifies some uppercase letters
Identifies numbers 1–10
Writes first name legibly
Copies two-part figures
Can count items one by one
Plays cooperatively

First grade
Knows address and birthdate
Recognizes all letters (upper- and lowercase)
Knows the sounds made by some letters ("buh" for *B*, etc.)
Reads a few simple words
Understands concepts of "more" and "less"
Can engage in projects with another child
Understands jokes

• Has the child had adequate preschool exposure?
• Is the school ready for the child?

A. History. A developmentally oriented history is an important component of the workup. It is also helpful to have input from the child's preschool or day care center. The following questions can steer the investigation. The list is not exhaustive but suggests the types of triggers that allow the clinician to probe for language, motor, cognitive, and emotional problems.

B. Key clinical questions

1. *Has the child followed a normal developmental trajectory (e.g., normal motor, language, and socioemotional milestones)?*

2. *Has the child had preschool experience?*

3. *Were there any developmental or behavioral concerns in preschool?*

4. *Does the child know colors, numbers, and letters?*

5. *Does the child play well with peers?*

6. *Is the child toilet trained? Are there any babyish behaviors (e.g., thumb sucking, pacifiers, bottle, "blanky")?*

7. *Is the child's language intelligible?*

8. *Does he or she understand the point of simple stories?*

9. *Can he or she spend extended periods away from parents?*

10. *Can the child dress himself or herself (e.g., button buttons, tie shoes)?*

C. Physical examination. The physical examination should be thorough, with attention directed to the child's size and growth (would he or she be the smallest or largest child in the intended class?), head circumference, vision, hearing, any signs of organic illness, neurologic status, and neurodevelopmental maturation. It is particularly helpful to document handedness and the presence or absence of excessive overflow movements and discoordination on fine and gross motor maneuvers. While soft neurologic signs are not indicative of serious problems, when combined with other features of developmental delay they may indicate a more substantial problem that warrants further investigation.

D. Developmental testing. In the context of parental questioning about school readiness, developmental testing is very much in order. The use of formal developmental screening tools (such as the Denver Developmental Screening Test II

Table 56-2. Pros and cons of retaining children

Pro	Con
The child is youngest in class; retention will make him or her the oldest in the new class.	Somebody has to be the youngest. If December babies are retained, November babies will become the youngest.
If child has minor academic weaknesses, repetition of material may be of modest benefit.	Repetition of academic material with no new interventions. Bright children will be bored and may act out.
Child who is small, shy, and still showing babyish tendencies may catch up physically and emotionally.	Large children will "stick out" in younger grades
Older boys in junior high and high school have some advantages (sports, etc.)	

[DDST-II]) can assist the primary care clinician in deciding if extended assessment is required. Alternatively, the clinician may prefer to use an informal set of questions to review the need for further assessment. Whether such extended assessments are conducted by the primary care clinician or a referral is made to a local psychoeducator or psychologist, it is imperative that the child's strengths and weaknesses be reviewed in all developmental areas.

III. Management

A. Children with specific developmental disabilities. If the school readiness work-up turns up specific developmental findings, the management hinges on attending to these. Generally, the child can enter the age-appropriate grade (kindergarten or first grade) as long as the appropriate developmental services are obtained, either as adjuncts to their school placement or integrated into their regular school day.

B. Children with mental retardation. School entry is a common time for families to come to terms with the fact that their child is globally delayed or mentally retarded. Often the full extent of the child's problems have been minimized in the playlike environment of preschool or an early intervention program. Management strategies for these children should include specific interventions targeted to their educational needs, as well as continued socialization in the least restrictive environment.

C. Children with behavioral concerns. Two groups of children raise prominent behavior issues at the school entry point: those with acting-out behaviors and those who appear socially inept or shy. In most cases, adaptations can be made to accommodate both groups. Sometimes, however, a child's acting out may be so severe and dangerous that a special placement is warranted. Similarly, there are rare children who are so socially and emotionally withdrawn that placement in a therapeutic day care or transition environment is helpful.

D. Schools that are not ready for children. The stickiest management question is what to do when the school is not ready for the child. Some school systems do not have adequate resources for children with special behavioral, developmental, or medical needs. Some cannot offer the additional services that environmentally disadvantaged children require. Most cannot meet the new demands of the ever-enlarging immigrant population. In these situations, the primary care clinician often needs to take an advocate's stance and demand that the school provide more appropriate opportunities for the child.

E. Holding back. Another thorny issue is the notion that children who are the youngest in the classroom are at risk for poor early school performance and lifelong self-esteem problems. This theory has led to a common practice (particularly in middle-class communities) of holding "December babies" back an extra year in preschool or kindergarten, particularly if they are boys. The clinician should be involved in reviewing the pros and cons of such decisions (Table 56-2).

If possible, the family should obtain the birthdates of all the children in the class. If their child is truly much younger than all the others, having him or her enter a class with children closer chronologically may make sense. The child's size also should be considered. If he or she is already quite big and would stick out physically as the oldest and the biggest if held back, that might be a strong factor for going forward. The family should also review similar situations with other family members. What has been the pattern with cousins, siblings, uncles, and others? How have they fared? Finally, the cultural norm of the town or neighborhood must be recognized. If a quarter of the child's class is being "held back," this may be a normative rather than an unusual experience.

Bibliography

For Parents
Neville H, Halaby M. *No Fault Parenting*. Tucson AZ: Body Press, 1985.

Trelease J. *The New Read Aloud Handbook*. New York: Penguin Books, 1989.

For Children
Berenstein S, Bernstein J. *The Berenstein Bears Go to School*. New York: Random House, 1978.

Mayer M. *Little Critter's This Is My School*. New York: Golden Books. 1990.

Zeifert H. *Harry Gets Ready for School*. New York: Puffin Books, 1991.

For Professionals
Bryant DM, Clifford RM, Peisner ES. Best practices for beginners: Developmental appropriateness in kindergarten. *Am Educ Res J* 28:783–803, 1991.

DeMeis JL, Stearns ES. Relationship of school entrance age to academic performance. *J Educ Res* 86:20–27, 1992.

Dworkin PH. School readiness. *Curr Opin Pediatr* 3:786–791, 1991.

Palfrey JS, Rappaport LR. School placement. *Pediatr Rev* 8:261–270, 1987.

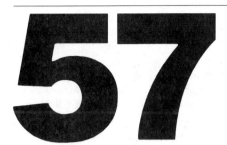

Self-Esteem

Robert B. Brooks

I. Description of the problem. Self-esteem plays a significant role in virtually every sphere of a child's development and functioning. Performance in school, the quality of peer relationships, the ease and effectiveness of dealing with mistakes and failure, the motivation to persevere at tasks, and the abuse of drugs and alcohol are behaviors influenced by a child's self-esteem. Given its importance and the number of children who are burdened by low self-esteem, it is a worthwhile goal of the primary care clinician to become knowledgeable about effective strategies to foster a child's sense of self-worth and competence.

Some clinicians have proposed that self-esteem is a product of the difference between our "ideal self," or how we would like to be and what we would like to accomplish, and how we actually see ourselves—the larger the difference, the lower our self-esteem. A broader definition was offered by the California Task Force to Promote Self-Esteem and Personal and Social Responsibility, which envisioned self-esteem not only in terms of "appreciating my own worth and importance" but also "having the character to be accountable for myself and to act responsibly toward others." This definition incorporates the respect and caring we show toward others as a basic feature of self-esteem, thereby lessening the possibility that self-esteem will be confused with conceit or self-centeredness.

A. Etiology/contributing factors

1. **Parent-child mismatch.** The development of self-esteem is a complex process that can best be understood as occurring within the dynamic interaction between a child's inborn temperament and the environmental forces that affect the child. "Mismatches" between the style and temperament of caregivers and children may trigger anger and disappointment in both parties. In such a situation children may come to believe that they have disappointed others, that they are failures, or that others are unfair and unkind. Low self-esteem is a common result unless parents are able to lessen the impact of these mismatches by understanding and appreciating their child's unique make-up and by modifying their own expectations and reactions so that they are more in concert with their child's temperament.

2. **Attribution theory.** Attribution theory is one promising framework for articulating the components of self-esteem by looking at the reasons that people offer for why they think they succeeded or failed at a task or situation. The explanations given are directly linked to an individual's self-esteem. It appears that children with high self-esteem perceive their successes as determined in large part by their own efforts, resources, and abilities. These children assume realistic credit for their achievements and possess a sense of personal control over what is occurring in their lives. In contrast, children with low self-esteem often believe that their successes are the result of luck or chance, that is, factors outside their control. Such a view lessens their confidence in being successful in the future.

   Self-esteem also plays a role in how children understand mistakes and failures in their lives. Children with high self-esteem typically believe that mistakes are experiences to learn from rather than to feel defeated by. Mistakes are attributed to factors within their power to change, such as a lack of effort on a realistically attainable goal. On the other hand, children with low self-esteem, when faced with failure, tend to believe that they cannot remedy the situation. They believe that mistakes result from situations that are unmodifiable, such as a lack of ability, and this belief generates

Table 57-1. Counterproductive coping strategies: Signs of low self-esteem

Behavior	Example
Quitting	Ending a game before it is over to avoid losing
Avoiding	Not even trying something for fear of failure
Cheating	Copying answers from someone else on a test
Clowning around	Acting silly to minimize feeling like a failure
Controlling	Telling others what to do
Bullying	Putting others down to hide feelings of inadequacy
Denying	Minimizing the importance of a task
Rationalizing or making excuses	Blaming the teacher for failing a test

a feeling of helplessness and hopelessness. This profound sense of inadequacy makes future success less likely because these children expect to fail and begin to retreat from age-expected demands, relying instead on self-defeating coping strategies.

Attribution theory has significant implications for designing interventions for reinforcing the self-esteem of children. It serves as a blueprint for asking the following questions: (1) How do we create an environment in homes and schools that maximizes the opportunity for children not only to succeed but to believe that their accomplishments are predicated in great measure on their own abilities and efforts? (2) How do we create an environment that reinforces the belief in children that mistakes and failure often form the very foundation for learning and growth—that mistakes are not only *accepted* but *expected?*

II. **Making the diagnosis.** The signs of low self-esteem and their emergence vary considerably. Children may display low self-esteem in situations in which they feel less than competent but not in those in which they are more successful. For instance, children with a learning disability may feel "dumb" in the classroom but may engage in sports with confidence. For some children, a sense of low self-esteem is so pervasive that there are few, if any, situations in which low self-esteem is not manifested.

With some children there is little question that their self-esteem is low. They say such things as, "I'm dumb," "I hate how I look," "I never do anything right," "I always fail," "I'm a born loser," "I'll always be stupid." Other children do not directly express their low self-esteem. Rather, it can be inferred from the coping strategies they use to handle stress and pressure. Children with high self-esteem use strategies for coping that are adaptive and promote growth (such as a child having difficulty mastering long division who asks for additional help from a teacher).

In contrast, children with low self-esteem often rely on coping behaviors that are counterproductive and intensify the child's difficulties. These self-defeating behaviors often signal that the child is feeling vulnerable and is desperately attempting to escape from the problematic situations. Commonly used self-defeating coping behaviors are listed in Table 57-1. Although all children at some time engage in some of these behaviors, it is when these behaviors appear with regularity that a significant problem with self-esteem is suggested.

III. **Management**

A. **Primary goals.** The strategies that follow have the greatest chance of being effective if adults convey to the child a sense of hope, caring, and support. These strategies should also take into consideration the child's "islands of competence," that is, areas that are (or have the potential to be) sources of pride and accomplishment. Caregivers have the responsibility to identify and build on these islands of competence, and, in so doing, a ripple effect may occur that prompts children to be more willing to venture forth and confront the tasks that have been problematic for them.

B. **Selected strategies for fostering self-esteem**

1. **Developing responsibility and making a contribution.** If children are to develop a sense of ownership and commitment, it is important to provide them with opportunities for assuming responsibilities, especially those that involve helping them to feel that they are capable and are contributing in some way to their world and that they are truly making a difference. For example:

   - Asking an 8-year-old to set the table at dinner or a 4-year-old to place his or her clothes in the laundry bag at the end of each day—requests framed as ways of helping the family.
   - Encouraging and helping a child to write a story about his or her learning disability to be used to increase the understanding of others about the challenges faced by children with learning problems.
   - Asking a sixth grader with low self-esteem who enjoyed interacting with younger children to tutor first and second graders in the school or to be a babysitter.
   - Enlisting children to participate in a "Walk for Hunger" charity drive.

2. **Providing opportunities for making choices and decisions and solving problems.** An essential ingredient of high self-esteem is the belief that one has some control over the events of one's life. To reinforce this belief, adults must provide children with opportunities to make choices and decisions and to solve problems that have an impact on their lives. These kinds of choices promote a sense of personal control and ownership. For example:

   - A clinician allowing a fearful child the choice of having his or her eyes or ears examined first so that the child is provided a sense of control.
   - Parents permitting a finicky eater to select (and eventually help prepare) the dinner meal at least once a week.
   - Having a group of elementary school students interview a town selectman, a police officer, and a lawyer as part of the process to decide whether skateboards should be allowed on school grounds, especially given the possible liability issues.
   - Parents asking their children whether they wanted to be reminded 10 or 15 minutes before bedtime that soon it will be time to get ready to go to bed.
   - A teenager deciding at what time parents may remind him or her to take medication, should he or she forget to do so.

3. **Offering encouragement and positive feedback and helping children to feel special.** Self-esteem is nurtured when adults communicate appreciation and encouragement to children, but such communication often fails to occur. Words and actions conveying encouragement and thanks are always welcome and energizing. They are especially important for children burdened by self-doubt. Even a seemingly small gesture of appreciation can trigger a longlasting, positive effect. For example:

   - Parents setting up a "special" 15-minute time in the evening with each of their two young children. The time can occur before each child goes to bed. The parents can highlight the importance of this time by calling it "special" and by saying that even if the telephone rings they will not respond to the call but instead will let the answering machine do so.
   - A primary care clinician sending a postcard to a child after an examination, saying how much she or he enjoyed seeing the child (as long as this is an honest sentiment).
   - Parents writing a brief note to their child commending the child for a particular accomplishment.
   - A recognition assembly in school in which student achievements and contributions are highlighted.

4. **Establishing self-discipline.** If children are to develop high self-esteem, they must also possess a comfortable sense of self-discipline, which involves the ability to reason and to reflect on one's behavior and its impact on others. The goal of discipline is to teach children, not to ridicule or humiliate them. If children are to take ownership for their actions, they must be increasingly involved in the process of understanding and even contributing to the rules, guidelines, limits, and consequences that are established. Adults must main-

tain a delicate balance between being too rigid and too permissive. They must strive to blend warmth, nurturance, and acceptance with realistic expectations, clear-cut rules, and logical consequences. In addition, if children are continuously misbehaving, the adults in their lives should attempt to understand why and focus on ways to prevent misbehavior from occurring in the first place. Examples of the effective use of discipline—including those that emphasize a preventive approach—are:

• Parents having difficulty getting a preschool child to bed. They yelled at him, but this only made matters worse. A consultation with a clinician revealed that the child was having nightmares and was frightened about going to bed. Greater empathy on the part of the parents and the use of a night-light, as well as placing a photo of the parents next to the child's bed, significantly lessened his anxiety and misbehavior.

• Parents not permitting their child to use the bike for several days after she had taken a bike ride on a dangerous street that she was not allowed to ride on (an example of the use of logical consequences).

• Parents asking a child who bounced a ball that broke a window in the house to help pay for the repairs.

5. **Teaching children to deal with mistakes and failure.** The fear of making mistakes and feeling embarrassed is a potent obstacle to meeting challenges, taking appropriate risks, and therefore, to the achievement of positive self-esteem. Caregivers should find ways to communicate to children that mistakes go hand in glove with growing and learning. Examples of helping children to deal more effectively with mistakes include:

• Parents who avoid overreacting to their children's mistakes and who avoid remarks such as: "Why don't you use your brain?" or "What a stupid thing to do!"

• Adults who share what they personally learned from mistakes and failures during their own childhood.

• A teacher who on the first day of the new school year asks students, "Who thinks they will probably make a mistake or not understand something in class this year?" Then, before any of the children can respond, the teacher raises his or her own hand. Acknowledging openly the fear of failure renders it less potent and less destructive and increases the child's courage to face new tasks.

Bibliography

For Parents
Bettner B, Lew A. *Raising Children Who Can.* Newton MA: Connexions Press, 1989.

Black K. How to boost your child's self-esteem. *New Woman Magazine* 22:116–123, 1992.

Briggs DC. *Your Child's Self-Esteem.* Garden City NY: Doubleday, 1970.

Brooks RB. *The Self-Esteem Teacher.* Circle Pines MN: American Guidance Service, 1991.

For Professionals
California State Department of Education. *Toward a State of Esteem: The Final Report of the Task Force to Promote Self-Esteem and Personal and Social Responsibility.* Sacramento: California State Department of Education, 1990.

Coopersmith S. *The Antecedents of Self-Esteem.* Palo Alto CA: Consulting Psychologists Press, 1981.

58

Sex and the Adolescent

Linda Grant

I. **Description of the problem.** Sexuality is present from birth. Its expression is the result of a complex interplay of biologic, psychological, interpersonal, and social factors, each with varying importance as the child grows up. In adolescence, the newly discovered ability to engage in sexual activity implies neither the cognitive and emotional maturity to deal with intimacy nor an understanding of its negative consequences (such as premature pregnancy and sexually transmitted diseases). It is the role of the primary care clinician to guide the adolescent in *responsible sexual decision making*.

A. **Epidemiology**

1. **Teenage pregnancy**
   - The United States has a higher rate of teenage pregnancy than any other industrialized country.
   - There are over 1 million pregnancies in 15–19 year olds annually. Approximately half of these are carried to term, and the other half are therapeutically or spontaneously terminated.

2. **Sexual experience**
   - There is no one profile of adolescent sexuality. Trends in coital initiation and continuation of sexual activity reflect differing ethnic and sex-specific rates. In general, the majority of adolescents are virginal at age 15 years; by age 19 years, approximately 55% of all whites and 75% of all blacks are coitally experienced.
   - Males consistently report earlier coital initiation than females.
   - Noncoital sexual behaviors vary by ethnic group. Studies indicate that white adolescents, in general, start with petting behaviors and move to greater intimacy in a sequential manner; black adolescents are more likely to engage in intercourse sooner and without much initial petting behaviors.

3. **Sexually transmitted diseases**
   - The 15–24-year-old age group has a higher rate of most sexually transmitted diseases (e.g., gonorrhea, chlamydia, pelvic inflammatory disease) than any other age group.
   - The rate of syphilis has increased by 28% for females in the past decade.
   - 25% of 20–29 year olds who have AIDS were infected during their adolescence.

B. **Developmental considerations**

1. **Dealing with body changes.** Adolescents must learn to be comfortable with their new physical identity. Puberty is a time when they come to terms with a changing body and bewildering emotions fueled by hormonal surges. The reproductive capacity is present before emotional and cognitive maturity have developed.

2. **Developing a separate identity.** The adolescent must develop an identity that is separate from the family. Sexual behavior is often viewed as a rite of passage into adulthood and as a way to become a distinct entity from the family. As adolescents separate from the family, they develop replacement relationships with their peers.

3. **Developing intimate relationships.** Another task of adolescence is to achieve the capacity to develop intimate and meaningful mutual relationships. Early

269

relationships may involve physical intimacy as a means of comparison and experimentation. Later, with the addition of formal operational thinking, emotional intimacy and reciprocity can be incorporated into relationships.

4. **Developing the ability to think abstractly.** Concrete operational thinking dominates early and mid-adolescence. Therefore, young adolescents are incapable of fully understanding the ramifications of their actions. This, coupled with a sense of infallibility and invulnerability, heightens the risk for sexual activity. Formal operational thinking, which develops around age 15 years, allows the adolescent to generate a more appropriate decision-making tree and to develop abstract thinking on moral values.

5. **Personality characteristics.** The degree of any risk-taking behavior in adolescence is mitigated by the individual's personality profile. In general those with low self-esteem, a tolerance for deviant behavior, and a propensity for sensation seeking are at highest risk. Those who place a high value on achievement and future orientation and who have strong religious beliefs are generally in lower-risk categories.

II. Making the diagnosis

A. **History.** The key to engaging adolescents is providing a trusting, confidential, nonjudgmental, and honest atmosphere. In order for adolescents to talk about their risk behaviors with the primary care clinician, they must be assured that disclosure will not compromise their relationships with their family, their friends, or the community. Adolescents often resist medical visits because they fear that the information will be shared with the parent. It is important to establish with them that what is said will be confidential and to inform them of any qualifying parameters. For example, when an adolescent's or another's safety is jeopardized (as in suicidal or homicidal ideation, physical or sexual abuse, and life-threatening illnesses), confidentiality may need to be breached. Informing the adolescent and his or her parent of these guidelines at the initial visit allows for a clarifying discussion of safety, communication, and trust. Clinicians should be aware of their state's statutes regarding mature and emancipated minors.

The sexual history should be part of a larger sociologic history that screens for all risk behaviors. The goal of a sexual history is to determine if there has been sexual activity and if so, the degree of health or emotional risk involved. Questioning needs to be direct and comprehensive. The clinician should make no *a priori* assumptions about the sexual activity, practices, or sexual orientation of any adolescent.

B. **Key clinical questions**

1. *Are you currently in a relationship?*

2. *Does this relationship include having sex?*

3. *What kind of protection do you use to avoid pregnancy and sexually transmitted diseases?*

4. *Have you ever had any sexually transmitted disease?*

5. *How many partners have you had?*

6. *How old were you when you first had intercourse?*

7. *What made you decide to have sex?*

8. *Has anyone ever forced you to have sex?*

9. *Have you ever been pregnant? What happened to the pregnancy?* or *Have you ever fathered a child?*

10. *Have you ever had sex with someone of the same sex?*

11. *Have you ever had rectal or oral sex?*

12. *Is sex an enjoyable experience for you?*

13. *Tell me what you know about AIDS.*

14. *What do you know about the different methods of birth control?*

15. *How do you feel about not being sexually active?*

C. **Physical examination**

1. **Pelvic examination.** A pelvic examination is appropriate in any adolescent who is sexually active, no matter what the age. There is some debate, however, as to when to initiate a pelvic examination in an adolescent who is *not* sexually active. Variables to consider include the patient's request, the nature of the gynecologic complaint, and the gynecologic versus chronologic age of the adolescent. For the young, virginal adolescent with a gynecologic complaint, external visualization and bimanual rectal palpation and/or pelvic ultrasound may be adequate.

   The development of a positive attitude toward pelvic examinations begins with the first. It is helpful to have the adolescent as involved as possible so that she feels in control of the process. For example, she can be asked if she wants to look at her cervix and external genitalia in a hand-held mirror. She should also be told that the examination will be stopped if she feels pain, and she should describe any discomfort. Each step should be anticipated so that there are no surprises.

   As the examination proceeds, the clinician should continue a relaxing and empowering dialogue, such as: "In order to see your cervix, the opening into your uterus, I need you to relax your muscles as much as possible. By taking deep breaths and focusing on relaxing your muscles, your vagina will open wider and the exam will be more comfortable."

2. **Male genitalia examination.** The male examination may be anxiety provoking for the adolescent, especially when the practitioner is female (as may be the pelvic examination performed by a male). Explanations and demonstrations of testicular self-examination as well as reassurance of normality help to relieve the anxiety. The male should be examined while standing, and it is helpful and educational to describe anatomic findings as a diversion during the examination. It is not necessary to comment on an erection unless the adolescent seems particularly embarrassed by it. The normality of the examination should always be stressed.

D. **Tests.** If an adolescent is sexually active, there should be routine screening for sexually transmitted diseases (STDs). In females this means at least yearly testing for gonorrhea and chlamydia. (However, screening intervals should take into account the epidemiology of the community.) Rectal and pharyngeal gonococcal cultures should be performed if there is a history of oral or rectal sex. A PAP smear should be performed annually. Males can be screened for asymptomatic STDs using urine dipstick testing for leukocyte esterase in areas of high STD prevalence. Both males and females should have syphilis serology testing. Adolescents should be aware of and have access to confidential and anonymous human immunodeficiency virus testing.

III. **Management**

A. **Anticipatory guidance.** Anticipatory guidance about sexual issues should be a part of routine health care maintenance throughout childhood (Table 58-1) and adolescence (Table 58-2). Thoughtful, knowledgeable, and developmentally appropriate parental guidance as well as preparation of young children allow for a more natural dialogue about sexual issues at puberty.

B. **Addressing adolescent sexuality**

1. **Primary goals.** The primary goals are to promote a healthy sexual attitude, to decrease sexual risk behaviors, and to assist parents in dealing with their child's sexuality.

2. **Developmental level.** Throughout adolescence, the progression of cognitive and emotional development influences sexual practices. A 13 year old deals with sexuality in a different way than does a 19 year old. The older teenager may better understand the repercussions of unprotected sex, be less dominated by the need for romantic spontaneity, and may begin to examine differential benefits and risks of various birth control methods. The younger teenager tends to be dominated more by immediate gratification, spontaneity,

Table 58-1. Preadolescent sexuality anticipatory guidance

Age	Sexuality issues and development	Parental concerns	Areas of anticipatory guidance
Pre-natal	Fetuses have been shown to suck their fingers in utero	"I don't care if it's a boy or girl as long as it's healthy"	Sex stereotyping: expectations for male-female differences in behavior are present even before birth. Awareness of this allows for later dialogue about expressions of individuality.
		"If it's a boy, what about circumcision?"	Discussing circumcision provides an introduction to discussing sexually related topics.
		"Should I breast feed?"	Breast-feeding discussions help emphasize importance of body contact. It is also important to stress importance of paternal body contact, cuddling, stroking.
2 wk	Temperament	"When I change the baby, his wee-wee stands up. Am I stimulating him too much?"	Use appropriate genitalia names (*penis, vagina, clitoris*) during the examination. This facilitates discussions as child ages.
			Infants and children enjoy and respond to touch but not with the same sexual/erotic context as adults. It is unlikely that normal touching is ever overstimulating at this age.
2 mo	Bonding	"I feel sexually aroused when I nurse."	Parents (both father and mother) may have erotic sensations and dreams about their child, especially in the first few months. This is normal. (Acting on one's fantasies with a child is not.)
		"My wife and I don't have a relationship like we used to."	The postpartum period is often a stressful time in a previously happy relationship. The clinician may be the only medical provider involved with the family at this point and can help the parents recognize and deal with the changes a new baby brings, including changes in sexual activity.
4–6 mo	Genital play initiation Body exploration	"My son plays with his penis when I change his diaper."	Exploration of the body (toes, fingers, genitalia) is a normal aspect of human development. Self-pleasuring (thumb sucking, genital manipulation) is a natural extension of this. Masturbation continues throughout life. Start discussions early.
9–12 mo	Avoidance of stigmatization	"I'm afraid to let my daughter go without a diaper at the beach because she plays with herself."	As with other social behaviors (e.g., eating, play) sexuality and its expression must be shaped into a social context. This is a process that starts at this age and proceeds gradually to ages 3–4 yr. Shame, doubt, and confusion result from inappropriate expectations.

Table 58-1 (continued)

Age	Sexuality issues and development	Parental concerns	Areas of anticipatory guidance
12–15 mo	Sex-stereo-typed play	"I bought my son a doll, but he only wants to play with trucks."	Most parents would like their daughters to achieve to their abilities and sons to be empathetic and caring. Responding to the child's individuality rather than trying to alter sex-specific behaviors is the appropriate path to this goal.
18 mo	Toilet training	"I want her out of diapers before this baby is born."	Toilet training should be initiated on the child's schedule of readiness, not the parents'.
2–3 yr	Anatomical comparisons	"He's asking questions. What should I say?"	Simple but accurate explanations are best. If a child wants to know more and if the answer is straightforward, he or she will generally ask more. Pregnancy is a fascination; sibling births provide opportunities to discuss reproduction as well as feelings. Toddlers are very much aware of the anatomical similarities with the same-sex parent and the contrasts with the opposite-sex parent. They identify their concept of gender role in this manner.
	Relationships	"My son saw my husband and I having sex. Is that bad for him?"	If intercourse is explained as a way that mothers and fathers have of showing affection and love, there is no psychological trauma for the child who interrupts his parents *in flagrante delicto*. Parents should initiate discussions of privacy and closed doors.
3–4 yr	Family flirtation	"My daughter flirts with my husband. Is this normal?"	Family members are the child's source of learning about human relationships. This is a time of magical thinking when children imagine marrying their opposite-sex parent. At this time children can begin to understand parental love for each other as different from a parent's love for a child.
	Sex play with peers	"I found my 4-year-old daughter with the 4-year-old neighbor boy without any clothes."	Sex play between children of the same or opposite sexes continues through childhood without harm, as long as adults remain calm when they discover their children in these games. Children at this age can begin to understand the difference between such play with same-age children and such play with adults or older children.
4–6 yr	Sexual appropriateness	"When can I teach my child about good and bad touching?"	Children at this age can understand that their bodies are their own, that sex play between adults and children is not appropriate, that children have a right to say "no" to an adult's touching if it makes them feel funny or uncomfortable or if they don't understand what's happening.

Table 58-1 (continued)

Age	Sexuality issues and development	Parental concerns	Areas of anticipatory guidance
	Modesty	"My son and daughter share a room. Is this a problem?"	The beginnings of privacy were taught with early body exploration. No matter how relaxed a child's family has been about bodies, the child's natural modesty at this age should be respected.
6–10 yr	Intimacy	"I've taken showers with my daughter since she was an infant. Should I stop this?"	Each family needs to decide what they are comfortable with and to discuss it. As long as feelings can be discussed openly, there should be no conflict or feelings of rejection if parent-child bathing is discontinued. There are many other comfortable ways for families to show affection.
			Children and parents sometimes find it comfortable to acknowledge that fantasies are common and are not a problem unless acted upon.
	Fantasy versus reality	"My 9-year-old son seems to have a crush on a 14-year-old neighbor boy. I'm concerned he might be gay."	Same-sex crushes are a normal part of development for both males and females and help consolidate gender identity. Discussion helps both child and parent appreciate normal development. Most who will continue with same-sex experiences recognize their homosexuality at this age.
	Out-of-home influences increase	"I won't let him watch the Playboy channel on cable so he goes next door and watches it."	Media influences are so pervasive that isolated censorship generally does not work. Open discussion of sexual themes in movies, magazines, and songs can help parents open conversations about attitudes that they are not comfortable with and allows their children to express their viewpoints.

and peer approval. Male-oriented methods of contraception (e.g., withdrawal and condoms) tend to be more popular with the younger age group, while middle adolescents opt for pharmacologic management, whether oral, implant, or injectable. As adolescents mature, they develop comfort with their own bodies and a better ability to assess a situation. The challenge is to interest adolescents in using condoms, in addition to whatever other method of birth control they may use.

3. **Empowerment.** Whether it is "saying NO" or requesting that a partner use a condom, all adolescents need to hear that it is their right with whom, when, and how they express their sexuality. The clinician should help them understand that sex should never be something that is "done" to them. The practitioner can role-play situations to assist these concepts. For example, he or she can strategize empowered constructive responses to typical lines, such as "It doesn't feel as good with a rubber" or "If you really loved me you'd do it with me," or "What? You're still a virgin! I can't believe it!"

4. **Sexuality and a partner.** Involving a partner in the visit can help to facilitate joint sexual decision making and may improve compliance with safer sexual practices. Males often have no understanding of the nature of a pelvic examination. Observation of the examination can be a powerful reinforcer of mutual sexual responsibility.

Table 58-2. Anticipatory guidance for adolescent sexuality

Age	Sexual areas of concern	Risk factors	Anticipatory guidance
Early adolescence, early puberty: 10–12 yr	Pubertal changes	Self-image	Gynecomastia is normal in adolescent males as is breast asynchrony in females. Such body disproportions distort adolescents' image of themselves.
			Early maturers, particularly females, need special guidance to avoid low self-esteem and premature sexual advances.
		Hormonal influences	Masturbation is a normal behavior that relieves sexual tension. Fantasies are normal while masturbating. Masturbation is a choice—teens can choose to do it or not.
Late puberty: 12–14 yr	Initiation of sexual activity without intimacy	Concrete thought Cannot perceive long-range implications of current actions	Discussions of sexual choices should emphasize that it is all right to say "no"; discussions regarding contraceptive use need to emphasize more immediate as well as long-term benefits (e.g., in addition to pregnancy prevention, oral contraceptives may relieve dysmenorrhea).
Midadolescence: 14–17 yr	Intimacy related to sexual romanticism rather than genuine commitment	Looks to peer group for support as he or she separates from family	Parents should be encouraged to continue sexual dialogue begun in latency. They should know their own values (what sex is for; who it is for; what makes it enjoyable; what makes it exploitive). Parental values should be shared with opinions, rather than judgments. Parents should respect teens' decisions.
	Sporadic or absent use of birth control; sexual experimentation	Formal operational thinking, variably applied	Teens begin to understand future implications of current actions; they know that use of birth control will protect from unwanted pregnancy, condoms will protect from sexually transmitted diseases.
		Risk taking and sense of omnipotence	Risk taking should be discussed. Once a young woman risks unprotected intercourse without becoming pregnant, she is likely to risk it again. Other risk behaviors such as drunk driving and drug use may have a negative interactive effect on sexual decision making.

Table 58-2 (continued)

Age	Sexual areas of concern	Risk factors	Anticipatory guidance
Late adolescence: 17–21 yr	Intimacy involves commitment	Family conflicts resolving as independence established	Teen begins to plan for future, including marriage and family.
		Comfort with bodies and gender identity	Relationships involve a mutual reciprocity. Counseling involves understanding of female sexual response, couple discussions of feelings.

Source: Adopted from Grant L, Efstratios D. Adolescent sexuality. *Pediatr Clin North Am* 35: 1988.

5. **Promoting condoms.** If an adolescent is sexually active, condom use should be promoted at every opportunity, no matter what the nature of the office visit is.

6. **Abstinence as a healthy choice.** An adolescent needs to hear that abstaining from sexual activity is normal and is becoming increasingly common, and that masturbation and noncoital petting are acceptable ways to relieve sexual tensions safely.

7. **Contraceptive choices.** What might work for one adolescent may not work for another, irrespective of developmental level. The best contraceptive is one that will be used; the adolescent is often the best judge of which method will work best for him or her.

8. **"Teachable moments" in daily life.** Broadcast and written media offer frequent examples of sexual subject matter. News events cover stories on sexual assault and controversies over gay and lesbian issues. Rock stars use explicit language in their lyrics, and actors have explicit love scenes. Parents and clinicians should be encouraged to use these examples to initiate conversations with their children and patients around these experiences.

9. **Advertising in the waiting room.** Adolescents may need an impetus to begin discussions of sexual issues. Availability of factual sexual information in the waiting room (e.g., posters, pamphlets, books, or fact sheets) will alert the adolescent that it is acceptable to raise these issues.

10. **School-based teaching.** School systems have become increasingly active in dealing with many adolescent behavioral issues, including sexuality. Condom availability and distribution programs, for example, have been incorporated into some health programs and have been shown to support sexual responsibility. The pediatric practitioner is in an ideal position to advocate for these services in his or her school system and help dispel the myths that open discussions of sexuality contribute to sexual risk taking.

IV. Clinical pearls and pitfalls
- A clinician must come to terms with his or her own sexuality. A clinician who is uncomfortable with gender issues or explicit sexual questions cannot effectively counsel. A practitioner who is unwilling to discuss sexuality issues objectively should have appropriate referral sources so that patients are not denied information. Alternatively, this practitioner should not see adolescent patients.
- Teenagers need guidance, not directives. A practitioner should express his or her opinions in a nonjudgmental way and allow adolescents the legitimacy of their own opinions.
- Do not assume that all sexual relationships are heterosexual. Providing literature in the waiting room on gay, lesbian, and bisexual health issues signals that the practitioner is comfortable in discussing same-sex experiences.
- The parent-practitioner relationship needs to be renegotiated prior to puberty so that parents understand confidentiality issues. Practitioners and parents should be partners in educating about sexuality.

• Sexuality is not a joking matter. Too often, adults deal with their own discomfort about sex by making jokes. Discussions with adolescents should always be serious but not somber.

Bibliography

For Parents
American Academy of Pediatrics. *A Bibliography of Educational Materials for Children, Adolescents and Families*. Elk Grove Village IL: American Academy of Pediatrics.
Order from Department of Publications, 141 NW Point Boulevard, PO Box 927, Elk Grove Village IL 60007.

Bell R. *Changing Bodies, Changing Lives*. New York: Random House, 1980.

Calderone M, Johnson EW. *The Family Book About Sexuality*. New York: Harper & Row, 1981.

Gordon S, Gordon J. *Raising a Child Conservatively in a Sexually Permissive World*. New York: Simon and Schuster, 1985.

Madras L. *What's Happening to my Body? Book for Boys*. New Market Press, 1988.

Madras L. *What's Happening to my Body? Book for Girls*. New Market Press, 1988.

TLC—Talk Listen Care Kit. Boston. Harvard Community Health Plan Foundation, 1989.
HCHP Foundation, 27 Mica Lane, Wellesley MA 02181. Can be ordered by calling (800)-TLC-KITT.

For Professionals
Grant LM, Efstratios D. Adolescent sexuality. *Pediat Clin North Am* 35:1988.

Hardy J. Premature sexual activity, pregnancy, sexually transmitted diseases: The pediatrician's role as counselor. *Pediatr Rev* 10:September 1988.

Hayes CD (ed). *Risking the Future: Adolescent Sexuality, Pregnancy and Childbearing*. Washington DC: National Academy Press, 1987.

59

Sexual Abuse
Deborah Madansky

I. **Description of the problem.** Sexual abuse is defined as the engagement of a child in sexual contact or activities that the child cannot comprehend, for which the child is developmentally unprepared and cannot give informed consent, and/or that violate societal, legal, and social taboos. The activity occurs for the gratification of the older individual and may include forms of anal, genital, and oral contact to or by the child, and exhibitionism, voyeurism, or using the child for the production of pornography. Force is often not involved, but coercion or threats may be.

A. **Epidemiology**
- The true prevalence is unknown since most cases go unreported. In retrospective surveys of adults, about 25% of women and 15% of men report sexual contact with an adult during childhood or adolescence.
- 40% of reported cases of child abuse and neglect involve sexual abuse.
- 75% of reported victims are female, but there is evidence that male victims are less likely to report.
- Male perpetrators are more common.
- The vast majority of perpetrators are known to the child.
- Sexual abuse crosses all socioeconomic, ethnic, and racial lines.

B. **Contributing factors.** Children at higher risk are those with a diminished capacity to resist or disclose, such as preverbal, developmentally delayed, or physically handicapped children, and children in dysfunctional or reconstituted families.

II. **Making the diagnosis**

A. **Presentations of child sexual abuse**

1. **Acute assault.** A child presenting within 72 hours of an assault should be referred to an emergency room, where forensic specimens may be collected.

2. **In the pediatric office**

a. The child is **referred by protective services or law enforcement** for a medical evaluation as part of an investigation.

b. The child is **referred by a family member** who is aware of or suspects sexual abuse.

c. The child is **seen for a routine examination** or medical and behavioral complaint where the differential diagnosis includes sexual abuse.

B. **Signs and symptoms**

1. **Specific indicators**

a. **Genital or rectal pain, bleeding, trauma, or infection.**

b. **Sexually transmitted diseases** (Table 59-1).

c. **Developmentally inappropriate sexual behavior in young children,** such as engagement in intercourse, oral sex, or sexual coercion.

d. **Compulsive masturbation.**

2. **Behavioral indicators** are nonspecific and similar to symptoms due to other stressors:

a. **Fears and phobias,** especially of circumstances similar to the abuse.

Table 59-1. Implications of commonly encountered sexually transmitted diseases for the diagnosis and reporting of sexual abuse of prepubertal infants and children

STD confirmed	Sexual abuse	Suggested action
Gonorrhea[a]	Certain	Report[b]
Syphilis[a]	Certain	Report
Chlamydia[a]	Probable[c]	Report
Condylomata acuminatum[a]	Probable	Report
Trichomonas vaginalis	Probable	Report
Herpes 1 (genital)	Possible	Report[d]
Herpes 2	Probable	Report
Bacterial vaginosis	Uncertain	Medical follow-up
Candida albicans	Unlikely	Medical follow-up

[a] If not perinatally acquired.
[b] To agency mandated in community to receive reports of suspected sexual abuse.
[c] Culture only reliable diagnostic method.
[d] Unless there is a clear history of autoinoculation.
Source: Reprinted with permission from the American Academy of Pediatrics Committee on Child Abuse and Neglect. Guidelines for the evaluation of sexual abuse of children. *Pediatrics* 87(2):254–260, 1991.

    b. Nightmares and other sleep disturbances.

    c. Appetite disturbance or eating disorders.

    d. Enuresis or encopresis.

    e. Change in behavior, attitude, or school performance.

    f. Depression, withdrawal, or suicidality.

    g. Excessive anger, aggression, or running away.

    h. Promiscuous behavior or substance abuse.

  3. Some children may have **posttraumatic stress disorder,** whose diagnostic criteria include having the following symptoms for at least 1 month's duration:

    a. Reexperiencing the traumatic event, such as in recurrent dreams, flashback memories, or repetitive traumatic play.

    b. Persistent avoidance of certain stimuli or numbing of general responses.

    c. Persistent symptoms of increased arousal, such as difficulty falling or staying asleep, irritability or angry outbursts, difficulty concentrating, hypervigilance, exaggerated startle, or physiologic reactivity to a memory of the event.

C. History

  1. The **parent or guardian** should be interviewed alone regarding his or her concerns, the child's disclosures or complaints, and a review of the child's medical, developmental, emotional, and behavioral status. The clinician should ask specifically about:

    a. The child's disclosures.

    b. Content of sexual play with peers, adults, or dolls.

    c. Masturbation or genital fondling.

    d. Genital complaints or symptoms.

    e. Toileting difficulties.

    f. Sleep disturbances (difficulty falling asleep, night waking, nightmares).

    g. Behavioral difficulties or changes.

    h. School performance.

2. The **child** should be interviewed, unless he or she has already been interviewed or is too young or unwilling to talk. Follow this sequence.

    a. Interview the child alone, and record the child's statements. (The parent may be the perpetrator, or even if not, children often are uncomfortable speaking to a parent.)

    b. Sit at eye level and take time to establish rapport with neutral topics (e.g., ask about the child's living situation, pets, school, favorite activities, etc.).

    c. Gear the discussion to the child's developmental level, and use his or her own terms for body parts. (For young children, dolls or line drawings may be helpful.)

    d. Introduce the topic of possible sexual abuse in a general way, such as, "Is there anything that you feel uncomfortable about that you would like to talk about?" or "I know you have had to leave your family and are now in a foster home. Can you tell me how that happened?" If these opening questions do not result in a spontaneous account, inquire more specifically, "Has anyone touched you or bothered you in a way that made you feel uncomfortable?" or "Lots of children come to see me because someone touched them in a way they didn't like. Did that ever happen to you?" If the child says, "Yes," then ask, "What happened?" Use nonleading questions, such as *what, who, where,* and *when.* Avoid any demonstration of emotion, pressure, or correction of the child. Have a "then what happened/ tell me more" approach.

    e. Be aware that **disclosures may take place during the physical examination** as the affected body parts are examined.

    f. Document what the child says verbatim in the record. Videotaped interviews are usually conducted by protective services or law enforcement and are probably unwise in the pediatric office.

    g. Reassure the child that it was okay to tell you, and whatever happened was not his or her fault.

D. Physical examination. Do a complete physical examination. This allows a familiar context for the child, opportunities for further rapport, and screening for other problems.

    1. **Genital examination**

        a. Be aware of examination positions (supine frogleg, prone knee-chest, lithotomy) and techniques (labial separation, labial traction).

        b. Use a good light source with magnification, such as an otoscope head, hand-held or headpiece lens, magnifying fluorescent light, or colposcope.

        c. Be aware of genital anatomy and normal developmental variations:

            (1) All girls are born with a hymen.

            (2) Newborn hymens are fleshy and redundant secondary to maternal estrogen effect.

            (3) Prepubertal hymens have thinner tissue.

            (4) Pubertal hymens are thickened and petaled from renewal of the estrogen effect.

            (5) Transverse hymenal opening diameter should be measured in prepubertal girls. Four millimeters is normal up to age 4 years. Add about 1 mm/year until puberty. The measure varies with position, amount of traction, kind of hymen, relaxation of child, and time elapsed since abuse.

d. Be aware of normal anatomic variations

   (1) Most hymens fit into one of five categories: crescentic (posterior rim), circumferential (annular), fimbriated (redundant), sleevelike, or septate.

   (2) Nontraumatic variations include periurethral and perihymenal bands, small hymenal mounds adjacent to vaginal ridges, perineal midline raphe, and hymenal flaps.

e. Be aware of abnormal findings not due to sexual abuse (straddle injuries, genital hemangiomas, lichen sclerosis, urethral caruncles, urethral prolapse).

f. Prepare the child prior to the examination with an explanation and/or demonstration on a doll.

g. Boys should receive a careful inspection of the penis, urethral meatus, scrotum, and surrounding skin.

h. Prepubertal **girls** require a careful inspection of the vulva, unless internal trauma is suspected (which requires a pelvic exam under anesthesia). Pubertal girls require a complete pelvic with a speculum.

i. Genital findings consistent with sexual abuse

   (1) Acute: lacerations, abrasions, ecchymoses, edema.

   (2) Chronic: scarring of hymen or other genital structures; absent hymen, attenuated hymen, distorted hymen, or U- or V-shaped indentations in posterior or lateral portions of the hymen; significantly enlarged hymenal diameter.

2. Anal examination

a. Be aware of **normal anal anatomy and variations,** including smooth areas at 6 and 12 o'clock (keyhole effect), erythema, midline skin tags, increased pigmentation, venous congestion, anal dilation with feces in the rectum.

b. Findings consistent with sexual abuse

   (1) Acute: lacerations, edema, abrasions, ecchymoses, fissures that come out to the skin.

   (2) Chronic: scars, dilation 20 mm or more without rectal feces, altered anal contour.

E. Laboratory tests

1. When indicated by the history or physical findings, culture for **gonorrhea** and *Chlamydia* in the throat, anus, and vagina/urethra.

2. Serologic tests for syphilis and human immunodeficiency virus (HIV) should be performed if the history warrants (taking into account of the incubation periods: up to 3 months for syphilis; up to 6 months for HIV).

3. Symptomatic children should be investigated for other genital infections, such as trichomonas, herpes, condyloma acuminata, *Gardnerella vaginalis,* and *Candida.*

4. Consider a **urinalysis** and **urine culture.**

5. Consider a **pregnancy test** for pubertal girls.

III. Management

A. Primary goals. The goals of management are to provide medical treatment for injuries or infections, arrange for psychosocial support for the child and family, and protect the child from further abuse by reporting to child protective services (Table 59-2).

B. Ongoing role of the practitioner

1. Help guide the family toward healing.

a. Provide or arrange crisis intervention counseling.

Table 59-2. Guidelines for making the decision to report sexual abuse of children

Data available			Response	
History	Physical	Laboratory	Level of concern about sexual abuse	Action
None	Normal examination	None	None	None
Behavioral changes	Normal examination	None	Low (worry)	± Report;* follow closely (possible mental health referral)
None	Nonspecific findings	None	Low (worry)	± Report;* follow closely
Nonspecific history by child or history by parent only	Nonspecific findings	None	Possible (suspect)	± Report;* follow closely
None	Specific findings	None	Probable	Report
Clear statement	Normal examination	None	Probable	Report
Clear statement	Specific findings	None	Probable	Report
None	Normal examination, nonspecific or specific findings	Positive culture for gonorrhea; positive serologic test for syphilis; presence of semen, sperm, acid phosphatase	Definite	Report
Behavioral changes	Nonspecific changes	Other sexually transmitted diseases	Probable	Report

* A report may or may not be indicated. The decision to report should be based on discussion with local or regional experts and/or child protective services agencies.
Source: Reprinted with permission from the American Academy of Pediatrics Committee on Child Abuse and Neglect. Guidelines for the evaluation of sexual abuse of children. *Pediatrics* 87(2):254–260, 1991.

    b. **Alert the family to their possible behavioral and emotional reactions,** especially if the family constellation is disrupted.

    c. **Encourage a sense of physical security for the child after the disclosure;** reassure children who were threatened with harm that there is no danger.

    d. **Parents should neither try to make children forget nor pry into details,** but rather be open to children's negative or positive expressions about the experience.

    e. **Help parents avoid overprotection and maintain normal routines, physical affection, and limit setting** whenever possible.

    f. **Help parents remember the needs of the rest of the family and themselves.**

  2. **Monitor the child and family adjustments over time.** As the victim enters each succeeding developmental stage, new questions and feelings may arise.

  3. **Be aware of local resources,** such as parent groups, offender treatment, victim witness advocates, and children's groups available to the family.

C. Criteria for referral

  1. **A clinician who does not have sufficient evidence** to report to child protective services but is still concerned should refer to an experienced mental health provider for a full sexual abuse evaluation.

  2. **A clinician who cannot conduct a complete medical evaluation** (or if the initial evaluation raises questions) should refer to a pediatric specialist in sexual abuse.

  3. **All sexually abused children should be referred to an experienced mental health provider** to evaluate the need for ongoing treatment. Even children without overt symptoms may harbor negative or confused feelings that may be revealed only in the context of a full evaluation.

IV. Clinical pearls and pitfalls
- Rely on the history for the diagnosis; most sexually abused children have no physical findings. This is because they were fondled, engaged in oral sex, or had minor injuries that healed quickly. Even hymenal tears can heal without a trace.
- Take the child's statements and behavior seriously. The incidence of genital complaints is higher than the incidence of genital findings in sexually abused children.
- Children who imitate adult sex acts or molest other children are highly suspect. (Normal sex play among peers is, "You show me yours, and I'll show you mine.")
- Make sure the parent(s) have adequate support; the child's adjustment is related to family adjustment.
- Sexually abused children may feel like "damaged goods" and need reassurance that their bodies are fine. Even if there is damage, the clinician can still honestly say that something is healed or will heal quickly.

Bibliography

For Parents
Crow P, Butler J. *Helping Children Recover from Sexual Abuse: A Guide for Parents.* Portland OR: Emanuel Hospital and Health Center, 1991.

MacFarlane K. *Please, No, Not My Child—Coping with Sexual Abuse of Your Preschool Child.* Los Angeles: Children's Institute International, 1983.

For Children
Freeman L. *It's My Body.* Seattle: Parenting Press, 1987.
For preschoolers.

My Very Own Book About Me. Spokane: Rape Crisis Resource Library, 1982.
For school-aged children.

Davis L. *The Courage to Heal Workbook.* New York: Harper & Row, 1990.
For adolescents.

For Professionals

American Academy of Pediatrics. Committee on Child Abuse and Neglect. Guidelines for the evaluation of sexual abuse of children. *Pediatrics* 87(2):254–260, 1991.

Chadwick DL et al. *Color Atlas of Child Sexual Abuse.* Chicago: Year Book Medical Publishers, 1989.

Heger A, Emans SJ (eds). *Evaluation of the Sexually Abused Child.* New York: Oxford University Press, 1992.

Jones DPH, McQuiston M. *Interviewing the Sexually Abused Child.* Denver: C. Henry Kempe Center for the Prevention and Treatment of Child Abuse and Neglect, 1986.

Shyness

Jonathan M. Cheek

I. **Description of the problem.** Shyness is the tendency to feel tense, worried, or awkward during social interactions, especially with unfamiliar people. This definition reflects three categories of shyness symptoms: somatic anxiety, cognitive anxiety, and observable behavior.

A. **Epidemiology**
  - Although transient situational shyness is virtually universal, about 30–40% of school-aged children and adults in the United States label themselves as shy.
  - There is a developmental peak for shyness during adolescence, when 60% of the girls and 48% of the boys in seventh and eighth grades identify themselves as shy.
  - Less than 50% of the children who first became shy during later childhood and early adolescence still consider themselves to be shy by age 21.
  - 75% of college students who say they were shy in early childhood continue to identify themselves as shy persons.

B. **Clinical features.** In early childhood, shyness is usually manifested as the relative absence or inhibition of normally expected social behaviors. The child appears excessively quiet, with diminished social participation. For shy children, the normal peaks of stranger anxiety (9 months) and separation anxiety (18 months) do not fade away. In later childhood and early adolescence, the cognitive symptoms of shyness, such as painful self-consciousness and anxious self-preoccupation, begin to become a significant component of this personality syndrome.

Longitudinal research indicates that shyness that continues into adulthood can create significant barriers to satisfaction in love, work, recreation, and friendship. Shy adults tend to be more lonely and less happy than those who are not shy. Childhood shyness does not, however, predict psychopathology in adulthood and should be considered part of the normal range of individual differences in personality and social behavior.

C. **Etiology**

   1. **Temperament.** Shyness is one of the few temperamental traits whose precursors in infancy are often clear. About 15–20% of infants typically respond to a new situation or stimulus (e.g., an unfamiliar toy, person, or place) by withdrawing and becoming either emotionally subdued or upset (crying, fussing, and fretting). It has been speculated that this pattern of inhibition to novelty is related to a lower threshold for arousal in sites in the amygdala. Infants with this highly reactive temperament in the first year of life are more likely to be wary or fearful of strangers at the end of the second year and are also more likely to be described as shy by their kindergarten teachers.

   2. **Transactional model.** Behavioral inhibition in infancy does not lead invariably to childhood shyness. Parents who are sensitive to the nature of their inhibited child's temperament, who take an active role in helping the child to develop relationships with playmates, and who facilitate involvement in school activities appear to ameliorate the impact of shyness on the child's subsequent social adjustment. Childhood shyness is a joint product of temperament and socialization experiences within and outside the family.

   3. **Late-onset shyness.** Many of the children who first become troubled by shyness between the ages of 8 and 14 do not have the temperamental predisposition for behavioral inhibition. Late-developing shyness is usually

caused by adjustment problems in adolescent social development. The bodily changes of puberty, the newly acquired cognitive ability to think abstractly about the self and the environment, and the new demands and opportunities resulting from changing social roles combine to make adolescents feel intensely self-conscious and socially awkward.

The inability of some adolescents to outgrow late-developing shyness has been linked to several factors. Research on the timing of puberty indicates that early-maturing girls and late-maturing boys suffer more severe social adjustment problems with their peers. Moving to a new neighborhood or school can disrupt the development of social skills, which are most easily practiced in safe and familiar surroundings. Shy adolescents need to experience positive social relationships in order to develop a healthy level of self-esteem. If parents, siblings, teachers, or peers tease and embarrass the shy adolescent, he or she may develop the self-image of being an unworthy and unlikable person.

Sex role socialization puts different pressures on adolescent girls and boys. Teenage girls experience more symptoms of self-conscious shyness, such as doubts about their attractiveness and worries about what others think of them, whereas teenage boys tend to be more troubled by behavioral symptoms of shyness because the traditional male role requires initiative and assertiveness in social life.

II. Recognizing the issue

A. Signs and symptoms. The child's visit to a primary care clinician is itself a prototypical shyness-eliciting situation, so signs of fearfulness and inhibition should be easily detectable.

B. Differential diagnosis. Some people prefer to spend time alone rather than with others but also feel comfortable when they are in social settings. Such people are **nonanxious introverts,** who may be unsociable but not shy. The opposite of shyness is social self-confidence, not extroversion. The problem for truly shy people is that their anxiety prevents them from participating in social life when they want to or need to.

C. History: Key clinical questions

1. *Is your child usually shy and withdrawn in new situations and when meeting new people?* An affirmative answer rules out the possibilities that the child is just nervous about the visit or is just in a sensitive mood on that particular day.

2. *Are you worried that your child is too shy to make friends or to do well in school?* Answers that indicate severe anxiety reactions, phobias, or withdrawal similar to mild forms of autism are red flags for more severe pathology. Some parents, particularly those who are somewhat shy yet have adapted well themselves, will label their child as shy but not see it as a problem. They are often sufficiently sensitive to the issue that no further intervention may be necessary.

3. *Do you feel disappointed or embarrassed that your child can't seem to be more outgoing or adventuresome?* Research suggests that an affirmative answer indicates the potential for significant long-term adjustment problems for shy children. For example, the feelings of disappointment in some fathers that their shy sons are not "masculine" enough can be a particularly painful problem. It is important for the parents of a shy child to understand the nature of the temperament and to help their child develop on his or her individual pathway, rather than attempting to enforce a personal or cultural ideal that will never be a good fit for the shy child.

III. Management

A. Advice to parents. The goals of intervention in this case are essentially proactive and preventative in nature: helping the shy child to achieve better adjustment in his or her current and future social life. It is worth noting that retrospective interviews with painfully shy adults frequently contain complaints that doctors and teachers had ignored their childhood shyness. They expressed the wish that some adult had become an ally or advocate by validating their problem and persuading their parents to help them deal more effectively with their shyness at an early age.

1. **Do not overprotect or overindulge.** Allow the shy child to experience moderate amounts of challenge, frustration, and stress rather than rushing to soothe away every sign of anxiety. With emotional support from parents and gradual exposure to new objects, people, and places, the child will learn to cope with his or her own special sensitivity to novelty. Gently and consistently nudge (but do not push) the child to continue gaining experience with new things.

2. **Respect the shy temperament.** Talk with the child about feeling nervous or afraid. Once the reality of these negative feelings has been acknowledged, encourage the child to talk about what can be gained from trying a new experience in spite of being afraid (an example from the parent's own childhood might be particularly helpful). Progress is usually slow because shy feelings may remain even after a particular shy behavior has been overcome. Sympathy, patience, and persistence are needed.

3. **Help the child deal with teasing about being shy.** Shy children are highly sensitive to embarrassment and need extra comfort when they have been the victim of teasing. They also need more support and encouragement to develop positive self-esteem than do children who are not shy.

4. **Help the child to build friendships.** Inviting one or two playmates over to the house lets the child experience the security of being on home territory. Sometimes a shy child will do better when playing with children who are slightly younger.

5. **Talk to teachers.** The child's teacher can be an important ally, but teachers sometimes overlook the shy child or incorrectly assume that excessive quietness indicates lack of interest or lack of intelligence.

6. **Prepare the child for new experiences.** Take the child to visit a new school or classroom before school starts. Help the child rehearse (e.g., by practicing for show-and-tell or an oral book report). Role-play anticipated anxieties, such as what a party or the first day of summer camp will be like.

7. **Find appropriate activities.** Help the child get involved in a club or after-school activity that can expand social contacts with others who share similar interests and enthusiasms. Be careful not to impose what you would like, or wish you had done as a child, onto a child who has different likes and dislikes.

B. **Advice to the shy child.** Shy children usually appreciate being made to feel that their problems of social anxiety are understood sympathetically by an adult and that they are not alone in experiencing these feelings. It is important not to minimize the significance of shyness but rather to emphasize to the child the increased enjoyment of social rewards that can be obtained if he or she begins to participate more actively in social life.

C. **When to refer.** If the parents of a child troubled by shyness appear to lack confidence in their ability to implement the advice, it may be appropriate to suggest a referral to a mental health professional.

Bibliography

For Parents

Publications

Chess S, Thomas A. *Know Your Child.* New York: Basic Books, 1987.

Cheek JM, Cheek B. *Conquering Shyness.* New York: Dell Trade Paperback, 1990. *For shy teenagers and their parents.*

Organizations

Anxiety Disorders Association of America, 6000 Executive Boulevard, Rockville MD 20852; (301) 231-9350.

For Professionals

Cheek JM, Melchior LA. Shyness, self-esteem, and self-consciousness. In H Leitenberg (ed), *Handbook of Social and Evaluation Anxiety*. New York: Plenum, 1990.

Jones WH, Cheek JM, Briggs SR (eds). *Shyness: Perspectives on Research and Treatment*. New York: Plenum, 1986.

Rubin KH, Asendorpf JB (eds). *Social Withdrawal, Inhibition, and Shyness in Childhood*. Hillsdale NJ: Erlbaum, 1993.

61

Sleep Problems

Barry Zuckerman

I. **Description of the problem.** Sleep behaviors are the result of a complex interaction of physiologic and caretaking factors. Knowledge of sleep physiology and its developmental changes is important for the primary care clinician, both to understand and to explain common sleep problems to families.

A. **Sleep physiology**

1. **Patterns.** In normal sleep, the child cycles between rapid eye movement (REM) and non–rapid eye movement (NREM) sleep. REM sleep is characterized by jerky rapid eye movements, absence of motor movements, an irregular pulse and respiratory rate, groaning, and dreaming. Because it is the lightest sleep stage, many infants and children awaken during REM sleep. NREM is a much deeper stage of sleep, which is subdivided into stages 1–4 (the deepest state).

2. **Cycling of stages.** During sleep, the child cycles between NREM and REM sleep. Each NREM/REM cycle lasts 50–60 minutes in infants, increasing to 90 minutes by school age. An 8-hour sleep contains 5–8 NREM/REM cycles (each a potential opportunity for waking during REM sleep).

3. **Duration of sleep**

a. **Newborn infants** sleep approximately 16 hours per day, **6 month olds** about 14.5 hours, and **12 month olds** about 13.5 hours.

b. Nighttime sleep becomes consolidated, generally lasting 6–8 hours, by **age 4 months** and 10–12 hours by **age 6 months.** Neither the introduction of solid food nor weight is associated with sleeping through the night.

c. By **age 9 months,** 84% of infants awaken at least once in the night. Most, however, return to sleep without parental intervention. Children who require help in returning to sleep are identified as nighttime wakers.

B. **Epidemiology**
- Sleep problems (such as night waking and resistance to sleep) occur in 20–30% of infants and young children.

C. **Etiology**

1. **Factors associated with problems of night waking**

a. **Perinatal problems** (e.g., prematurity, perinatal asphyxia)

b. **A difficult temperament** (e.g., lower sensory threshold, less adaptable)

c. **Breast feeding** (waking decreases with weaning)

d. **Night feeding** (children need a nighttime feeding only until age 4–6 months)

e. **Co-sleeping with the parents.** It is unclear whether parents take children with sleep problems to bed or taking children to the parental bed causes sleep problems. In cultures that accept co-sleeping (e.g., African-American), parents are less likely to describe sleep problems compared to cultures that are less accepting of co-sleeping.

f. **Family stress**

  g. Maternal depression (causal connection is not well established).

  h. Maternal employment (in some but not all studies).

 2. Sleep-onset associations. The manner in which a child falls asleep influences whether he or she is able to return to sleep after a nocturnal awakening or requires parental attention. Some parents inadvertently "teach" their child to associate falling asleep with their presence. If children fall asleep in their parents' arms and/or while being fed, they are unable to return to sleep after an awakening until those same conditions (e.g., mother's presence) are present.

 3. Separation issues. When children are first put to bed or when they reach wakefulness during REM sleep, they may cry out for their parent. Parents, especially mothers, may not be able to tolerate being separated from their infant and have a low threshold to intervene. Such ambivalence around separation can perpetuate night waking problems.

D. Resistance to sleep

 1. Autonomy. By 9 months of age (and particularly during the second year), children are motivated to control their bodies and the environment. Letting go of daytime exploration and excitement is difficult, leading to resistance to sleep and the old adage: *Adults want to fall asleep; children want to stay awake.*

 2. Inappropriate expectations for sleep. Every child has a different need for sleep. Some children are simply not tired at the arbitrarily imposed bedtime and vociferously resist exhortations to "just go to sleep!"

II. Recognizing the issue. Because of the disruption of their own sleep, many parents are motivated to discuss sleep problems with the primary care clinician. Night waking should be considered a problem only if the parents deem it one.

A. History: Key clinical questions

 1. During infancy

  a. *How do you know when your child is awake?* During REM sleep many children groan and move around. Some parents take this as a signal that the child is awake and intervene. Parents need to give the infant an opportunity to return to sleep by himself or herself.

  b. *How do you put your child to sleep?* If a child's sleep-onset associations involve being held or fed, or both, the infant will need similar care to fall asleep following a nocturnal awakening.

  c. *Do you feed your infant when he or she awakens? How much?* Beyond age 6 months, children do not need a feeding at night to thrive.

  d. *Have you been away from your baby? Have you and your spouse gone out by yourselves? When you are away, do you think and worry about your baby all the time?* Some parents have significant separation issues with their infant that lowers their threshold to intervene during a nighttime wakening. Such separation issues need to be addressed before a management plan can be successful.

 2. Toddlers

  a. *Do you have other problems with your child?* For children with pervasive behavioral problems, management should first address problems occurring during the day and not at night, when everyone is fatigued and tense.

  b. *Are you frustrated about not being in control? Do you believe your child is in charge? Do you get into power struggles with your child?* These questions assess parental acceptance of their child's autonomy strivings and help to see if power struggles are at the root of the sleep problems.

  c. *Are you afraid that the sleep problem is part of a larger, more significant problem?* Some parents are especially anxious because of the worry that the sleep problem is the sign of a much deeper and more significant psychological or medical problem.

    d. *How much of a problem is this for you?* Sleep problems are a family problem: they rarely have a direct negative impact on the child. If the family is not disturbed by the problem, they are unlikely to have the motivation and resolve to follow through with management strategies.

B. Behavioral observations. Clinical assessment of the parent-child interaction can provide helpful information. An anxiously hypervigilant parent or one with many somatic concerns about the child, for example, may suggest separation difficulties. An overly intrusive parent may suggest a high level of anxiety or difficulty accepting the child's autonomy. At the other extreme are parents who appear oblivious to the child's behavior; here the problem may be maternal depression and/or preoccupations with their own rather than their child's needs.

C. Physical examination. The primary care clinician should ensure that no occult medical problem (e.g., serous otitis media) underlies the sleep disturbances.

III. Management

A. Information for parents

    1. **Explain sleep cycles,** especially the likelihood of movement, vocalizations, and awakening during hourly periods of REM sleep. Parents need to provide infants the opportunity to return to sleep.

    2. **Describe the concept of sleep-onset associations,** especially in the first year. Explain that the problem is not that their infant wakens at night (since most infants do); the problem is that the infant *requires the presence of a parent to fall back asleep.* Ensure they understand the idea by asking the parents what their own sleep-onset associations are (e.g., on side, two pillows, firm mattress) and whether they ever have a problem sleeping in a new environment. Temperamentally adaptable infants (and adults) usually do not have problems with sleep-onset associations.

    3. **Children can go 8–10 hours a night without being fed by age 6 months.** They can be conditioned to awaken by nighttime feeding.

    4. **Identify and address separation concerns,** especially if they are associated with the vulnerable child syndrome (see Chapter 89).

B. Night waking

    1. **Specific strategies**

        a. **There is no magic cure for sleep problems,** but parents should know that with consistency, resolve, and a little time, most will improve.

        b. **Instruct the parents to put the child to bed while still awake** (including naps) and allow him or her to find independent sleep-onset associations. The conditions in which the child first falls asleep (e.g., no parent present) will then be present when the child awakens at night. Parents can still hold, rock, and feed their child before bed; the trick is to stop such measures before the child actually falls asleep.

        c. **Decrease the amount of milk given at a night feeding** over a 10-day period, or else add more and more water to the bottle, so that after 1 week it contains only water.

        d. **Address separation issues for the child** by the incorporation of a transitional object between ages 4–12 months. This could be a blanket, a doll, or some other favorite object. When the child wakes at night, the presence of the object may help the child master separation.

        e. **Bedtime routines can address autonomy strivings.** A child has the opportunity to "control" the type and sequence of a limited number of activities prior to getting into bed. This includes washing up, getting dressed, kissing parents, and reading a story.

        f. For **persistent night waking,** the parent must short-circuit the expectations for their help in falling asleep.

	Monday	Tuesday	Wednesday	Thursday	Friday	Saturday	Sunday
Time woke in morning							
Times and lengths of naps during day							
Time went to bed in evening							
Time settled in bed in evening							
Issues in settling to bed and what you did							
Times and lengths of waking at night and what you did (what was successful and what was not)							

Figure 61-1. Sample sleep diary.

(1) **For the older child.** The issue should be addressed during a planned discussion during the day. If parents are frustrated and no one is sleeping well, have the parents put a mattress or sleeping bag on the floor next to their bed for the child. Over the course of 2–3 weeks the child will have adjusted to the new rules. When that happens, the mattress or sleeping bag can start moving from the parents' room toward the child's room.

Some parents enjoy cosleeping with their child. This practice is the rule in most nonindustrialized cultures of the world. In most cases, parents can be reassured that it is not harmful for their child to sleep with them as long as they are comfortable with it.

(2) **For the younger child.** The parents should institute a gradual (over 1–2 weeks) program of reducing contact with the child after a nocturnal awakening. For the first few nights, for example, the parent can stand next to the bed with a hand on the child rather than picking the child up. Then the parent can sit next to the bed without physical contact. In the following stages, the parent should not talk or make eye contact with the child. Finally, the chair can be moved progressively farther from the bed until it is outside the room.

C. **Resistance to sleep.** Parents should be instructed that it is their responsibility to put their child to bed, but it is the child's responsibility to get himself or herself to sleep. Setting a time to go to bed with clear rules (e.g., no eating, no getting out of bed) is a reasonable request. The actual falling asleep should not be the parents' concern. If a child needs only 7 hours of sleep, there is no reason to try to increase its duration.

If the issue is that the child sleeps very late and then is not sleepy at night, instruct the parent to awaken the child ½ hour earlier every morning, until the desired time is achieved. This will lead to increased fatigue earlier in the night.

D. **Backup plans**

1. A **sleep diary** (Fig. 61-1) can help parents and clinician better understand the child's sleep patterns and parental responses. A sleep diary not only provides information for the clinician but can help to boost the parents' awareness of the dynamics of the sleep problem.

2. **Rule out family dysfunction, maternal isolation, or maternal depression.** Explore feelings of separation and autonomy struggles.

Bibliography

For Parents

Ferber R. *Solve Your Child's Sleep Problems*. New York: Simon and Schuster, 1985.

Weissbluth M. *Healthy Sleep Habits, Happy Child*. New York: Fawcett Columbine, 1987.

For Professionals

Lozoff B, Wolf AW, Davis NS. Cosleeping in urban families with young children in the United States. *Pediatrics* 74:171–182, 1984.

Adair R et al. Reducing night waking in infancy: A primary care intervention. *Pediatrics* 89:585–588, 1992.

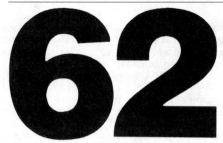

Stuttering

Barry Guitar and
Gayle Belin-Frost

I. Description of the problem. Stuttering is a disruption of speech, characterized by repetitions, prolongations, or complete blockages. These may be accompanied by physical struggle, frustration, and fear of speech. The term *disfluency* is often used synonymously with *stuttering,* but also may refer to the hesitations common in the speech of normal children who are learning to talk.

A. Epidemiology
- The prevalence of stuttering is 1% among school-aged children, slightly lower in adults, and slightly higher in preschool children.
- The incidence is 5%.
- The difference between prevalence and incidence figures reflects the tendency for children who stutter to recover, usually before puberty.
- The male-female ratio among preschool children is about 2:1 and rises to 4:1 in adulthood, suggesting that females are more likely to recover.

B. Familial transmission/genetics.
Parents who stutter are more likely to have children who stutter; this is especially so for women who stutter. A multifactorial (polygenic) model has been suggested to account for the transmission.

C. Etiology/contributing factors

1. **Environmental.** A home or school environment that places high demands on a child's performance can contribute to stuttering. Examples include pressure to speak more rapidly, articulately, or with more advanced language than the child is able or pressure to succeed socially, academically, or athletically. Stuttering may also be exacerbated by stressful but normal life events, such as the birth of a sibling, separation from a parent, or a family move.

2. **Organic/transactional.** Predispositions to stuttering include an inherited or acquired difficulty in speech motor coordination and a temperament that reacts to stress with excess muscular tension and effort.

3. **Developmental.** Stuttering usually appears between ages 18 months and 5 years. In most children, early symptoms will resolve. In others, the signs and symptoms may worsen from (1) easy repetitions with minimal awareness, to (2) rapid and physically tense repetitions with evidence of frustration, to (3) blockages of speech, accompanying struggle behaviors, and avoidance of words and speaking situations.

II. Making the diagnosis

A. Signs and symptoms/differential diagnosis.
See Table 62-1.

B. History: Key clinical questions

1. *How long have you been aware of your child's stuttering?* If the child has stuttered for more than 6 weeks, suspect a potential chronic problem.

2. *How have the disfluencies changed since they began?* If there has been an increase in effort, emotion, or avoidance associated with stuttering, it is worsening.

3. *What is your child's stuttering like at its worst?* Many children who stutter do not do so in the clinician's office. It is important to have the parents describe the signs and symptoms that have caused them concern.

Table 62-1. Signs and symptoms of normal disfluency and stuttering

	Normal disfluency	Mild stuttering	Severe stuttering
Speech behavior	Occasional brief repetitions of sounds, syllables, or short words (*li-li-like this*)	Frequent long repetitions of sounds, syllables, or short words (*li-li-li-like this*) Occasional prolongations of sounds	Very frequent and often very long repetitions of sounds, syllables, or short words Frequent sound prolongations and blockages
Other behavior	Occasional pauses, hesitations, or fillers Changing of words or thoughts	Repetitions and prolongations associated with blinking, looking to side, and physical tension around mouth	More evidence of struggle, including pitch rise in voice Extra words used as "starters"
When most noticeable	Comes and goes when child is excited, tired, sick, talking to inattentive listeners	Comes and goes in similar situation but is more often present than absent	Present in most speaking situations More consistent
Child's reaction	Usually none apparent	May show little concern or some frustration and embarrassment	Embarrassment and fear of speaking
Parent's reaction	Varies from none to a great deal	Some concern but not a great deal	Considerable degree of concern
Referral decision	Refer only if parents quite concerned	Refer if continues for 6–8 wk or if parental concern justifies it	Refer as soon as possible

   4. *Is the child bothered by his or her stuttering?* If so, the child will soon react to the stuttering with physical tension and struggle and should be referred.

 C. Tests. Ask the child several direct questions (e.g., name, age, address) that must be answered without substitution or circumlocution. This is likely to elicit disfluency or avoidance if the child is a stutterer.

III. Management

 A. Primary goals. The family must understand that the child is doing the best that he or she can with speech and will only get worse if they criticize or correct. Rather, they should find ways of reducing stress on the child.

 B. Information for the family

   1. It should be emphasized to the parents that **they did not cause the problem.**

   2. The **etiology** may be a slight difference in brain organization that favors some skills (e.g., drawing) but creates more hesitancy in speech, especially during childhood.

   3. The **onset of stuttering** may be associated with a spurt in speech and language development or increased stress.

   4. Parents should know that if the child is frustrated by the stuttering, **they should occasionally acknowledge it in an accepting, encouraging way.** They can also assure the child that if she or he would like help with it, there are people who can help.

C. Initial treatment strategies

1. As much as possible, **parents should talk with their child in a slow, relaxed manner,** using short sentences and simple vocabulary to promote fluency.

2. **A brief period should be set aside each day at a regular time when one parent can interact alone with the child.** The parent should use a slow speech rate and follow the child's lead in choosing topics of conversation and play activities. The aim is to give the child a sense of being the center of attention for a brief period.

3. **Family should institute turn taking in competitive speaking situations,** such as dinner table conversations.

4. **Parents should occasionally make a comment expressing empathy,** such as "Lots of kids get stuck on their words sometimes. I know it makes talking hard, but it's okay, and you can take as long as you like."

5. **Attempts should be made to slow the pace of life in the home,** including the pace of conversations. After the child says something, parents should pause for a second or two before responding.

D. Criteria for referral

1. **The child is stuttering with physical tension and is showing concern or frustration.** He or she should be referred immediately.

2. **Initial strategies have been tried for 1 month without appreciable lessening of the stuttering.**

3. **Referral should be made to a speech-language pathologist** certified by the American Speech-Language-Hearing Association, preferably one who specializes in stuttering. (The Stuttering Foundation of America can suggest a nearby professional.)

IV. Clinical pearls and pitfalls

- Most parents blame themselves. The clinician can reassure them that they did not cause their child's stuttering, but they can play a big part in their child's ability to cope with it.
- Most children outgrow stuttering, especially if parents can reduce psychosocial pressures and increase acceptance of the child as she or he is now.
- Parental attitudes and treatment programs that put a high premium on completely fluent speech probably interfere with recovery. Effective programs help the child speak in a more natural way, with less effort and struggle, but do not aim for perfection.

Bibliography

For Parents

Organizations

National Stuttering Project, 2151 Irving Street, Suite 208, San Francisco CA 94122-1609; (800) 364-1677.

Stuttering Foundation of America, PO Box 11749, Memphis TN 38111; (800) 992-9392.

Publications

Conture E, Fraser J. *Stuttering and Your Child: Questions and Answers.* Memphis TN: Stuttering Foundation of America, 1989.

Cooper E. *Understanding Stuttering: Information for Parents.* Chicago: National Easter Seal Society, 1979.

For Professionals

Guitar B. Is it stuttering or just normal language development? *Contemp Pediatr* February:109–125, 1988.

Guitar B, Conture E. *The Child Who Stutters: To the Pediatrician.* Memphis TN: Stuttering Foundation of America, 1991.

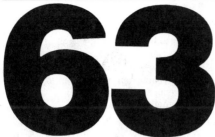

Substance Abuse in Adolescence

Karen Hacker

I. Description of the problem. The hallmarks of addiction to drugs and alcohol are compulsivity (the abuser has lost control and is unable to stop using the substance) and dysfunctionality (the abuse has a damaging effect on relationships, work, school, parenting, etc.). It is best regarded as a chronic disease with frequent exacerbations and remissions and with a lethal potential.

A. Epidemiology
- 25% of 12–17 year olds and 50% of 18–25 year olds report having used illicit drugs.
- The use of drugs and alcohol peaks at ages 16–18 years and declines after age 22 years.
- Males more than females.
- Seen in all socioeconomic strata.
- In 1991, 8 million seventh to twelfth graders drank weekly.
- Of high school seniors in 1989, 65% had used alcohol in the past month, 33% reported binge drinking (more than five drinks in a row) in the past 2 weeks, 66% had tried cigarettes, and 18% smoked daily.

B. Comorbidities

1. **Motor vehicle accidents** are the leading cause of death in 15–19 year olds. Excessive drinking is considered responsible for 50% of motor vehicle fatalities. Failure to wear seat belts is also associated with substance use.

2. **Homicide and suicide** (the second and third leading causes of death in adolescents) are also associated with drug and alcohol use.

3. Teenagers who use drugs and alcohol at an early age are **more likely to begin having sex** within the following year than those who do not use.

4. Alcohol and substance use may **decrease the likelihood of using condoms.**

C. Etiologies/contributing factors

1. **Risk factors.** The major risk factors for substance abuse in adolescents include:

   a. **Gender (male>female).**

   b. **Earlier age of onset.**

   c. **Parental or sibling alcohol/drug use.**

   d. **Peer drug use.**

   e. **School failure.**

   f. **Low self-esteem.**

   g. **External locus of control.**

   h. **Poor relationship with parents.**

   i. **Depression, anxiety.**

   j. **Lack of social conformity.**

   k. **Low religious commitment.**

Table 63-1. Levels/phases of substance abuse

Level/phase	Feeling	Use	Signs and symptoms
I. Use	Learns the effect of alcohol/drugs, low tolerance	Infrequent and responsible: special occasions, religious ceremonies, social	Few, first episode of intoxication
II. Misuse	Seeks the effect of alcohol/drugs, losing control and choice	Regular use/pattern, mostly weekends Using without parental permission	May develop hangovers, unexplainable mood swings Lies regarding use Schoolwork begins to suffer; tardiness, truancy
III. Abuse/ harmfully dependent (early stage of addiction)	Preoccupied with alcohol/drugs; losing control and choice	2–3 times per week and on weekends Establishes rituals for use and plans next use Promises to cut down but fails All friends are users	Repeated injuries Weight loss or gain Blackouts Shortened attention span Depression, suicidal thoughts Legal problems: Shoplifting, vandalism, driving while intoxicated School failure: suspension; fights with parents, may be abusive
IV. Addiction/ harmfully dependent (middle and late stages of addiction)	No longer has control over alcohol/drugs; living for the substance	Compulsive use and high tolerance Binge use, reckless use Solitary use increases Spends large amounts of time getting substances	Weight loss, tremors, blackouts, withdrawal symptoms, deteriorating health Personality change, paranoia, depression, impaired memory Commits crimes, assault, stealing, dealing drugs Suspension or expulsion from school Home life deteriorates, stays away from home

2. **Developmental factors.** Adolescence is a time of transition in which the child is struggling to achieve adulthood and establish his or her identity. As physiologic and emotional changes are taking place, the adolescent (particularly between ages 15–19 years) begins to experiment with risk-taking behaviors. There is an increased reliance on and identification with peers rather than family. Taking risks may bring peer acceptance and independence and help to forge one's own identity. These normal developmental processes make adolescence a particularly vulnerable time in which to experiment with substance abuse.

II. **Making the diagnosis.** The stages of adolescent alcohol and drug abuse or addiction can be broken down into four levels/phases (Table 63-1).

A. History. It is important to establish a trusting relationship with the adolescent. Confidentiality should be guaranteed (unless the drug use is of clear and immediate danger), and questions should be asked without the parent present. The provider must always balance a desire to protect the adolescent by disclosing substance abuse to the family with the negative effect such disclosure may have on the clinician's therapeutic relationship with the adolescent.

1. **Key clinical questions.** Questions about substance abuse should be incorporated into a more general psychosocial history that probes home, family, activities, peer interactions, substance use, and sexuality. Questions should be asked in a matter-of-fact, nonjudgmental way with a tone of wanting to help, not condemn, the patient.

   a. *Do you smoke cigarettes?* If the answer is yes, *How often do you smoke: a pack a day or more, a pack every other day, a pack a week?* Cigarette smoking is addictive and also an important indicator of other drug use.

   b. *How often do you drink? Never? Special occasions? Once a month? Once a week? Two to three times a week? Four or more times a week?* Asking forced-choice questions about use and amount will help pinpoint actual use. Teenagers tend to binge drink on weekends rather than use daily.

   c. *How much do you usually drink, when you drink? One or two drinks? Three or four drinks? Five or more drinks?*

   d. *If you often take other drugs, is it once a month? Once a week? Every day?* Quantifying use is important in determining the effect that alcohol or drug use may have on the individual.

   e. *What drugs have you ever taken?* Knowing exactly what drugs have been used is important for assessing signs and symptoms and level of current use.

   f. *When was the last time that you took any drugs?* A historic perspective is important in quantifying the frequency of use.

   g. *What do drugs or alcohol do for you?* This information will help the clinician determine the rationale and context within which the adolescent is using substances.

   h. *Do you think any of your friends have a drug or alcohol problem?* Peer use is a strong determinant of adolescent drug or alcohol use.

   i. *Has your drinking or drug use ever caused you any trouble or concern?* This question helps in assessing the patient's level of denial or self-awareness of the issue.

   j. *Does anyone in your family have a problem with drugs or alcohol? If so, who?* It is important to assess the family history of addictions in order to determine risk.

B. Physical examination. It is rare to see any physical effects of drugs and alcohol abuse during adolescence. However, evidence of a specific substance used may be noted in an individual who is high or is an active user (Table 63-2).

C. Tests. Urine and blood toxic screens are a tool for diagnosis, but their use may damage the potential for a therapeutic relationship between clinician and patient. Who is asking for the test? Who has access to test results, and what will be done with them? Has the adolescent consented to testing? The clinician must balance the need for diagnostic certainty with the potential loss of ability to help the patient deal with the problem.

III. Management

A. Primary goals. The primary care clinician should strive to:

1. **Identify** those at risk for substance abuse.

2. **Prevent** future alcoholism or drug addiction.

Table 63-2. Alcohol and drug uses and effects

Drug	Administration	Effects	Withdrawal	Test
Alcohol	Oral	Depressant Slurred speech "Drunken behavior" Loosening of inhibitions	Anxiety Tremors Convulsions Delirium tremens Hallucinosis, possible death	Liver enzymes test may be elevated Blood alcohol level for acute intoxication
Depressants (barbiturates, benzodiazepines)	Oral	Slurred speech Disorientation Drunken behavior	Anxiety Insomnia Tremors Convulsions Possible death	Urine toxic screen up to 1 wk after last use
Stimulants (cocaine, crack, amphetamines)	Oral Smoked Injected Sniffed	Increased alertness Excitation Increased pulse, blood pressure Hunger depressant Insomnia	Apathy Somnolence Irritability Depression Sinus congestion	Urine toxic screen up to 3 d after last use
Cannabis	Smoked Oral	Euphoria Relaxed inhibitions Increased appetite	Insomnia Hyperactivity Occasionally reported	Urine toxic screen up to 1 mo after last use in heavy users
Opiates (heroin, morphine, opium)	Injected Smoked	Euphoria Drowsiness Respiratory depression Constricted pupils Nausea	Watery eyes Flulike syndrome Tremors Chills, sweating Cramps	Urine toxic screen up to 4 d after last use
Hallucinogens (LSD, mescalin, peyote, PCP)	Oral Smoked	Hallucinations Illusions Nausea Anxiety, psychosis/paranoia	Withdrawal symptoms not reported	Urine toxic screen up to several weeks after last use of PCP 12 hr after LSD

3. **Intervene** to diminish drug abuse and the associated mortalities and morbidities.

4. **Treat** those who are alcoholics or drug abusers.

B. **Strategies.** Chemical dependency is a chronic disease, and relapses, failures, and repeated attempts at sobriety are expected. It may take multiple encounters before the adolescent trusts the clinician and begins to acknowledge the problem. A provider may need to engage other persons in the teenager's life (e.g., family, friends, teachers) for any intervention to be successful.

1. For seriously addicted adolescents, **referral for inpatient detoxification and/or outpatient substance abuse treatment** will be necessary.

2. In the case of adolescent substance users whose use does not put them at severe risk but who are clearly experiencing problems, **early intervention strategies** can be used. These involve defining the problem, education, brief

counseling, and negotiating follow-up and treatment. For many, referral to outpatient resources may be appropriate.

3. **Prevention strategies**

   a. **Ask questions about substance use** and maintain a nonjudgmental tone so that the patient feels safe to raise the issue.

   b. **Teach responsible problem solving, decision making, and refusal skills** by rehearsing various scenarios with the adolescent and role-playing how to avoid drug taking in a socially acceptable way.

   c. **Educate the patient** about the hazards, social unacceptability, and media influences on substance abuse. Have brochures, pamphlets, and other materials about drug use in the waiting room.

IV. **Clinical pearls and pitfalls**
   • Addiction is a chronic illness with remissions and exacerbations.
   • The adolescent's family may be the greatest enabler of the chemical dependency.
   • Unless an adolescent can recognize the problem and break through denial, treatment is very difficult.
   • Always double the amount an adolescent says he or she uses.
   • Common adolescent use patterns include polydrug use on weekends and vacations.

Bibliography

For Parents

Publications
Falco M. *The Making of a Drug-Free America: Programs That Work.* New York: Times Books, 1992.

Organizations
Alateen, 1372 Broadway, New York NY 10018-0862; (212) 302-7240.

Alcoholics Anonymous, General Service Office, PO Box 459, Grand Central Station, New York NY 10163; (212) 686-1100.

Johnson Institute, 7151 Metro Boulevard, Minneapolis MN 55435; (612) 944-0511.

National Clearinghouse for Alcohol and Drug Information, 1776 East Jefferson Street, Rockville MD 20852; (301) 468-2600.

For Professionals
Rogers P. Chemical dependency. *Pediatr Clin North Amer* 34: 1987.

Schaefer D. *Choices and Consequences.* Minneapolis: Johnson Institute, 1987.

Werner M. *Adolescent Substance Abuse, Risk Factors and Prevention Strategies* Maternal and Child Health Technical Information Bulletin. Washington DC: US Government Printing Office, 1991.

64

Suicide

Karen Norberg

I. Description of the problem. Threatened suicide is one of the most serious emergencies in pediatrics, not only because of the risk to life but because of the serious distress communicated by a threat or gesture of suicide. **Completed suicide** refers to a self-directed action that results in death. **Suicide attempt** or **suicide gesture** refers to intentional behavior that the child believes might result in self-harm (whether or not this assessment is medically realistic and whether or not the intention actually includes death). **Suicidal ideation** refers to self-reported thoughts about self-harm (not necessarily accompanied by action).

A. Epidemiology
- In the United States roughly 1% of adolescents aged 12–15 years has made at least one suicide gesture.
- 1% of suicide gestures are lethal. The rate of completed suicides is 13.2/100,000 among young adults aged 15–24 years (peak is at age 20 years) and 0.8/100,000 among children aged 5–14 years. These rates reflect a steady increase over the past three decades.
- School-aged children report suicidal thoughts as often as adolescents, but the likelihood of actual self-harm increases with age.
- Girls are about two times more likely to attempt suicide as boys, but boys are three to four times more likely to complete suicide, largely because of the greater lethality of their chosen methods.

B. Contributing factors. Risk factors for higher lethality are listed in Table 64-1. Others include:

1. Life stresses/social communication

  a. Suicide attempts are most often precipitated by **crises** for which the child or adolescent fears rejection (e.g., arguments with girlfriend or boyfriend, school failure, unplanned pregnancy, identification of gay sexual orientation).

  b. Most attempts have a **strong communicative intent,** expressing a wish to change a situation or relationship.

  c. A past history of significant life stresses, and especially a history of traumatization, multiple losses, or parental abuse or family violence, greatly increases the likelihood of suicidality.

2. Developmental

  a. Completed suicide in children **under age 10 years** is rare; however, children as young as age 4 or 5 years may make a gesture (e.g., wrapping a cord around the neck) during which they may specifically state a wish to die.

  b. Children **over age 10 years** have a generally realistic understanding of what might be harmful or lethal. This change in cognition may explain the increased risk of actual intentional self-harm as children get older.

3. Substance abuse

  a. Of older adolescents who attempt suicide, **30–70% have a history of significant alcohol or drug abuse.**

Table 64-1. Risk factors predicting greater lethality of suicide attempts in children and adolescents

Intent
Wishes for death
Did not expect otherwise to gain from gesture
Specific, realistically lethal plan
Rescue/discovery was not expected

Method
Higher lethality: guns, hanging, use of motor vehicle, jumping from a great height
Lower lethality: overdose, wrist cutting, attempted suffocation

Concurrent problems
Alcohol intoxication (increases impulsivity)
Major depression
Psychosis
Serious physical illness
Previous suicide attempts

Social environment, trauma
Recent loss or disappointment
Sexual assault, other trauma or abuse
Suicide in relative or acquaintance
Social isolation
Rejection, lack of support from family

---

      b. Acutely, **the use of alcohol and drugs increases the likelihood of acting on impulse** and interferes with judgment.

      c. **Chronic and significant alcohol or drug use may be associated with multiple other social and family stressors.**

    4. **Environmental**

      a. **"Contagion."** Suicide and suicide attempts appear in clusters, especially in circumstances that dramatize or intensify the effects of a suicide gesture as an attempt to communicate. Publicizing a real or fictional suicide in newspapers or on television, for example, has been reported to increase the suicide rate by 7–10% among adolescents and young adults.

      b. **Lethality of opportunity.** Access to lethal methods affects the rate of completed suicide. Increased lethality of gestures among older adolescents is related to increased access to alcohol, motor vehicles, and guns.

II. **Assessing the risk.** Among adolescents who complete suicide, about half have had a known history of depression, alcohol abuse, psychosis, or previous suicide attempt. Most adolescents who succeed in suicide have given some sign or warning shortly before the event—a note, a gesture, or a verbal statement to someone important to them—that in retrospect might have offered an opportunity for intervention. In general, **all suicide gestures and suicidal ideation should be immediately evaluated by a mental health professional.** The primary care clinician can serve the adolescent as a known and trusted professional in the initial assessment of the situation.

    A. **Interview with the child.** If possible, the interview with the child or adolescent should take place in a quiet, private area, without interruptions. Details of the interview depend on the urgency of the situation and the developmental level of the child. Table 64-2 provides key clinical questions for such an interview.

    B. **Interview with parents.** Information should be gathered from as many other informants as possible. Although care must be taken to protect the confidentiality of the adolescent, it is ethical and necessary to communicate with the family,

Table 64-2. Questions for assessing suicide intent in children

---

Present episode
Can you tell me what happened? What happened next?
Did you [try to/want to] hurt yourself?
How did you [plan to] hurt yourself?
Was anyone else nearby at the time? Expected?
Had you been drinking or using other drugs?

Motivation: death
What did you think would happen if you tried to hurt yourself?
What did you want to have happen?
Did you think you would die? Get hurt badly?
Have you ever tried to hurt yourself before? What happened?

Concepts of death
What do you think happens when a person dies? Do you believe in life after death?
What did you think would happen if you died?
Have you known anyone who has died? Who? How did they die?
Do you have a wish to join them in death?
Have you pictured what your funeral would be like? Who would be sad?

Motivation: communication
Why did you want to hurt yourself?
Did you want to frighten someone?
Did you want to get even with someone?
Did you wish someone would rescue you?
Did you hear voices telling you to hurt yourself?
Did you change your mind afterward? How do you feel now?

Motivation: family, school stresses
Do you feel very sad or upset about anything?
Has anything upsetting happened that you have had trouble telling someone
   about?
Did you or do you feel that your family does not care about you?
Have you had a fight with someone important to you?
Do you have difficulty in school? Do you worry about school?
Do you get into fights at school? Do other kids tease you?
Do your parents punish you much? Do you argue with your parents?
Do your parents fight with each other?
Have you been separated from your parents? When?
Has anyone important left or stopped seeing you? Who?
Is anyone in your family sick? Who?
Is anyone else in your family sad or upset? Who?

Motivation: hopelessness and depression
Have you been thinking about death for a long time?
Do you often blame yourself for things?
Do you cry a lot? Do you prefer to stay by yourself?
Do you have trouble paying attention in school?
Do you have trouble sleeping or eating? Do you feel tired a lot?
Do you feel that things are likely to get better?

Table 64-3. Criteria for referral of suicidal children or adolescents

Refer for hospitalization if
The child has made a medically significant gesture.
The child expresses a strong intent to harm himself or herself, verbally or through ongoing behavior.
The child is uncommunicative or unwilling to give convincing reassurances of safety.
Hospitalization may not be required if
Strong social supports and supervision are available.
The gesture was not medically serious.
The gesture seems to have accomplished its communicative intent.
The patient is willing to give assurances that he or she will call someone rather than act on further suicidal feelings.
Follow-up treatment is available.

even against an adolescent's wishes, in a life-endangering situation. Issues to be explored include:

1. **The family's knowledge of current stresses in the patient's life.**

2. **The family's attitude toward the patient** (supportive or devaluing?) and the status of ongoing conflicts between parent and child.

3. **Any parental history of suicide, alcoholism, drug abuse, depression, or family violence.**

4. **The willingness of the family to seek help for the patient.**

C. **Behavioral observations.** The child's behavior may give clues about the presence of depression or anxiety. Emotional expressiveness and general cooperation may indicate the child's desire for help and may provide clues about the dependability of the child's promises not to hurt herself or himself in the future.

III. **Management.** Any child or adolescent who has made a gesture of intentional self-harm or who is expressing a strong wish to hurt himself or herself should be seen by a mental health professional for consultation.
Table 64-3 lists criteria for hospitalization.

A. **Primary goals.** The primary goals of management are to assess the need for acute hospitalization and to make the appropriate referrals. Long-term goals may include changes in family patterns of communication, identification of the contribution of chronic stressors or past traumas, and treatment of underlying depression and other causes of despair.

Bibliography

Lewis M. Psychiatric assessment of infants, children, and adolescents. In H Lewis (ed), *Child and Adolescent Psychiatry.* Baltimore: Williams and Wilkins, 1991.

Shaffer D. et al. Preventing teenage suicide: A critical review. *J Am Acad Child Adolesc Psychiatry* 27(6):675–687, 1988.

Terr L. Childhood traumas: An outline and overview. *Am J Psychiatry* 148:10–20, 1991.

65

Temper Tantrums

Robert Needlman

I. Description of the problem. Temper tantrums are easier to recognize than to define. They typically include crying, yelling, stamping, or other violent displays of anger or frustration. Less dramatic behaviors include persistent complaining, whining, or petulance.

A. Epidemiology
- 50–80% of 2–3-year-old children have tantrums at least weekly and 20% at least daily.
- 60% of 2 year olds with frequent tantrums will continue to have them at age 3 years. Of these, 60% will continue at age 4 years.
- The prevalence of explosive "tempers" remains approximately 5% throughout childhood.
- Severe tantrums are often accompanied by other significant behavioral problems, such as disturbed sleep or overactivity.
- Tantrums are not related to gender or social class.
- There is no known genetic or familial predisposition.

B. Etiology/contributing factors
1. **Developmental.** Tantrums occur when negative emotions of anger or frustration exceed the child's ability to control them. In toddlers, the conflict between the drive for autonomy and continued dependence creates frustration and emotional distress. What to put on, what to put in the mouth, where to go, and when to leave are some of the many decisions that toddlers want to make independently but cannot. Language, a crucial means of emotional expression and self-regulation, is usually too immature to be of much help. In older children, tantrums may be a learned behavior, reinforced by parental compliance or, paradoxically, by the intense negative attention they elicit.

2. **Temperamental.** Temperament plays an important role. Intense children tend to express their feelings dramatically; persistent children are prone to longer displays; children with irregular sleep or hunger patterns are likely to have their needs frustrated more often.

3. **Environmental.** Tantrums may be associated with a number of environmental factors, including overcrowding and limited access to the outdoors. Familial risks for increased tantrums include marital stress, domestic violence, parental depression, substance abuse, frequent corporal punishment, and an inability to set firm limits.

4. **Organic.** Recurrent upper respiratory infections, respiratory allergies, disturbed sleep, hearing loss, speech and language delays, and attention deficit hyperactivity disorder (ADHD) are all associated with increased tantrums. Tantrums may also be increased in autism, traumatic brain injury, and severe mental retardation.

II. Recognizing the issue

A. Signs and symptoms.
The clinical features that differentiate normative tantrums from problem tantrums are listed in Table 65-1

B. History: Key clinical questions
1. *What exactly happened the last time your child had a tantrum? What set it off? What did your child do? How did you respond? Was that a typical*

Table 65-1. Clinical features of problem tantrums

A high degree of parental concern, anger, or sadness. Tantrums are a problem if parents think they are.

The parent does not volunteer anything positive about the child.

The child is older than age 4 years or less than age 1 year.

Tantrums occur three times a day or more or last more than 15 minutes.

Tantrums occur regularly in school.

Tantrums are associated with intentional damage to valuable objects, attacks on others, or self-injurious behavior.

There are multiple other behavioral problems (e.g., sleeping, learning, peer interactions).

---

episode? A play-by-play account of a specific, recent episode can provide critical information about what the parent means by "a tantrum" and about its antecedents and reinforcers. Be sure to ask about delayed consequences (such as punishments the next day or special treats that may be offered because the parent feels upset about having gotten so angry).

2. *How often do tantrums result in your child's getting what he or she wants?* When parents capitulate following particularly long tantrums, they inadvertently teach the child to carry on for longer and longer periods. In behaviorist jargon, behaviors maintained by intermittent reinforcement are particularly resistant to extinction.

3. *Do the tantrums occur at school, as well as at home?* Children usually manage to "pull it together" around peers. Tantrums in school may suggest that the child is experiencing a higher level of stress in school due to difficulties in learning or social functioning. When a child behaves well in school but not at home, attention needs to be directed to the patterns of family relationships.

4. *Do the tantrums get in the way of normal family functioning?* Tantrums require prompt attention if they cause parents to avoid going shopping, hiring babysitters, or inviting friends to their home.

5. *Does the child have other behavioral problems, such as overactivity, enuresis, or aggressive behaviors directed against peers or siblings?* A pattern of multiple behavioral problems suggests the need for a more comprehensive psychological evaluation.

6. *How do you feel when your child is having a tantrum?* If parents report extreme anger, shame, or guilt, these feelings need to be addressed for intervention to succeed.

7. *When does the child go to sleep? Are there tantrums around bedtime? Does the child snore, breathe irregularly, sleep restlessly, or wake frequently?* Sleep problems suggest overtiredness as a possible contributor. Irregular bedtimes and bedtime tantrums may indicate a lack of structure or a failure of parents to set firm limits.

8. *When the child is happy, how does he or she show it? Are all emotions expressed intensely? Does the child stick with a challenge until it is mastered, or is he or she easily distracted?* These questions explore temperamental contributors. In the absence of other concerning features, an intense, persistent child who occasionally has intense, long tantrums may be normal.

9. *Does the child have tantrums more with the mother or with the father?* Family relationships may play a role in maintaining the tantrums. If tantrums occur more with one parent (usually the mother), it may be because that parent is more ambivalent about limit setting. It may also be that the other parent is subtly undercutting the partner's authority.

C. **Behavioral observations, physical examination, and tests.** Provision of a few age-appropriate toys allows observation of the child's play skills (an indication of cognitive level and attention) as well compliance with the instruction to clean up. There are no specific physical findings, but signs of allergy ("shiners," the allergic crease), chronic otitis, or enlarged adenoids (mouth breathing) may be helpful. A written record of tantrums (tantrum log) noting time, duration, precipitants, and consequences can help to document the extent of the problem and any improvement.

III. Management

A. Primary goals

1. **Identify contributing factors and, when possible, remedy them.**

2. **Relieve parents' distress by helping them to understand their child's behavior and by correcting unrealistic expectations and fears.**

3. **Widen the focus of attention** to include the long-term emotional well-being of the identified child and the quality of family relationships.

B. Initial treatment strategies

1. **"Child-proof" the home,** in order to reduce the number of times the parent is forced to say "no."

2. **Allow young children to make frequent small choices,** all within the realm of the acceptable (e.g., "Do you want to drink your milk from the blue cup or the red one?").

3. **Limit frustrations by paying attention to the child's temperament and rhythms:** active children may need time to run around every day; slow-to-warm-up children need time to get used to a new environment; children who are hungry every day at 4:30 P.M. need a before-dinner snack.

4. **"No" should be absolute.** Many parents say "no" when they really mean, "I don't think so." When the child protests sufficiently, the parent backs down, thereby rewarding the tantrum. Children quickly distinguish between "hard NO's" ("NO playing with sharp knives") and "soft no's" ("no cookie before dinner"), and rarely have tantrums about the former. Parents need to learn to pick their fights carefully and then plan to win.

5. **Ignoring** is an effective way to turn off tantrums or, at least, avoid reinforcing them. In some cases, however, walking away from a young child in the middle of a tantrum may make the child feel even more out of control and may escalate the tantrum. Additionally, when parents first begin to ignore tantrums, the tantrums may intensify for a period of days or weeks before subsiding. Specific instructions to parents about how to react can be helpful, for example, "Stand 5 feet away. Keep doing whatever you were doing. Do not speak, or speak only in a neutral tone of voice. If your child is near a hard object, move it or move the child. Do not let the child hurt himself or herself or anyone else."

6. **Ensure that the tantrums do not threaten self-esteem by deprecating statements after the tantrum.** Parents should talk about "losing control" rather than "being bad," and avoid talking excessively about the tantrum afterward.

C. Criteria for referral.

If these strategies do not lead to quick improvement, more extensive evaluation may be indicated. Treatment will be dictated by the assessment of etiology. In some cases, effective interventions might include suggesting that the parents find a play group or other social supports. Referral may be necessary for treatment of parental depression, substance abuse, domestic violence, or other family dysfunction.

Bibliography

For Parents
Turecki S, Tonner L. *The Difficult Child.* New York: Bantam Doubleday, 1989. *Practical and sensitive advice, with an emphasis on temperament as major determinant of children's behavior.*

Ginott H. *Between Parent and Child*. New York: Macmillan, 1965.
Still one of the best guides to talking with children, giving clear messages, and effective positive and negative feedback.

Brazelton B. *Toddlers and Parents*. New York: Bantam Doubleday Dell group, 1974.
The chapter focusing on tantrums is particularly insightful and readable.

For Professionals
Needlman R, Howard B, Zuckerman B. Temper tantrums: When to worry. *Contemp Pediatr* 6(8):12–34, 1989.

Campbell SB. *Behavior Problems in Preschool Children*. New York: Guilford, 1990.
A comprehensive treatment worthy of study.

Temperamentally Difficult Children

Stanley Turecki

I. **Description of the problem.** A "difficult child" is a normal young child whose innate temperament makes him or her hard to raise. Inherent in this definition is a view of normality that is broad; children are different and do not have to be average in order to be normal. For a child to be considered temperamentally difficult, a basic criterion has to be met: the child's constitutionally determined personality traits cause significant problems in child rearing.

Temperament is the *how* of behavior, rather than the *why* (motivation) or the *what* (ability). For example, three equally motivated and able children may approach a homework assignment quite differently, depending on their behavioral style. One will begin on time and work steadily to completion, the second will delay and procrastinate but then work very persistently, and the third will jump in immediately and quickly lose patience.

The scientific acceptance of the concept of temperament owes much to the pioneering work of Stella Chess and Alexander Thomas, and their New York Longitudinal Study, in which they identified nine temperamental characteristics evident from infancy or early childhood. A range exists for each category. Table 66-1 lists the difficult aspects of each temperamental trait.

Difficult children are not all alike. Some are impulsive, distractible, and highly active; others are shy and clingy. Some throw loud tantrums; others whine and complain. Some can hit, kick, or even bite; others are verbally defiant. Some are unpredictable in their eating or sleeping habits; others are sensitive to noise, textures, or tastes. Most difficult children have trouble dealing with transition and change, and almost all are strong-willed and extremely stubborn.

A. **Impact on the family.** The concept of a difficult temperament should always be combined with that of goodness of fit—the match or compatibility between a child and his or her environment. Behavior that presents a problem to one family may be readily accepted by another. For example, a child's idiosyncratic and strongly held tastes in clothing and food would only trouble a fashion- and nutrition-conscious parent. A highly active, impulsive, excitable 6-year-old girl would be considered an energetic tomboy if she lived on a farm with four older brothers but be diagnosed as suffering from attention deficit hyperactivity disorder if she were the only child of finicky older parents living in a cramped city apartment.

Truly difficult children are, above all, hard to understand. Their behavior confuses and upsets the most experienced parent or teacher. The tried-and-true methods of child rearing simply do not work, so that effective discipline is replaced by inconsistency, power struggles, excessive punishment, or overindulgence. Parents will say that nothing works or that the child controls the family.

The primary caregiver of such a difficult child (usually the mother) is generally bewildered, overinvolved, and exhausted. She may feel guilty, inadequate, and victimized. Often such children are somewhat easier with their fathers, who may become increasingly critical of the mothers.

Marital strain is common; a fragile but potentially viable marriage may be ruptured by the stress of a difficult child. In addition, individual vulnerabilities of adult personality may be accentuated, resulting in parental syndromes of anxiety, depression, or substance abuse. The siblings are often expected to behave in an excessively adult manner, and their needs can be neglected as the household increasingly revolves around the difficult child.

Table 66-1. Description of difficult traits

Trait	Child's behavior
High activity level	Very active, restless, fidgety; always into things; makes you tired; "ran before he walked"; easily overstimulated; gets wild or "revved up"; impulsive, loses control, can be aggressive; hates to be confined.
Distractibility	Has trouble concentrating and paying attention, especially if not really interested; doesn't "listen"; tunes you out; daydreams; forgets instructions.
High intensity	Loud and forceful whether miserable, angry, or happy.
Irregularity	Unpredictable; can't tell when he'll be hungry or tired; has conflicts over meals and bedtime; wakes up at night; moods are changeable; has good or bad days for no obvious reason.
Negative persistence	Stubborn; goes on and on nagging, whining, or negotiating if wants something; relentless, won't give up; gets "locked in"; may have long tantrums.
Low sensory threshold	"Sensitive"—physically, not emotionally; highly aware of color, light, appearance, texture, sound, smell, taste, or temperature (not necessarily all of these); "creative," but with strong and unusual preferences that can be embarrassing; clothes have to feel and look right, making dressing a problem; doesn't like the way many foods look, smell, or taste; picky eater; bothered and overstimulated by bright lights and noisy settings; refuses to dress warmly when the weather is cold.
Initial withdrawal	Shy and reserved with new people; doesn't like new situations; holds back or protests by crying or clinging; may tantrum if forced to go forward.
Poor adaptability	Has trouble with transition and change of activity or routine; inflexible, very particular, notices minor changes; gets used to things and won't give them up; has trouble adapting to anything unfamiliar; can want the same clothes or foods over and over.
Negative mood	Basically serious or cranky; doesn't show pleasure openly; not a "sunny" disposition.

B. Epidemiology
- 15–20% of young children are temperamentally difficult.
- Highly active, impulsive, difficult children are more likely to be boys. All other temperamentally difficult traits are as likely to be seen in girls as in boys.
- There is no correlation with birth order, intelligence, or social class.

C. Etiology. Temperament refers to dimensions of personality that are largely constitutional in origin. Genetic factors definitely contribute. Pregnancy and delivery complications may be somewhat more common in the histories of difficult children. Some of these children are allergic, with a propensity to develop ear infections. Uneven language and learning skills development are not uncommon. Many difficult children are intelligent but socially immature. All of these factors suggest a biologic basis for a difficult temperament.

II. **Making the diagnosis.** A pathology-oriented model is limiting and often counterproductive. There is no "difficult child syndrome," just as there is not a definitive "test for hyperactivity." Much more valid in dealing with problem behaviors in young children is a model that focuses on individual differences and goodness of fit. The aim is to describe the child's behavior, temperamental profile, and strengths, as well as areas of vulnerability.

A. **History.** Questioning the parent about the manifestations of a child's difficult temperament and its impact on the family is the key to identification. The clinician should inquire about the parents' approach to discipline, the child's school functioning, and the presence of secondary manifestations, such as fearfulness, nightmares, excessive anger, and emotional oversensitivity. Impaired self-image is seen in poorly managed difficult children.

B. Differential diagnosis. A difficult temperament is evident from an early age and is relatively stable and consistent over time. A child whose behavior has become difficult may be going through a developmental stage or reacting to stress. An example is a youngster who begins to misbehave after his or her parents separate.

C. Behavioral observations. Some problem behaviors are readily apparent in the office visit: impulsivity, hyperactivity, disruptiveness, clinging and withdrawal, tantrums, aggressiveness, or undue sensitivity to pain. However, a child may be stubborn, irregular, negative and cranky, intense, sensitive to light and taste, or poorly adaptable. When a parent reports such "nonvisible" difficult behavior that is not apparent during the office visit, the clinician should not assume that the parent is inventing or causing the problem.

III. Management. The difficult child's adjustment can be greatly enhanced by the ongoing involvement of the primary care clinician. The central therapeutical goal is to improve the compatibility between a child and the significant persons in his or her life.

A. General issues

   1. Erroneous perceptions can be corrected. The parents of very difficult children invariably feel victimized and often assume that the child's behavior is intentional. Parents need to understand that their children are not enemies who are "out to get them." Seeing the problem behavior as temperamentally determined rather than willful disobedience allows the parent to deal with it far more neutrally.

   2. The caregivers need support and understanding, especially when the child's behavior is difficult at home but unremarkable at school or in the clinician's office.

   3. Practical advice can be offered on issues such as school selection and communication with teachers. The parents may need guidance on how to share responsibility more evenly, how to deal with other family members, and how to respond to the often-plentiful advice offered from several quarters that tends to make parents (particularly single parents) feel defensive and inadequate.

B. Principles of adult authority. The fundamental goal for the parents of a difficult child is to replace the power struggles, frustration, and wear-and-tear of an ineffective disciplinary system with an educated, rational, kind, accepting, yet firm attitude of adult authority. Inevitably, habitual patterns of negative interaction have developed. It is the parents' job to initiate the necessary changes to improve the fit between their child-rearing style and their child's temperament. Several shifts in attitude are involved in making such a change.

   1. Parental leadership. It should be clear to everyone that the parents are in charge. Certainly the child's opinion should be solicited when appropriate, but the ultimate decision lies with the parents. The model is that of the excellent supervisor at work: approachable, supportive, clear in expectations, and very much in charge.

   2. Strategic planning and planned discussions. The automatic, often excessively punitive, reactions to the child's behavior must be replaced with a system that emphasizes structure and predictability. Decisions about rules, new procedures or routines, and consequences should be made privately by the adults and then presented to the child. Such a planned discussion always takes place away from the heat of the moment. The child is calmly, clearly, and deliberately told what will be expected from now on. Both parents, if possible, should be present at such a meeting. The attitude is kind but serious. The parents should be concise and avoid moralizing, lest they lose the child's attention. The child should be viewed to some extent as a junior collaborator in the planning to improve the family atmosphere and input elicited. At the end of a planned discussion, the child needs to repeat the key points to make sure she understood them and is then encouraged to "do her best." Asking a young child, at a calm time, to try hard to meet a specific and reasonable expectation is a very powerful statement. Generally planned discussions can be used with children as young as age 3 years.

3. **Rational punishment.** Going hand in hand with planned discussions is the clear, firm enforcement of consequences for unacceptable behaviors that are within the child's control and important enough to warrant taking a stand. In a typical vicious cycle, a mother may find herself punishing and saying "no" repeatedly, but no parent can possibly be effective in such circumstances. Most difficult children need less punishment, rather than more, and this can be achieved through consistency, structure, and routines in everyday life.

The important first step for parents is to recognize and address major unacceptable behaviors and ignore the myriad minor irritations that take place every day with a very difficult child. Ideally, a punishment should be administered briefly and without anger. Its main objective is to show the child that the parents are serious about stopping the behavior. Simplicity and predictability are important; a variety of punishments are unnecessary. With a younger child, parents can show seriousness by facial expression and tone of voice.

C. **Management strategies.** Management, as distinct from punishment, is used when the adult decides that the misbehavior is temperamentally based; the child, in effect, "can't help it." The parent's attitude, while still firm, is much more sympathetic and kind. The basic message is, "I understand what's happening. I know you can't really control yourself, and I am going to help you with this." Sometimes behavior falls into a gray area, where it is not clear whether it is deliberate. In such instances, it is best for the parent to make the emotionally generous decision and help rather than punish the child.

Management suggestions designed to promote the child's success can be geared to particular temperamental characteristics. Strategies should be explained to the youngster during a planned discussion.

1. **The impulsive child.** A child who is easily excited can lose control in an overly stimulating environment and misbehave or become aggressive. The most common mistake parents and teachers make is to wait for the youngster to strike out and then lecture or punish, instead of intervening early.

If the child is easily excited, it is important to recognize the signs of escalation—for example, moving more rapidly, talking in a louder voice, or laughing excessively. The adult should try to step in before the child gets out of hand. This technique is called **early intervention.**

Some youngsters can be distracted. Others need a **time-out** (not as punishment, but as a cool-down period away from the action). A parent can teach the child to self-manage by saying, for example, "You're getting too excited. Let's do something quiet until you calm down."

2. **The highly active child.** High-energy children can become restless when they are confined to the dinner table or a classroom seat. They may begin to fidget or have difficulty paying attention. This behavior can be managed once the adults in charge **recognize the signs.** A restless youngster can be permitted to leave the dinner table and walk around between courses; a sympathetic teacher could ask the child to run an errand. Building vigorous physical activity into their daily routine is also helpful.

3. **The irregular child.** Most people fall easily into a regular rhythm of sleeping and eating, but some are naturally irregular. Battles can result when parents insist that a child who is not hungry must eat or that a youngster who is not tired must sleep. One strategy is to **differentiate between bedtime and sleep time, mealtime and eating time.**

It is reasonable to require a child to be in bed by a certain hour or to join parents and siblings at dinner. However, parents should not force a youngster to sleep when he or she is not tired. or to eat when he or she is not hungry. To avoid overburdening the family chef, a child with an irregular appetite can be taught to fix simple snacks, such as fruit, cold cereal, or yogurt.

4. **The poorly focused child.** Some children are easily distracted by their environment or even by their own thoughts. As a result, they appear to be not

paying attention or, if they miss instructions, disobedient. Parents and teachers can manage the problem by **making eye contact** in a friendly way before giving such a child directions. Instructions should be kept brief and simple.

5. **The child who resists change.** Some youngsters have difficulty with transitions. A poorly adaptable or shy child may be distressed by anything new. Other children focus so intently that they are locked into one activity and refuse to move to another. When they are asked to shift gears, they may cling, have a tantrum, or otherwise react negatively.

    If the issue is poor adaptability, parents can help by **preparing the child for change.** Even a simple warning, such as, "Finish playing with your trains, because we have to go shopping in 10 minutes," can be effective. Shy children require time and sympathetic understanding. A parent might say, "I know it's hard for you to get accustomed to new things, so I won't leave until you're used to being here."

6. **The stubborn child.** Persistent, stubborn children can be extremely frustrating for parents and teachers. With these children, adults can take a stand early and terminate the confrontation. This technique is called **bringing it to an end.** A parent should not try to reason with a stubborn expert negotiator. Instead, the discussion should be ended. However, it is common for parents of a stubborn child to engage in a constant battle of wills and say "no" all the time. They should be encouraged to say "yes" more often, especially when the issue at hand is not really important.

7. **The finicky child.** Certain children are particular because they have heightened sensitivity to touch, taste, smell, sound, temperature, and colors. Parents may get into arguments because a youngster insists on wearing the same comfortable green corduroy pants day after day or refuses to eat the inexpensive brand of frozen pizza that the rest of the family enjoys. Parents should be advised to **respect a child's preferences** when possible and to seek compromises that avoid unnecessary power struggles.

8. **The cranky child.** Parents can be distressed and angered by a child who is generally negative, somber, or pessimistic. Treats that would delight most children scarcely rate a smile from this youngster. The harder the parent tries (and fails) to make him or her happy, the greater the tension becomes. A suggestion for parents is to **accept the child's nature** and not to expect a level of enthusiasm that she or he cannot give.

D. **Criteria for referral.** The decision to refer to a mental health professional is often determined by the primary care clinician's interest in behavioral issues, expertise in parent guidance, and time availability. Assuming the presence of all these, a referral would still be needed in the case of an extremely difficult child, when the vicious cycle of ineffective discipline is longstanding, or when a clinical syndrome is suspected or can be identified in the child or other family members.

Bibliography

For Parents
Brazelton T. *Touchpoints*. Reading MA: Addison-Wesley, 1992.

Chess S, Thomas A. *Know Your Child*. New York: Basic Books, 1987.

Turecki S. *The Difficult Child*. New York: Bantam, 1989.

For Professionals
Carey, WB, McDevitt S (eds). *Clinical and Educational Applications of Temperament Research*. Amsterdam: Swets and Zeitlinger, 1989.

Chess S, Thomas A. *Temperament in Clinical Practice*. New York: Guilford Press, 1986.

Thomas A, Chess S. *Temperament and Development*. New York: Brunner-Mazel, 1977.

Turecki S. *The Emotional Problems of Normal Children*. New York: Bantam, 1994.

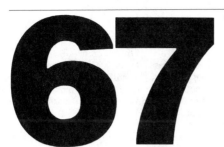

Thumb Sucking

Kerline Vassell

I. **Description of the problem.** Most infants engage in sucking that is not directed toward nutrition. They may use a pacifier or other object or fingers or toes, primarily as a means of self-soothing.

A. **Epidemiology**
- Seen in the fetus as early as age 18 weeks.
- 80% of all infants suck their fingers or thumbs.
- 30–45% of preschool children and 5–20% of children age 6 years and older continue to engage in thumb sucking.
- Most long-term thumb sucking began before age 9 months.
- Slightly more prevalent in girls than boys.
- More prevalent in children of higher socioeconomic status.
- 32–55% of children who suck their thumbs or fingers have an attachment object, such as a blanket, toy, piece of cloth, or their own hair.

B. **Etiology.** Some believe thumb sucking is a learned habit. Others, especially psychoanalysts, believe thumb sucking is an expression of infantile sexuality and that it reflects emotional disturbance when it persists beyond infancy. Most believe thumb sucking is a means of self-comforting. It may help to relieve stress and calm a child in response to environmental challenges. Alternatively, because of its self-calming effects, thumb sucking may occur only when the child is falling asleep, tired, bored, frustrated, unhappy, hungry, or insecure.

C. **Negative sequelae**

1. **Dental.** The most common adverse consequences of thumb sucking (especially if it persists beyond age 4 years) are dental, in particular malocclusion of both primary and permanent dentition. It may also lead to temporomandibular problems, anterior overbite, open bite, posterior crossbite, narrowing of the maxillary arch due to buccal wall contraction, mucosal trauma, atypical root resorption, and abnormal facial growth. The risk is highest among children who suck persistently, day and night.

2. **Abnormal digits.** With chronic thumb sucking, a digital hyperextension deformity can occur that may require surgical correction. Also seen are callus formation, irritant eczema, paronychia, and herpetic whitlow.

3. **Psychological effects.** Because thumb sucking is viewed as immature and socially undesirable, it may result in impaired parental and peer relationships. Parents and peers may criticize, ridicule, tease, and/or punish the child who sucks her or his thumb, and these reactions may adversely affect the child's self-esteem.

4. **Accidental poisoning.** Children who thumb or finger suck are at higher risk of accidental poisoning (e.g., lead poisoning) compared to those who do not.

II. **Making the diagnosis.** Thumb or pacifier sucking becomes a problem at any age when it interferes with normal developmental achievements, social interactions, or exploration of a nonstressful environment. As the child gets older, thumb sucking may provide secondary gain because of the attention that parents and others pay to it.

A. **Physical examination.** The examination may reveal a wrinkled, red digit with or without callus formation. Oral examination should be performed to look for malocclusion and other dental complications.

III. Management

A. Primary goals. The primary goals of treating thumb or pacifier sucking are to prevent the dental complications and potential adverse effects on the parental-child relationship, social relationships, and the child's self-esteem. In general, no intervention is needed until about age 4 years because most children spontaneously stop as they develop other self-regulatory strategies and because most adverse sequelae do not emerge until this age.

B. Initial treatment strategies

1. Identify stressors. Before treatment is instituted, the habit's adaptive function should be recognized. Once the emotional and psychological triggers are identified, alternative coping strategies (such as verbalizing the feelings) can be introduced.

2. Empower the child. If treatment is to be successful, the child must be actively involved, cooperative, and, most important, interested in stopping. Parents should be counseled that threats and punishment should not be used as these may result in increased resistance and thereby prolong the habit. They must remain patient and understanding, and provide emotional support without criticism as they accept that it is the child's, not their, task to overcome the habit.

a. Before age 4 years. Thumb sucking is normal as long as it does not interfere with social or developmental functions. The behavior should be ignored and no special attention given to it, lest it accrue secondary gain. If the child appears bored, he or she should be distracted without mentioning or showing concern about the thumb sucking. The child should be praised when not sucking his or her thumb.

b. After age 4 years. If thumb sucking is persistent and problematic, several behavioral modification and positive reinforcement techniques can be used:

(1) Gentle reminders such as a chart or calendar that the child uses to keep track of this progress.

(2) Rewards such as stickers, extra story time, special treats, or extra time with parents for suck-free days.

(3) Praise when the child is not thumb sucking.

(4) A change in the habit from a pleasurable experience to an obligatory one. A certain time (10–15 minutes) should be set aside each day for the child to go to his or her room and be *required* to suck all ten fingers for this amount of time or to spend 10–15 minutes just sucking the thumb. For some children, thumb sucking then loses its appeal.

(5) A bitter-tasting substance (available over the counter) is applied to the thumb each morning, every night, and each time the child is noticed thumb sucking. If thumb sucking does not occur after 1 week, the morning application is stopped. After another week, the afternoon application is stopped. After another week without thumb sucking, the nighttime application is also discontinued. If thumb sucking recurs, the process is repeated. This strategy is especially effective when children want to stop but put their thumb into their mouth without thinking. In fact, it must be emphasized that the liquid is a reminder to help the child stop, not a punishment.

(6) If thumb sucking occurs primarily at night, **gloves, thumb splints, or socks** can be used to remind the child. An elastic bandage can also be used. It is wrapped around the straightened elbow at bedtime. When the child raises hand to mouth, the bandage exerts pressure and reminds the child not to thumb suck. The child should be responsible for remembering to apply the glove or bandage and should not be reminded.

    C. Criteria for referral. If behavioral modification fails, the child may be referred to a pediatric dentist for an intraoral application such as a palatal bar or crib that interferes with placement of the thumb in the palatal vault.

IV. Clinical pearls and pitfalls
- Do not worry about thumb sucking until the child is at least age 4 years.
- Ensure the cure is not worse than the disease. In some cases, orthodontic wear is a small price to pay for a relaxed parent-child interaction and positive self-esteem.

Bibliography

For Parents

Brazelton TB. *Touchpoints: The Essential Reference.* Reading MA: Addison-Wesley, 1992.

Garber SW, Garber MD. *Good Behavior.* New York: St. Martin's, 1982.

Ilg FL, Ames LB, Baker LB. *Child Behavior: The Classic Child Care Manual from the Gesell Institute of Human Development.* New York: Harper Collins, 1981.

Schmitt BD. *Your Child's Health* (2nd ed.) New York: Bantam Books, 1991.

For Professionals

Adair SM. When thumbsucking becomes a problem. *Contemp Pediatr* 8(4):75–81, 1986.

Friman PC. *Thumbsucking in Childhood; Feelings and Their Medical Significance* (Ross Laboratories); Vol. 29-No 3, 1987.

Friman PC, Schmitt BD. Thumb sucking: Pediatricians' guidelines. *Clin Pediatr* 28(10):438–440, 1989.

Leung AKC. Thumb sucking. *Amer Fam Phys* 44(5):1724–1728, 1991.

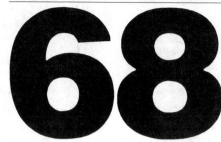

Tics and Tourette's Syndrome

Larry Scahill and
Donald J. Cohen

I. **Description of the problem.** Tourette's syndrome (TS), a chronic movement disorder of childhood onset, is characterized by multiple motor and phonic tics. Motor tics are typically quick, clonic movements involving the eyes, face, neck, and shoulders, with eye blinking, facial grimacing, and head jerking being most common. Tics may also involve other muscle groups and may include slower, more purposeful or dystonic movements. Phonic tics are typically brief vocalizations (such as repetitive throat clearing, grunting, or other noises) but may also include complex sounds such as words, parts of words, short phrases, or, occasionally, obscenities.

A. **Epidemiology**
- Transient tics, which do not persist over time, are relatively common compared to the frequency of TS. Estimates of prevalence for transient tics in the general population of school-aged children are 5–15% with a 3:1 ratio of boys to girls.
- The prevalence of TS is estimated to be 1 in 1000 for boys and 1 in 10,000 for girls.
- Neither ethnicity nor socioeconomic status is considered to have a significant effect on the relative risk of tics or TS.

B. **Familial transmission.** Data from family-genetic studies suggest that TS is inherited as a single autosomal dominant gene with incomplete penetrance and variable expressivity. The range of expression appears to include TS, chronic motor or chronic vocal tics, and some forms of obsessive-compulsive disorder. Whether transient tics and other behavioral manifestations (such as hyperactivity, inattention, or impulsiveness) are part of the TS phenotype remains controversial.

C. **Etiology.** The precise etiology of TS is unknown. The observation in the 1970s that the potent dopamine blocker haloperidol reduced tics has directed much attention to central dopaminergic systems. Noradrenergic, endogenous opioid, and serotonergic systems have also been implicated in the pathophysiology of TS. The consistent observation that boys are more likely to be affected than girls has also led to speculation about the potential role of androgens in the pathophysiology of tic disorders.

Twin studies demonstrate that monozygotic twins are far more likely to be concordant for TS than are dizygotic twins. Even concordant monozygotic twins, however, may not be equally affected, indicating that environmental factors may influence the phenotypic expression of the gene.

Adverse perinatal events and infectious agents have been proposed as contributing environmental factors. Stimulant drugs and sympathomimetic decongestants may aggravate tic symptoms and should be used with caution in children with TS. Finally, intolerant environments that fail to recognize the involuntary nature of tics may impose undue pressure on the child to suppress tics, which may increase tic severity.

II. **Making the diagnosis**

A. **Types of tic disorders**

1. **Transient tic disorders** refer to tic symptoms that last less than 1 year.

2. **Chronic tic disorders** refer to motor or phonic tics (but not both) of at least 1 year's duration.

3. **TS** is defined by the occurrence of both motor and phonic tics that persist for more than 1 year. In addition, there are frequently a shift in the anatomical site of the motor tics and a changing repertoire of motor and phonic tics that typically wax and wane in severity.

   Motor tics generally precede the emergence of phonic tics, and parents often describe the replacement of one tic with another. Eye blinking, which may herald the onset of a tic disorder in a 6- or 7-year-old child, may subside after several months, only to be followed by head jerking or incessant throat clearing.

   The tics of TS can be suppressed for brief periods of time. Thus, it is not unusual to hear reports that the child has frequent tics at home and relatively few tics in school. Older children and adults often describe a physical sensation or an urge ("like having to sneeze") prior to having a tic, but this may not be expressed by younger children. To make the definitive diagnosis of TS, the primary care clinician should secure consultation from a pediatric neurologist, child psychiatrist, or multidisciplinary clinical service specializing in tic disorders.

B. **Differential diagnosis.** There are no definitive diagnostic tests for TS. The clinician therefore must rely on history and observation to make the diagnosis. The list of diagnoses to be considered in the clinical evaluation of a child with a possible tic disorder includes other movement disorders, pervasive developmental disorders, obsessive-compulsive disorder, and rare metabolic disorders (e.g., Hartnup or Wilson's disease) that may be accompanied by tics.

C. **History: Key clinical questions.** In many cases, the child and family may have coined a word such as *twitches, habits,* or *noises* to describe the tics. It is often useful to borrow the term when taking the history. Specific questions include:

   1. *Can you recall when the twitches first started?* It is important to trace the onset and course of tics.

   2. *Can you recall which tic came first?* The goal is to chart the course of tic symptoms over time.

   3. *Have you ever made any sounds, such as repetitive throat clearing or grunting?* Diagnosis of TS requires a history of phonic tics.

   4. *Do other kids in school ever ask you about your twitches or sounds?* Whether tics are noticed by others is a crude indicator of severity.

   5. *Have you ever been teased because of your twitches?* Teasing often suggests that the tics are interfering with socialization.

   6. *Do you ever try to control your twitches? What happens?* In TS, tics can be suppressed for brief periods of time.

   7. *Has anybody else in the family ever had twitches or repetitive behaviors?* The presence of a positive family history of tics helps confirm the diagnosis of TS.

   8. *Is there anybody in the family who has to check things over and over, clean things excessively, or rearrange things over and over?* It is useful to screen for obsessive-compulsive symptoms, which may be an alternative expression of the putative TS gene.

D. **Behavioral observations.** Many children try to suppress their tics during a clinical consultation. Thus, failure to observe tic symptoms during the office visit should not preclude the diagnosis of TS. The clinician should watch for motor and phonic tics, as well as the child's activity level, interpersonal skill, linguistic competence, thought processes, affect, and attentiveness. Video recordings of the child can be instructive.

E. **Physical examination.** Other than tics, children with TS usually have a normal physical examination. A routine neurologic examination may reveal mildly abnormal coordination and "soft signs," suggesting a general neuromaturational delay. Neurologic consultation is indicated when the routine examination is markedly abnormal.

F. Tests. There are no specific diagnostic studies for TS. Tests and procedures are used to rule out other diagnoses (e.g., electroencepalogram for seizure disorders, MRI scan for brain tumors). Standardized questionnaires such as the Child Behavior Checklist for the parent and the Conner's Teacher Questionnaire can be used to assess the child's overall adaptation and school adjustment. Psychological testing is indicated when there are questions about a learning disability.

III. Management

A. Primary goals. The most important aim of treatment for a child with TS is to promote the child's optimal development: prevent social isolation, maintain age-appropriate interests, foster success in school, and reinforce positive family relationships. Education remains the most effective strategy to meet these goals by promoting understanding and tolerance within the child's environment. For example, many parents and teachers need help understanding the involuntary nature of tics. Some parents may even express irritation that the child is not trying hard enough to suppress the tics. Also, as with other chronic conditions, successful treatment often requires going beyond the condition itself and attending to the child's response to the disorder. The clinician needs to be watchful of the child's overall adjustment and may need to collaborate with educators and mental health professionals.

B. Information for the family. Many families feel relieved after the diagnosis of TS has been made because they at least have an explanation for the child's difficulties. But other questions, such as whether all of the child's problems can be attributed to TS, whether TS is progressive, and whether other children in the family will develop the disorder, often emerge.

Parents should be reminded that the tics of TS are involuntary. By contrast, impulsive behavior should not be regarded as outside the child's control and should be subjected to appropriate limit setting. Families should also be informed about the natural history of TS, which tends to wax and wane in severity and to decrease in severity with age.

C. Initial treatment strategies. The first line of treatment in most cases is education, which may include the child, the family, and the school. Specific goals of treatment depend on the source of major impairment: tics, obsessive-compulsive symptoms, or problems associated with attention deficit hyperactivity disorder (ADHD). Treatment is often multimodal and multidisciplinary and may involve education, parent training, individual or group therapy for the child, special education programming, and pharmacotherapy. Depending on the severity of the disorder and available services for a particular child, the primary care clinician may act as the coordinator of such a multidisciplinary team or as a collaborator with specialized clinical services.

D. Follow-up care. Medication is indicated for tics when they interfere with daily activities. Three medications are currently used to treat tics: haloperidol, pimozide, and clonidine. The goal of pharmacologic therapy is to reduce the number, frequency, and intensity of tics. Complete control of tics, however, is rarely achieved without producing unwanted side effects.

Medication might also be considered when a child's tic disorder is compounded by the presence of obsessions and compulsions or symptoms of ADHD. In severe cases, clinically significant symptoms may be present in all three areas: tics, obsessive-compulsive, and ADHD. Such children may require treatment with more than one medication because no single agent is likely to be effective for all three symptoms. The primary care clinician should always consider referral to a child psychiatrist, pediatric neurologist, or specialty clinic for tic disorders prior to starting medication. In many cases, once pharmacotherapy has been initiated, the child can be followed by the primary care practitioner with periodic consultation.

Bibliography

For Parents

Organizations
Obsessive Compulsive Foundation, PO Box 70, Milford CT 04660; (203) 878-5669.

Tourette Syndrome Association, 42–40 Bell Boulevard, Bayside NY 11361; (718) 224-2999.

Publications
Bronheim S. *An Educator's Guide to Tourette Syndrome.* Bayside NY: Tourette Syndrome Association, 1990.

Haerle T (ed). *Children with Tourette Syndrome: A Parents' Guide.* Rockville MD: Woodbine House, 1992.

For Professionals
Chase TN, Friedhoff AJ, Cohen DJ (eds). *Advances in Neurology.* New York: Raven Press, 1992.

Cohen DJ, Bruun R, Leckman JF (eds). *Tic Disorders and Tourette's Syndrome.* New York: Wiley, 1988.

Cohen DJ, Riddle MA, Leckman JF. Pharmacotherapy of Tourette's syndrome and associated disorders. *Psych Clin North Am* 15:109–129, 1992.

Kurlan R (ed). *Handbook of Tourette's Syndrome and Related Tic and Behavioral Disorders.* New York: Dekker, 1993.

Toilet Training
Steven Parker

I. **Description of the problem.** Toilet training is one of the great developmental challenges of early childhood. After 2 years of a devil-may-care attitude to the social niceties of the process of excretion, polymorphous pleasure in diaper changes and perineal cleansing by caregivers, and indifference to voluntary sphincter control, in Selma Fraiberg's phrase: "The missionaries arrive . . . bearing culture to the joyful savage." Armed with Dr. Spock rather than the Bible, the adults try to cajole the skeptical child into making a dramatic developmental leap without clear benefits. It is a difficult sales job and is best attempted only after the child exhibits developmental readiness to understand and master the complex physiologic and psychological tasks of toilet training (Table 69-1). This "child-centered" approach, described by Brazelton in 1962, is the most commonly used in the United States and almost always effective.

A. **Epidemiology**
- In the United States, 26% of children achieve daytime continence by age 24 months, 85% by age 30 months, and 98% by age 36 months.
- Nighttime continence usually occurs within a few months after daytime control is achieved.
- The average time to successful toilet training is 3 months.
- Girls are usually faster than boys in achieving control.

II. **Management.** Suggestions for parents on toilet training strategies are set out in Table 69-2.

A. **Information for parents.** A number of key principles should be discussed with the parents.

1. **There is usually no hurry or benefit to early toilet training.** Although the process can be initiated in response to outside pressures (e.g., day care requirements), there are good reasons to try to wait until the child is developmentally prepared.

2. Like most other developmental challenges of childhood, **it is best to empower the child to take responsibility for achieving continence.** Since control of stool and urine will be achieved sooner or later, the most important outcome of toilet training is a boost in the child's self-esteem at mastering the task. It is a long-term goal that should never be sacrificed to the short-term strategies to achieve continence.

3. **Toilet training is not a contest; it proceeds by fits and starts with successes and frequent relapses; if the timing is wrong, it can always be postponed.** Say to parents: "I *guarantee* that your child will not walk off to kindergarten wearing a diaper."

4. **The parents should not transmit a sense of disgust toward the stool but treat it as a wonderful gift from the child.**

B. **Resistance to toilet training.** Some children resist toilet training, even if the parental technique is impeccable. The primary care clinician can make these suggestions to the parents.

1. **Do not fight, punish, shame, or nag under any circumstances.** Be sympathetic and try to understand the resistance from the child's point of view.

Table 69-1. Signs of developmental readiness for toilet training

Language skills
  Able to follow two-step independent commands (e.g., "Take off your pants and go to the bathroom")
  Uses two-word phrases (e.g., "bye-bye poop," "go potty")
Cognitive skills
  Imitates actions of caregivers (e.g., sweeps the floor)
  Understands cause and effect (i.e., is capable of understanding the reasons for mastering the actions involved in toilet training)
Emotional skills
  Desires to please parents-caregivers by complying with their requests
  Shows diminishing oppositional behaviors and power struggles
Autonomy/independence
  Shows drive for independence and autonomy in self-care activities (e.g., insists on feeding self, tries to take off own clothes)
  Evinces pride and possessiveness toward belongings ("*my* car" and eventually "*my* poop")
Motor skills
  Can ambulate with ease
  Is capable of pulling pants off independently
  Can sit still for 5 min without help
  Can somewhat control urinary/anal sphincter (e.g., urinates large amounts sporadically, rather than constant wetting)
Body awareness
  Shows awareness of wet or soiled diaper
  Manifests signs of urge to void or defecate (e.g., facial expression, goes off into a corner)

2. **Discontinue training for a few weeks or months if the child is emphatically negative.**

3. **Continue discussions with the child** about toilet training and emphasize the maturity demonstrated by such behavior.

4. **Encourage the child to imitate parents and siblings** by inviting him or her into the bathroom.

5. **Remind the child that it is her or his responsibility for this task,** not yours.

6. **Encourage the child to change his or her own diapers.** Remind the child how "yucky" it feels to walk around with a wet or soiled diaper.

7. **Matter-of-factly ask the child at the first sign of impending defecation if he or she wants to use the potty.**

8. **If the child appears afraid of painful stools, add prune juice or fiber to the diet to ensure soft stools.** Postpone potty training until fear of defecation subsides.

9. **Discuss what rewards the child would like in response to successful toilet training.** Try star charts to reinforce successful attempts.

10. **If the child is obstinately recalcitrant, is clearly capable of mastering the task, is developmentally and emotionally healthy, is more than age 3 years, *and* the lack of training is a significant problem for the family,** have a solemn ceremony of throwing away the diapers, announce that he or she is an official big boy or girl now, give encouragement to "do your best," and allow maturational urges to overtake autonomy issues.

Bibliography

For Parents
Brazelton TB. *Doctor and Child.* New York: Delta Books, 1970.

Fraiberg S. *The Magic Years.* New York: Charles Scribner's Sons, 1959.

Table 69-2. Ten steps to successful toilet training

1. Buy a potty chair, and place it in a conspicuous, convenient place. Tell the child, "This is your potty chair. This is where you will [use child's terms for urination and defecation]." Be sure to stress what a special and wonderful chair it is.

2. Allow the child to get used to the chair by sitting on it, fully clothed, for about 5 minutes a couple of times a day for about a week. Try to choose times that the child is more likely to have a bowel movement (e.g., after meals). Never force the child to sit on it.

3. Encourage the child to watch parents or siblings use the bathroom. Explain, "This is where we go potty." Let the child watch the excreta being flushed down the toilet and wave "bye-bye" to it (skip this if the flushing frightens the child).

4. Have the child sit on the potty with the diapers off. Do not urge or expect results, but if it happens, praise the child. Move the potty chair progressively closer and finally into the bathroom.

5. With the child, throw the stool from the soiled diaper into the potty. Tell the child that this is where the stool and urine should go. Then take the pail and dump the stool down the toilet. Wave "bye-bye poop" with the child.

6. Ask the child during the day, "Do you have to go potty?" to keep attention on bodily sensations. Observe the child for signs of impending urination or defecation. Say: "Let's take off your pants and go potty." Assist the child in disrobing and going to the potty chair. Sit for as long as the child wants. Praise success, but do not criticize failure ("Oh, you don't want to go. Okay. Maybe next time").

7. Reinforce positive features of potty training to child (e.g., "just like a big boy," "just like Mommy does," "You did it by yourself!"), and praise successes as they occur.

8. Once a semiconsistent pattern of voiding-stooling on the potty is established, ask the child if he or she wants to give up the diaper "like a big boy or girl" during the day. If yes, make a show of throwing them all away in the garbage and wave "bye-bye" to them. Admire the child for putting on training "big boy or girl" pants.

9. Once training is well established, try an over-the-toilet-seat chair.

10. Nighttime continence may take a few months to acquire after daytime dryness is achieved. There is usually no special strategy needed; simply ask your child when he or she would like to try training pants in the night.

Schmitt BD. *Your Child's Health.* New York: Bantam Books, 1987.

Spock B. *Baby and Child Care.* 1990.

For Professionals

Brazelton TB. A child-oriented approach to toilet training. *Pediatrics* 29:121–128, 1962.

Howe AC, Walker CE. Behavioral management of toilet training, enuresis, and encopresis. *Pediatr Clin North Am* 39:413–432, 1992.

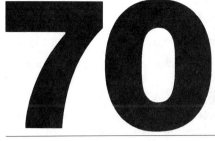

Unpopular Children

Melvin D. Levine

I. **Description of the problem.** Chronic rejection by peers condemns a child to a life of isolation, extreme self-doubt, and perpetual anxiety. The unpopular schoolchild is susceptible to daily embarrassment through both passive and active exclusion by classmates. Such a child must endure the inevitable painful refrain, "Sorry, this seat is saved." In many cases exclusionary comments and actions may be augmented by bullying and verbal abuse. It is regrettably true that many of the most popular children are able to boost their status among peers by being especially creative and demonstrative in their predatory acts against unpopular children. The victim's imposed isolation and constant fear of further humiliation is likely to take its toll on development and behavior.

A. **Contributing factors.** There are multiple pathways that may culminate in a state of unpopularity during the school years. In many instances, more than one factor may predispose a child to peer rejection. The following are among the common predisposing factors:

1. **Intrinsic social cognitive dysfunction,** such as a "learning disability," impairing social awareness, practice, and skill. Social cognitive dysfunction, probably the most common source of unpopularity, may mediate or interact with other factors to yield unpopularity in a child. Table 70-1 contains 18 of the most important subcomponents of social cognitive dysfunction. A clinician assessing a patient's social cognition can make use of such a list to pinpoint a child's troubles in specific subcomponents. This process may ultimately provide a basis for coaching the child in the social domain.

2. **Attention deficits.** Traits such as impulsivity, insatiability, and verbal disinhibition associated with attentional dysfunction engender unpopularity.

3. **Physical unattractiveness.** Children whose physical appearance is somehow displeasing to their peers have been shown to be vulnerable to social isolation.

4. **Poor gross motor skills.** Inferior athletic abilities may potentiate unpopularity.

5. **Language disability.** Children with expressive language problems may not be able to use verbal communication to control relationships and keep pace with the banter and lingo of peers.

6. **Autism and autism-like conditions.** Children who show signs of autism (including very mild forms, such as Asperger syndrome) display varying degrees of social cognitive dysfunction, which commonly incites peer rejection.

7. **Shyness.** Some youngsters who are chronically shy in their temperament and therefore avoid social contact may fail to gain the experience needed in the quest for popularity.

8. **Poor coping skills.** A lack of adaptability and problem-solving skills may cause some children to react to daily stresses and conflicts with maladaptive behaviors, such as aggression. Such behaviors alienate others and promote rejection by classmates.

9. **Eccentricity.** Children who are nonconformists or have unusual interests, speech patterns, tastes, or values may be rejected by their more conventional

Table 70-1. Social cognitive dysfunction: The troubled subcomponents

Subcomponent	Description
Weak greeting skills	Trouble initiating a social contact with a peer skillfully
Poor social predicting	Trouble estimating peer reactions before acting/talking
Deficient self-marketing	Trouble projecting an image acceptable to peers
Problematic conflict resolution	Trouble settling social disputes without aggression
Reduced affective matching	Trouble sensing and fitting in with others' moods
Social self-monitoring failure	Trouble knowing when one is in social trouble
Low reciprocity	Trouble sharing and trouble supporting/reinforcing others
Misguided timing/staging	Trouble knowing how to nurture a relationship over time
Poor verbalization of feelings	Trouble using language to communicate true feelings
Inaccurate inference of feelings	Trouble reading others' feelings through language
Failure of code switching	Trouble matching language style to current audience
Lingo dysfluency	Trouble using the parlance of peers credibly
Poorly regulated humor	Trouble using humor effectively for current context/audience
Inappropriate topic choice/maintenance	Trouble knowing what to talk about and for how long
Weak requesting skill	Trouble knowing how to ask for something inoffensively
Poor social memory	Trouble learning from previous social experience
Assertiveness gaps	Trouble exerting right level of influence over group actions
Social discomfort	Trouble feeling relaxed while relating to peers

peers who feel more comfortable with close replicas of themselves and harbor fears of contamination with "weirdness." Thus, a child who loves to learn about spiders or enjoys listening to Handel oratorios may be ostracized by more conventional classmates.

10. **Family patterns.** There exist self-contained families that do not value generalized popularity, or the family unit itself remains isolated either voluntarily or of necessity (perhaps due to genetic social cognitive dysfunctions).

B. **Secondary phenomena.** The clinical picture of an unpopular child is likely to be complicated by a chain of secondary phenomena, which may include extreme anxiety (or even depression), low self-esteem, and a repertoire of maladaptive defense tactics, such as excessive and inappropriate clowning, extreme controlling behaviors, or outright withdrawal. Often these children seek relationships with adults or with much younger children because they are unable to form alliances within their own age group. In some cases, school phobic behaviors or somatic symptoms may be encountered. Finally, it is not unusual for children who experience social difficulties at school to become aggressive, oppositional, and/or excessively demanding and dependent at home.

II. **Making the diagnosis.** Unpopular children merit careful clinical assessment. Their social difficulties may in fact represent the tip of an iceberg with respect to behavioral and developmental health. The causal factors and potential complications of unpopularity need to be sought through direct history taking, direct observations of the child's image and manner of relating, physical and neurodevelopmental examinations, and reports from teachers. Especially difficult cases may necessitate investigation by a multidisciplinary team.

Information can be gathered from several sources to detect the presence of subcomponents of social cognitive dysfunction listed in Table 70-1. The unpopular child should be interviewed alone to elicit her or his perspective. Nonthreatening questions may be posed to acquire insight into traumatic social scenarios at school. The most common interpersonal "hot spots" are the bus stop, the school bus, the playground, the bathroom, the gymnasium, and the area around lockers. Children can often recreate vividly the stressful scenes that unfold daily against these backdrops. The patient should be reassured that many other children have such difficulties and that it is safe and important to talk about them with an adult.

III. **Management.** The management of the unpopular child must take into consideration the multiplicity of factors operating to engender peer rejection. Associated neurodevelopmental problems (such as a language disability or an attention deficit) require appropriate treatment. The complications, such as somatic symptoms or depression, also demand targeted intervention. In addition, the child's individual social cognitive dysfunction must be addressed. Some possible management approaches to deal directly with a child's unpopularity are summarized below.

A. **Explain the social skill problems carefully to the child.** These may require multiple sessions; not all affected children can process such information readily.

B. **Have the parent of the child who needs social improvement accompany that child to an activity with other children.** Then, during a calm and private interlude, the parent can discuss the social interactions (especially the *faux pas* and transgressions) that occurred.

C. **Help the child locate one or two companions with whom to relate and begin to build skills.** It can be helpful if such peers share interests and perhaps some traits with the unpopular child.

D. **Inform the classroom teacher or building principal if a child is victimized by peer abuse in school.** It is the school's responsibility to make every effort to contain this activity. A strongly worded note from a primary health care provider may be vital in such cases.

E. **Help the rejected child develop skills, hobbies, or areas of expertise that can enhance self-esteem and be impressive to other children.** The management of such a child should always include the diligent quest for and development of such specialties. Ideally, such pursuits should have the potential for generating collaborative activities with other children.

F. **Never force these children into potentially embarrassing situations before their peers.** For example, an unpopular child with poor gross motor skills needs some protection from humiliation in physical education classes.

G. **Manage any family problems or medical conditions** through counseling, specific therapies (e.g., language intervention or help with motor skills), and/or medication (e.g., for attention deficits or depression).

H. **Identify social skills training programs within schools and in clinical settings.** Clinicians should be aware of local resources that offer social skills training to youngsters with social cognitive deficits. Most commonly this training makes use of specific curricula that are used in small group settings in a school or in the community.

I. **Reassure these children that it is appropriate for them to be themselves, that they need not act and talk like everyone else in school, that there is true heroism in individuality.** Clinicians, teachers, and parents need to tread the fine line between helping with social skills and coercing a child into blind conformity with peer pressures, expectations, and models.

Bibliography

For Parents and Children

Levin MD. *All Kinds of Minds*. Cambridge MA: Educators Publishing Service, 1993.

Levine MD. *Keeping a Head in School*. Cambridge MA: Educators Publishing Service, 1990.

Levine MD. *Educational Care*. Cambridge MA: Educators Publishing Service, 1994.

Osman B. *No One to Play With: The Social Side of Learning Disabilities*. New York: Random House, 1982.

For Professionals

Asher SR, Coie JD (eds). *Peer Rejection in Childhood*. Cambridge: Cambridge Press, 1990.

Cartledge G, Milburn JF (eds). *Teaching Social Skills to Children*. New York: Pergamon Press, 1980.

Coleman WL, Lindsay RL. Interpersonal disabilities: Social skill deficits in older children and adolescents: Their description, assessment, and management. *Pediatr Clin North Am* 39(3):551–568, 1992.

McTear MF, Conti-Ramsden G. *Pragmatic Disability in Childhood*. San Diego: Singular Publishing Group, 1992.

71

Violent Youth

Peter Stringham

I. **Description of the problem.** Parents are anxiously searching for sensible advice to keep their children safe in what they perceive as an increasingly violent world. Pediatric practitioners can suggest behaviors that will increase nonviolent problem-solving skills in their patients.

A. **Epidemiology**
   - The murder rate of men ages 15–24 years in the United States is 1/5000 (compared to 1/80,000 in England and 1/200,000 in Japan). Murder is the second leading cause of death (after auto accidents) in this age group.
   - The rate of assaults is many times the murder rate. For example, one in five American homes had a partner hitting the other in the last year.

B. **Etiology/contributing factors**

   1. **Environmental.** A host of environmental factors have been shown to contribute to violent behaviors in children and adults: a cold, inconsistent child-rearing environment; the experience of child abuse; excessive corporal punishment; witnessing violence in the home and community; viewing media violence; coping with socioeconomic disadvantage; and the use of alcohol and other drugs. Equally important, the presence of a gun can turn a violent impulse into a lethal event.

   2. **Developmental.** Constant exposure to environmental violence in an infant and young child can cause a disconnected, hypervigilant style of relating to adults and peers. Witnessing violence in the home, in the neighborhood, and on television teaches children that the way to solve conflicts is through violence. Some parents teach their children that violence is the best way to resolve conflict. Violent individuals tend to believe that violence is *the preferred* way to handle most conflict. They tend to experience the world as harsh and interpret ambiguous situations to be laden with hostility. They view people as either victims or bullies and have few other strategies for resolving potentially violent conflicts. Many have developed an impulsive style of acting without assessing the situation or the consequences of their actions.

II. **Making the diagnosis**

A. **History: Key clinical questions.** The goal of the history is to assess the risk that the child is (or will become) violent. As in other aspects of clinical care, the best way to determine the risk for violence is to ask the right questions about violence in the home, disciplinary techniques, violent encounters in the community, and personal behaviors and attitudes. Clinical judgment must be exercised in pursuing these lines of questions; there is no need to ask all questions at each visit or for every patient.

   1. **For parents**

      a. **Domestic violence**

         (1) *How do you and the baby's father get along? How often do you have yelling or screaming fights? How about pushing or shoving fights?* If answers are negative, no other questions are necessary.

         (2) *Any injuries? What was it about? Tell me about your worst fight. Tell me about your last fight. Are you afraid? Are you safe now? Do*

you know what to do if you are not safe? Is there a gun in the house? At subsequent visits, the clinician can inquire about how couple is getting along.

b. **Gun in the house**

   (1) *Is there a gun in any place where your child spends time? What kind? What is it for? Is it loaded?*

c. **Discipline**

   (1) *How do you correct the child if he or she slaps or bites?* [For an older child] *How do you discipline this child if he or she misbehaves and has to be corrected?*

d. **Attitudes toward violence**

   (1) *If someone tries to pick on your child, what do you think he or she should do?*

e. **Street fighting**

   (1) *How many fights does your child get into? What are they about? What do you do about it?*

2. **For older children**

   a. **Attitudes toward violence**

      (1) *Violence is a big problem in this neighborhood. I think all people have to know how to handle themselves on the streets around here. What would you do if a kid wanted to fight you? Do you know how to get out of a fight?*

      (2) *Do you know why a kid would try to fight with you? What are they trying to get out of it?*

      (3) *If someone calls you a name, how do you respond?*

   b. **Street fighting**

      (1) *How many pushing or shoving fights have you had in the last year? What were they about? Anything serious? Any injuries? Have you ever been threatened with a weapon? How would you get out of a fight?*

   c. **Weapon carrying**

      (1) *Have you ever carried a weapon for self-protection? Are there guns or knives in any of the places you hang out?* This may not be a necessary question if the clinician has identified very little violence in the patient.

   d. **Home environment**

      (1) *How many times were you hit at home in the last year? How did that make you feel?*

   e. **Partner violence**

      (1) *Have you ever had a pushing or shoving fight with a girlfriend [boyfriend]?*

B. **Assessing the risk for violence.** In assessing the degree of risk for the family and patient, a 4-point scale can be utilized: Class 0 = no real risk for violence; Class I = minimal risk for violence; Class II = moderate risks for violence; Class III = significant risk for violence.

   1. **Domestic violence**

      a. **Class I.** Physical fights in the past, but none now. Parent expresses no fear. There is some coercion by the spouse (e.g., telling the woman where she can go, who her friends can be).

      b. **Class II.** Some physical fighting but no injuries. The woman denies fear and says she is safe.

c. **Class III.** There have been injuries, fear, a gun in house, or threats to patient or to children.

2. **Street-fighting teenagers**

a. **Class I.** Few nonserious fights, does not know how to get out of a fight or tough neighborhood, no serious threats, no weapon carrying.

b. **Class II.** Minor injuries, many fights (more than four a year), threatened with knife or gun, likes to fight, no severe criminal behavior, no violent gang, no gun carrying. (If several of these factors exist, the teenage might be in class III.)

c. **Class III.** Many fights, likes fighting, serious fights, would never walk away from a fight, in a violent gang, dealing cocaine, carries a gun, strongly believes that violence is the only response to perceived threats.

III. Management

A. Primary goals

1. **To teach beliefs and skills that enhance the child's ability to respond to stress and perceived threats in a nonaggressive way.**

2. **To help parents and patients to incorporate nonviolent behavior as an integral part of their self-image.**

3. **To decrease the environmental factors that increase violence.**

B. Initial treatment strategies

1. **Domestic violence**

a. **Class I.** Pediatric clinicians need basic skills for treating domestic violence, because medical people may be the only adults outside the family who have any contact with a coerced or battered parent.

Advocate that coercion be stopped and that fighting be discussed with spouse. Try to see if the mother could say to partner, "If you are upset and you say you are upset, I will try to help you. If you are upset and you attack me verbally or in any other way, that will put a lot of distance between us." Does she need more services?

b. **Class II.** The clinician must come down strongly on the side of nonviolence: *This worries me a lot* or *You may be in danger* or *You do not deserve to be hit* or *This might be getting out of control. Are you safe now? Do you know what to do if you don't feel safe?* The clinician can give the telephone number of a domestic violence hot line, attempt to refer to counseling specifically to discuss domestic violence, and possibly try to talk to the spouse. The last may work only if there is a good rapport with the husband and the clinician is confident that the talk will not engender more abuse.

c. **Class III.** The mother should not leave the office until the clinician feels she is safe. Other professionals can be involved in the assessment or identification of resources. The clinician should not try to intervene with the batterer, as this may cause more harm. The police may need to be involved.

2. **Promoting nonviolent discipline**

a. **Ask about disciplinary techniques early on and suggest to parents:** *Your child will soon begin getting into everything. I recommend that the major rule in your house be: "No hurting anyone." It is confusing to a child to say not to hurt anyone and then to hit the child yourself. If your child hits, you can say, "No hitting anyone; it hurts" and try to distract the child or move her or him to another activity.*

b. **If a parent prefers corporal punishment or slaps the child in the office, the clinician should not chastise the parent or offer a judgmental, self-righteous sermon. He or she can explain that discipline is important but that hitting a child does not work as well in the long run as alter-**

native techniques (see Chapter 11) and may cause some unanticipated long-term problems.

3. **Teenagers with street violence.** All the described interventions are in the office, but they can be adapted to larger groups and to the community. Clinicians should try to involve parents, schools, and community leaders to promote nonviolence in the larger community.

   a. **Class 0 (Prevention)**

   (1) **The key to intervention** with children and violent teenagers is to help them see that people who fight are trying to use victims to solve frustrations that are unrelated to the victim.

   (2) **Teach the teenager to walk away from potential fights** with such street-tested interventions as saying: "I don't have anything against you. This isn't worth fighting about. I don't want to fight with you about this. If you have a problem with me, I'll talk to you, but I don't want to fight with you." Nonviolent interventions deal with the aggressor's tendency to misread others as more hostile than they are, and help the aggressor find a face-saving way to end the conflict nonviolently.

   (3) **With young children,** walk them through this exercise: "Why would a kid come up to you and say, 'You're ugly; so's your mother'? He is probably saying that because he wants to fight you. When some kids are upset, they try to make themselves feel better by fighting. Do you know any kids like that? Pretend I'm a kid your age. If I came up to you and said, 'I feel really upset. I would feel better if you talked to me for 5 minutes,' what would you say? Most kids say, 'Sure.' What would you say if I said, 'I feel really upset. I would feel better if I could fight with you.' Will you fight with me then? So if a kid says, 'You're ugly and so's your mother,' what he really means is 'I feel really upset and I think I would feel better if you fight me.'"

   b. **Class I**

   (1) **Express worry about the child's safety:** *You have told me that you would not walk away from a fight, and that worries me.* If this is a younger child, the worries can be expressed to the parents. (Parents may be advocating street fighting because they think this will make their child safer.)

   (2) **If suggestions to avoid fighting are viewed as impractical,** the clinician can truthfully say: *You are right; I don't know everything about your friends and neighborhood. What kinds of things might work there? I see a lot of kids, and I am always looking for new ways to help them stay safe. If you can think of things that will work, I want to know about them.*

   c. **Class II**

   (1) **Express concern to the child:** *Your exam shows you are healthy and well. You are growing up to be a strong person. You have told me that you fight a lot. I am worried about this.*

   (2) **Try to teach the connections among depression, frustration, anger, and violence,** both from the victim's and the bully's points of view. Help the patient handle frustrations in a manner that is as satisfying as violence is but less risky (e.g., sports, music, being creative, talking to a trusted person).

   (3) **Present dilemmas** to help the patient see that he or she has nonviolent beliefs and skills on which to build: *Your best friend's aunt is in the hospital. You feel really sorry for your friend and would like to help him out. He begins to yell at you, "You always thought you were better than me. You've always looked down on me. Let's step outside and settle this." You really like this guy and feel sorry for him. What could you do?* The clinician can help the child to struggle through a solution, suggest other possibilities, and remind him or

her that the same strategies that might work with a friend can also work with a stranger.

(4) Address weapon carrying: *You told me you used a switchblade to feel safe. That worries me. Do other kids know that you carry a knife? If they knew and had a disagreement with you and thought it might turn into a fight, do you think they might get a weapon? What might happen? After a fight, don't you always try to have someone settle it anyway and make peace?*

(5) Try to teach a nonimpulsive approach to an ambiguous situation: *When most guys are approached by a kid who wants to fight, they ask themselves, "Why is this guy trying to fight me? Is he upset? Is he drunk? Have I caused this in any way?" Then they ask, "Am I sure he has no weapon?" Then they ask, "If I wanted to calm him down, what could I do?" After they have answered all those questions, they decide whether to fight.*

d. Class III

(1) The clinician should try to find *anything* **the patient wants his or her help with.** An intervention will be successful only if the clinician has established some alliance. Many of these patients are very distrustful and emotionally disconnected. The clinician can try the class II street-fighting intervention as a way of giving the child new skills that might be useful in areas where he or she is alone and no one knows his or her reputation.

(2) If there is evidence of violence toward a girlfriend, say: *When a woman begins to fear a man, love slowly dies. The woman takes away her trust and support. If they are having sex, the woman cannot relax and the man has no chance of pleasing her. He will turn into a bad lover. That's sad; you have to feel sorry for a guy like that.*

Bibliography

Alpert E, Freund K. *Partner Violence: How to Recognize and Treat Victims of Abuse— A Guide for Physicians*. Waltham, MA: Massachusetts Medical Society, 1992.

American Academy of Pediatrics—Committee on Adolescents. Firearms and adolescents. *Pediatrics* 89:784–787, 1992.

Prothrow-Stith D. *Deadline Consequences: How Violence Is Destroying Our Teenage Population and a Plan to Begin Solving the Problem*. New York: Harper Collins, 1991.

Sege R. Adolescent violence. *Curr Opin Pediatr* 4:575–581, 1992.

Straus M, Gelles R, Steinmetz S, *Behind Closed Doors: Violence in the American Family*. Garden City NY: Anchor Books, 1980.

Violence: A Compendium from JAMA, American Medical News, and the Specialty Journals of the American Medical Association. Chicago: AMA, 1992.

I. **Description of the problem.** Children who witness violence on the street and in the home are silent victims. Although it is clear that children who are the *victims* of violence (e.g., child abuse and sexual abuse) suffer severe and long-lasting consequences, there is accumulating evidence that *witnessing* violence is also damaging to children. Because their scars are emotional and not physical, the primary care clinician may not fully appreciate their distress and miss an opportunity to provide needed interventions.

A. **Epidemiology**

1. **Community violence**
   • More than a third of New Orleans school-aged children had witnessed severe violence; 40% had seen a dead body.
   • 10% of children under age 6 years in inner-city Boston had seen a knifing or shooting.

2. **Domestic violence**
   • 3 million children witness domestic violence every year. Clinical experience suggests that witnessing violence in the home may be even more harmful to children than is exposure to community violence.

II. **Making the diagnosis**

A. **Symptoms.** Children who witness severe or chronic violence may suffer psychological trauma and may develop symptoms of posttraumatic stress disorder (PTSD) (Table 72-1). Although young children often will not fully meet these criteria, certain behavioral changes are often seen (e.g., sleep disturbances, social withdrawal, aggressive behavior, and increased anxiety about separations from caretakers).

B. **History: Key clinical questions.** It is important for the primary care clinician to inquire about violence in the lives of all children. Questions may be prefaced by a statement that assures the family members that they are not being singled out for this line of questioning and that the clinician considers the topic of violence to be within the scope of problems to be addressed in a medical visit. Additionally, the clinician has communicated that violence and exposure to violence are a risk to the child's well-being and are a legitimate focus of concern during the clinical visit.

1. *I know that there is a lot of violence in our world these days. I have begun to ask all of my patients about their experiences with violence. I would like to ask you a few questions.*
   • *Are you ever worried about your child's safety?*
   • *Has your child seen frightening things?*
   • *What does your child watch on television? Are you concerned about what your child is watching on television?*
   • *Has your child witnessed violence on the streets or in the neighborhood?*
   • *Has he or she witnessed violence in the home?*
   If there are disclosures of witnessing violence, the following questions will explore how the child may have been affected.

2. *What happened? What did the child see or hear?* The clinician should elicit the story from both the child and the parent. It is preferable to hear the child's story first and, if possible, separately. Children's accounts of traumatic

Table 72-1. Symptoms of posttraumatic stress disorder

Numbing of responsiveness to the outside world
  Constriction of emotions
  Reduced involvement with play
  Dissociative states
  Foreshortened view of the future
Intrusive recollections of the traumatic event
  Flashbacks or intrusive recollections
  Reenactment through play
  Avoidance of traumatic cues
  Difficulties with concentration
Autonomic disturbances
  Hyperarousal, hyperalertness
  Sleep disturbances
  Distractibility

events give important clues about how they viewed the event, how they perceive their role, and what kind of meaning they make of the event. Since children frequently misunderstand or misperceive a sequence of events, the child's account provides important information about how to correct misperceptions.

3. [To the child] *When and how often do you think about what happened? Do thoughts come to you while you are in school? What do you do when these thoughts occur?*

4. *Are there sleep difficulties? What kind? Nightmares? Difficulties sleeping alone?*

5. *Does the child seem less interested in play or school? Does the child worry more?*

6. *What behavioral changes have you observed in the child? Is the child fearful of being apart from you or other caretakers?*

III. Management

A. Counseling the parents. This aspect of the intervention is much more difficult if the child is living with ongoing domestic violence. Maximizing safety may be a difficult task because the mother may be unable to leave the batterer. In cases of domestic violence, it is necessary to help the woman assess the safety of her children and herself. This discussion should convey the clinician's concern about the impact of violence on the child and mother. He or she should help to formulate a plan the mother can use in the event of future violence, including the telephone numbers of the local domestic violence hot line and battered women's shelter. A referral for counseling should be attempted. More typically, many families of children who have witnessed violence can be effectively counseled by the primary care clinician. Counseling for parents should include the following components:

1. A careful **review** of the facts and details of the violent event.

2. **Information** about the expectable symptoms and behaviors associated with witnessing violence.

3. **Assistance** in restoring a sense of stability to the family in order to enhance the child's feelings of safety (e.g., by establishing consistent routines, assistance in accessing concrete supports such as housing, benefits).

4. **Strategies** to encourage the child to express feelings about the event (e.g., verbally, through drawings or play).

5. **Assurance** that it is not a forbidden topic for discussion. It is helpful to the child to be able to talk about it within the family. Without overfocusing on the incident, parents can communicate their willingness to talk to the child about what has happened.

B. Counseling the child. For some children the process of telling their story in detail is in itself therapeutic. The child has a chance to reflect on the event, to try out new coping strategies, and to receive empathic and supportive feedback. By asking sensitive and detailed questions, the clinician models for the parents how to talk to children about frightening or unpleasant events. Thus, the primary care clinician's role with the child is to:

1. **Review** the facts and details of the traumatic event and help the child accurately understand what has happened.

2. **Give the child a forum to share worries, fears, and anxieties and to help the child accommodate to the trauma.**

C. Criteria for referral. The child or family should be referred in the following circumstances:
• The symptoms have persisted for more than 6 months.
• The trauma was particularly violent or involved the loss of a parent or caretaker.
• The caretakers are unable to be attuned empathically to the child.
• The child is in an unsafe environment.
Referral should be made to mental health specialists who are familiar with treating children who have experienced trauma. Specialized treatment for these children may include psychological debriefing through play therapy, behavioral/cognitive strategies to decrease sensitivity to traumatic reminders, and pharmacological interventions.

Bibliography

For Parents

Publications

Garbarino J. *Let's Talk about Living in a World with Violence.* Chicago: Erickson Institute, 1993.

Monahan C. *Children and Trauma: A Parent's Guide to Helping Children Heal.* New York: Lexington Books, 1993.

Organization

National Council on Child Abuse and Family Violence, (800) 222-2000.
Operates a help line with information about local resources for battered women. Also provides literature on request.

For Professionals

Eth S, Pynoos RS. *Post-traumatic Stress Disorder in Children.* Washington DC: American Psychiatric Press, 1985.

Garbarino J, Dubrow N, Koestelny K, Pardo C. *Children in Danger: Coping with the Consequences of Community Violence.* San Francisco: Jossey-Bass, 1992.

Groves B, Zuckerman B, Marans S, Cohen DJ. Silent victims: Children who witness violence. *JAMA* 269(2):262–264, 1993.

Jaffe PG et al. Children's observations of violence, parts 1 and 2: Critical issues in child development and intervention planning. *Can J Psychiatry* 35:466–476, 1990.

Udwin O. Annotation: Children's reactions to traumatic events. *J Child Psychol Psychiatry* 34:2, 115–127, 1993.

Family Issues

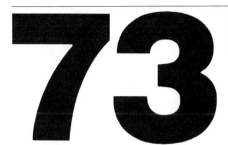

Adoption

Nancy Roizen

I. Description of the problem

A. Epidemiology

- Approximately 2% of the population is adopted—52% by nonrelatives and 48% by relatives.
- For parents adopting because of infertility, the rate of conception after adopting is 8–14%.
- The outcomes of adoptions are considered good to excellent in 70%, unclear in 20%, and bad in 10%.
- In 3% of adoptions, problems lead to discontinuation of the adoption.
- In special-needs adoptions, discontinuation occurs in 11–14%.
- Placement with one or two parents is equally successful.
- In general, the younger the child is at the time of adoption, the more successful is the adoption.

II. Primary care clinician's role: information gathering

A. Preadoption.
During the preadoption process, the clinician should obtain important information from the birth parents and medical records. Since adopted children are somewhat more likely than the general population to have attention deficit hyperactivity disorder, fetal alcohol syndrome, mental retardation, or congenital malformations, the clinician should specifically ask about a family history and look for indications of their presence in the child. The clinician should also obtain details about the birth parents' appearance, interests, and talents and the reason for placing the child for adoption, information that the adoptee may want later, in adolescence.

B. Postadoption.
Studies indicate that almost all adoptions have transitional problems. Parents have had idealized expectations about the child's behaviors that are not being realized. For instance, the adoptive parents may think that the child is too cuddly (or not cuddly enough), eats too much (or not enough), or does not signal needs clearly. The clinician should plan a follow-up visit within days rather than weeks of the adoption and keep close and frequent contact with the adoptive parents to monitor the goodness of fit between parental expectations and child behavior.

C. Older adoptee.
For the older adoptee, the clinician should seek additional information on the history and quality of the child's social attachments, history of adverse experiences (such as abuse, deprivation, neglect, rejections, and separations) and educational experience (including quantity, quality, and potential special needs).

III. Management

A. When to tell the child he or she is adopted.
The age at which parents should tell the adoptee about the adoption is somewhat controversial. The importance of the child's learning of the adoption from the adoptive parents cannot be overstated. To learn of adoption from someone else can cause an irreparable breach of trust. The clinician should strongly encourage parents to tell the child early, when he or she is an egocentric preschooler (age 3–4 or earlier) so the adoptee will never remember a time when he or she did not know the truth about his or her adoption. Following disclosure at the preschool age, most parents report a positive reaction from their child, and the adoption is clearly an acceptable topic of conversation from then on.

Table 73-1. Issues of adoption at different ages

Preschool
  "Where did I come from?"
  Life and death issues
  Generally accepting of being adopted
School age (7–11 years)
  "Why was I adopted when most people aren't?"
  Worried that their value as a person is less because they are adopted
  Concerns about being different
  Aware that they have lost someone who played an extremely important role in
    their life
  Imagines birth parents as rich, famous, and more attractive than adoptive
    parents
Adolescence
  Task of developing an identity and discovering how they are different and how
    they are connected to "their people"
  Concerns about family illness such as insanity and talents, and physical
    appearance of birth family
  Interest in meeting birth parents

B. **How to tell the child he or she is adopted.** The adoption story should be explained at the child's developmental level and include the following elements:

1. **The adoptive parents' motivation for adoption.**

2. **Acknowledgment of the important role of the birth parents in the creation of the child.**

3. **The information that the child was conceived, grew inside the birth mother, and was born just like all other children.**

4. **A suggestion that the decision of the birth parents to place him or her for adoption was in no way the fault of the child.**

5. **Acknowledgment that there are happy and sad feelings associated with adoption.**

6. **A statement of the adoptive parents' love for the child** and how happy they are that she or he joined their family

7. **The specifics of each adoption story will vary according to the circumstances.** The adoption story might be something like, "We could not make a baby ourselves, so we decided to adopt. You were made by another man and woman, your birth parents, and born to your birth mother, just like all other children. But your birth parents could not take care of a baby, so we adopted you. We're sure that they were sad that you were separated from them. You came to live with us, and we're happy we're a family."

C. **Sequence of developmental issues.** The adoptee's understanding of adoption changes as he or she develops. At different ages the child will focus on different issues and need access to different information to answer questions (Table 73-1).

1. During the **preschool** age, children are interested in the facts of how they were born and came to be part of their families. A picture book that depicts the story can be very helpful.

2. Around **ages 7–11 years,** the child begins to appreciate the uniqueness and implications of his or her adoptive status. The child's questions, however, may be viewed by the adoptive parents as a potential rejection. The clinician needs to reassure them that the emergence of the child's questioning is part of the normal development sequence and may herald even tougher questions. Children at this age may imagine their birth parents to be richer, more famous, and otherwise more attractive than their adoptive parents. For this reason, many adoptive parents share letters from and pictures of the birth parents with the child. If the birth parents are known to the child but not

as his or her birth parents, the elementary school years are an opportune time to reveal this information to the child.

3. In the **early adolescent search for identity,** the adoptee may begin to seek more specific information about the birth parents. Teenagers master the task of developing an identity by discovering how they are different from every other human being and how connected they are to "their people." Having more than two parents makes this task more complicated. If little is known about the birth parents, the adolescent may create an idealized picture of them.

4. In the **late adolescent period,** the adoptee may muse about marriage and children and become even more interested in the biologic and medical status of the birth parents. Concerns about family illnesses such as insanity may surface. Adolescents, with rare exceptions, should have all the available information about their origins to help them make sense of their life.

D. **Adoptees' questions about birth parents.** As the child asks more probing questions about the birth mother and why she did not keep him or her, the answers should afford the opportunity to develop a positive attitude about her. In a discussion of this issue, a parent could say, "Your mother chose adoption because she felt unprepared to raise a child, any child, at that time." The adoptive parent could go on to explain that the birth mother felt unprepared for reasons related to a lack of money, maturity, and resources. The adoptive parent should never imply that the reason for the adoption had anything to do with something the child did.

Often there is little information available about the birth father. As the child realizes that there most certainly was a father involved, she or he also realizes that he too has abandoned her or him. An adoptive parent could say to the child, "Your birth father was most likely overwhelmed by the situation and thought that he was not entitled to be more involved. He probably thinks about you and wonders about how you are doing." As with discussions about the birth mother, the child should be encouraged to think positively about the birth father.

In some cases, the birth parents had problems, such as alcoholism, drug abuse, child abuse, or mental illness, that led to the adoption. These circumstances need to be discussed and explained in an understanding way, such as: "Your parents needed help but did not know how to ask for it. So their problem with alcoholism was a signal that they needed help and needed someone else to care for their child."

E. **Outsiders and adoption.** People may ask personal questions about an adopted child out of curiosity or because the child looks different from the adoptive parents. Parents should never hide the fact that a child is adopted but always respect the child's right to privacy with regard to the details about the birth parents and the circumstances of the adoption. Private details not to be shared might include genetic and social history or details that have not yet been shared with the child. One way to respond to such questions would be to say, "I don't want to go into all those details because I think it should be Jenny's choice when she's older what information she wants to share."

In the early elementary school years, the adoptee may be teased about being adopted. When this happens, the child needs to tell a sympathetic and supportive adult and be helped to develop a reply. The child needs to tell what happened and how he or she felt, responded, and would like to respond if it happened again. For instance, the child could be coached to say, "Yeah, I'm adopted. So what? So was President Ford!"

F. **Searching for the birth parents.** Some adolescents express an interest in meeting their birth parents; others may only be interested in knowing certain information (such as what they look like). About 40% of adoptees seek the identity of their birth parents or seek to locate and meet them. Studies show that following reunions with birth parents, the majority of adoptees have shown more positive relationships with their adoptive parents. The adolescent adoptee should be encouraged to postpone the search until young adulthood, when he or she may have the maturity and experience to put the adoption in proper and healthy perspective. Searching is time consuming and energy draining, and it may be confusing to try to establish relationships with biologic parents while trying to become independent of adoptive ones.

G. Special-needs adoptees. Special-needs or hard-to-place adoptees include certain minorities, children older than age 6 years, children with a chronic illness or a psychological problem, or children who must be adopted with a sibling. Discontinuation of the adoption is more likely if the child is older, if the child has made many moves, and if there is another child in the home (especially if the child is of the same age). Some special-needs children have been enormously deprived, and the behaviors caused by deprivation make special demands on a family. In preadoptive counseling, the clinician should explore the adoptive parents' readiness to assume the extra effort and time demanded in adopting a child with special needs.

H. Transracial or mixed racial adoption. The American Academy of Pediatrics recommends that a child be placed with a family of the same racial and cultural background whenever possible. However, minorities are overrepresented in the group of children available for adoption. In 1970, 35% of African-American adoptees were adopted by white families. By age 3 years, children are aware of differences in skin color and, by age 4 years, they are aware of racial groupings. Since every child needs a positive sense of racial and ethnic identity, adoptive parents have a responsibility to acquaint the child with his or her heritage and to integrate aspects of the child's heritage into the family's life (e.g., celebrating the holidays of the child's ethnic origin, making foods from the child's country of origin). Although various minority groups have long opposed adoption of minority children by parents of a different racial background, the few long-term follow-up studies of African-American children adopted by white parents do not show evidence of undue difficulties.

I. Open adoption. Open adoption is the sharing of information and/or communication between adoptive and biological families. One advantage is the ready source of information available as the child feels a need for it. The practice of open adoption has not been well researched, and the long-term effects on the child are not known.

Bibliography

For Parents

Publications
Bolles EB. *The Penguin Adoption Handbook: A Guide to Creating Your New Family.* New York: Penguin, 1984.

Melina LR. *Making Sense of Adoption: A Parent's Guide.* New York: Harper & Row, 1989.

Organizations
National Adoption Center; (800) TOADOPT
Information on adoption by local area.

Adoptive Families, 3333 Highway 100N, Minneapolis MN 55422; (800) 372-3300.
Provides a wonderful newsletter for adoptive families, full of information and articles.

For Professionals
Donovan DM, McIntyre D. Loss in the lives of children. In Donovan DM, McIntyre D (eds). *Healing the Hurt Child: A Developmental Contextual Approach.* New York: Norton, 1990.

Schwartz EM. Problems after adoption: Some guidelines for pediatrician involvement. *J Pediatr* 87:991–994, 1975.

Sokoloff B. Adoption and foster care—The pediatrician's role. *Pediatr Rev* 1:57–61, 1979.

Bereavement and Loss

Benjamin S. Siegel

I. **Description of the problem.** The death of a loved one (including pets) is a major crisis and stress in the life of a child. It is estimated that 5% of all children will experience the death of a parent by age 15 years, and 40% of junior and senior high school students have experienced the death of a friend their age.

   A. **Coping with loss.** The task of children who experience a great loss is to attempt to understand what happened and why the death occurred, to mourn the lost person in their own way and at their level of cognition and affective development, and to construct an enduring inner reality of that lost person and the lost relationship. Long-term mental health outcomes of bereaved children are influenced by:
   • The age at which the death takes place.
   • The person who has died (parent, sibling, friend, or relative).
   • The nature of the relationship between that person and the child.
   • The timing of the death (sudden, chronic, expected, unexpected).
   • The nature of the death (illness, suicide, sudden infant death syndrome, AIDS, murder, accident).
   It is useful to divide childhood into four major age categories to understand the child's knowledge of and emotional reaction to death and loss (Table 74-1).

   B. **Communication issues.** Most adults in our culture feel uncomfortable talking with children about death. Death is viewed as outside the normal cycle of life, something to be fought against and denied. This attitude is problematic when the adults who are most needed by children are in the midst of their own mourning and grief, so that their grief intensifies when their children question them or discuss the death. Other times, adults may wish to protect children from emotional distress by denying the loss altogether. Well-meaning adults may use euphemisms to explain about death, such as the metaphor of a "long journey" or "going to sleep," which may be confusing to children and make them afraid to go to sleep or fearful when a loved one is sleeping.
   Adults must help children to come to terms with difficult questions:
   • What is death?
   • Can it happen to me?
   • Can it happen to some other loved one?
   • Am I responsible for the death?
   • Who will take care of me now?
   • Why did the person die?
   • Where is the dead person now?
   • Why won't the dead person come back?

II. **Role of the primary care clinician.** The primary care clinician, especially one who has had a long-term relationship with the patient and family, is in an excellent position to provide initial counseling and appropriate referral (Table 74-2). Competence in this area requires not only the willingness to explore these issues with families but also an honest appraisal of one's own thoughts and feelings about the meaning of death.

III. **Management.** The most important goal for the provider is to help the parents address their thoughts and feelings about the loss and to encourage them to be emotionally available to their children. The provider should encourage the adult caretakers to communicate with the children and remember that accommodation and adaptation to the death of a loved one are a continual process, often lasting a lifetime. Children

Table 74-1. Cognitive and affective stages of grief and loss

Age	Cognitive understanding	Emotional/affective	Potential symptoms
Young children less than age 3 yr	Death is separation, abandonment, change	Feelings of loss	Sadness Fearfulness Poor feeding Sleep problems Irritability Developmental delay Regression Increased crying
Preschool (3–6 yr) Preoperational (prelogical) Magical thinking Fantasies Causation of thought* Egocentric	Realization that death exists Reversibility of death (ages 3–5) Death equals sorrow of others Death is temporary Death is catching Fear that sleep = death Loving someone is dangerous Dead people still eat and breathe	Guilt (I am responsible) Shame Fear of punishment because of my thoughts, feelings, and actions Fear of catching whatever caused the death Fear of other loved one's dying Anger at loved one Denial	Delayed grief Enuresis Encopresis Sleep disturbances Nightmares Temper tantrums Hyperactivities Loss of control of behavior
School age (6–11 yr) Concrete operations (logical) Problem solving	Death is permanent Death will not happen to me Biologic understanding of death Death is universal Dead people do not think, feel Dead people can sometimes look alive	Anger, sadness Guilt Some fear of retribution Denial	Somatic complaints Resistance to going to school Decreased school performance Inattention, fighting, daydreaming, failure to complete work Acting-out behavior
Adolescence (12+ yr) Formal operations (abstract logical)	Death as an inevitable universal process Death as irreversible Death can happen to me Idealization of dead person	Strong denial of death Anger Guilt Sadness Embarrassment Wanting to join the loved one (suicidal ideation) Grieving with peers	Delinquency Drug and alcohol abuse Somatic complaints Depression Suicide ideation Sexual acting out School failure

*The idea that one's thoughts or wishes can cause something to happen.

Table 74-2. Role of primary care provider

To acknowledge one's own feelings of sadness and loss

To demystify and explain the reasons for death at a level the child can understand

To encourage the child to ask questions and explore his or her fear and fantasies

To encourage the child to see the body of the person who has died if the child and adults feel comfortable, and to participate in the religious or cultural rituals of grief and mourning as practiced by the family

To explore hidden feelings and memories of the dead person

To explain to parents different stages of cognitive and affective development of children and anticipate specific kinds of grief reactions

To deal with and accept any of the displaced anger that family members may have

To monitor the grief reaction and refer for mental health consultation when appropriate

To support the child and family over time

---

confront the loss at each stage of development as they gain a greater understanding of the world and themselves, and they experience new feelings at each stage of development. Nurturing and support over time by family and friends are the best healing experiences for the bereaved child.

A. Very young children (to age 2 years)

1. **Encourage parenting figures to provide consistent care in a familiar environment** since children at this age react to death primarily with feelings of separation and loss.

2. **Familiar toys, appropriate transitional objects, and consistent caretaking are crucial.** Frequently, family members are involved in their own grief and have little energy to spend with the infant or toddler. A close relative or even a babysitter well known to the child could be engaged to provide the support of which others may be incapable.

B. Preschool (ages 3–6 years)

1. **The child's understanding.** Since children at this age are egocentric, they believe they may have caused the death. It is important to emphasize that the loved one has really died, that they did not cause the death, and that they will be taken care of. Sometimes the pain of the loss is simply too great for children to comprehend, and they behave as if nothing has happened. Or they become angry with whomever brought the bad news or angry with family members because they were not strong enough to prevent the death.

2. **Explanations.** Because children at this age believe that death is reversible, they may ask such questions as, "When is Daddy coming home?" or questions of bodily functioning, such as, "If Grandma is in the coffin underground, won't she get cold?" or "How will she breathe if she is all covered up?" These questions may be upsetting for grieving adults, who need to be encouraged to be quite direct and honest: "Tommy is dead. We will never see him again. We are all very sad." "I will try to answer your questions and would like to know what you think or feel when someone dies. I also want you to know that you will be taken care of at all times." Sometimes referring to a dead pet (if that had been in the child's experience) is a useful way to link the child's past loss to the present. Reading selected stories can also be useful.

3. **Participation in rituals.** Children at this age may go to funerals, or participate in any family rituals should they choose. They should be accompanied by an empathic adult who is well known to them and emotionally available to meet their needs. The direct experience about what happens at funerals prevents unrealistic fears and fantasies from developing and enhances long-term adaptation. If a child does not wish to go to the funeral or is overwhelmed by the crowd and the communal grief reaction, special times may be established for later visitation to the funeral home or gravesite. If children choose not

to participate, a clear, concrete description of what happened should be provided.

C. **School age** (ages 6–12 years)

1. **The child's understanding.** At this age children can understand biologic functioning. Adults should be encouraged to give more information about the reasons for the death (e.g., "His body stopped working completely," or "Her heart stopped," or "The lungs no longer worked," or "He died of cancer").

2. **Explanations.** Honesty, even about suicide or homicide, usually facilitates long-term adaptation.

3. **Grieving.** Parents should be encouraged to acknowledge their emotions to their children and give their children permission to express their own feelings. Grieving of parents and children may be dysynchronous. The child's grief reaction may appear just at the time that adults are getting over the acute mourning stage.

4. **Participation in rituals.** Children at this age should be encouraged to participate in all formal events, such as funeral services, burial services, memorial services, and other rituals dictated by religion or culture. The child needs an empathic person present and should not be forced to participate if he or she does not wish to.

D. **Adolescence**

1. **Adolescents mourn as adults do,** but they are new to the existential realization that death can happen to them. They also wish to participate in all activities.

2. **Adolescents can sometimes harbor guilt** that they may have been responsible for the death.

3. Peer relationships are very strong and **adolescents often prefer to be with their friends** rather than family members.

4. **Sometimes they develop idealized images of the loved one, occasionally want to "join" the loved one,** and have thoughts of suicide. Although suicidal ideation is a common symptom in bereaved adolescents, it is rare for adolescents actually to attempt suicide.

E. **School.** The task of telling schoolmates about the death is very important for the child. School officials should be informed. Teachers should be sensitive to abnormal grief reactions requiring referral. Special ceremonies and memorial services can be organized in the school setting. Close friends, teachers, guidance counselors, and school administrators often attend funerals. The primary care clinician might consider a role in school consultation for the grieving child.

IV. **Criteria for referral.** In order to help the child and the family, time needs to be set aside to address many of the issues mentioned. Some primary care providers feel that their role is to obtain a history and to refer to a mental health provider. Others, especially if there has been an ongoing relationship and they enjoy the role of counseling and education, can use that relationship to address immediate issues of grief and follow the child and family through the grief process. After the initial consultation at the time of the death, a 2- to 4-week and a 4- to 6-month follow-up consultation is appropriate.

A mental health referral is advisable when the provider feels uncomfortable by the feelings or questions generated during the consultation. Other reasonable criteria include distress for more than 6 months; intense, inconsolable grief; and poor functioning at home, in school, or with peers.

Bibliography

For Parents

Kübler-Ross E. *On Children and Death*. New York: Macmillan, 1983.

Grollman EA. *Talking about Death: A Dialogue Between Parents and Child* (3rd ed). Boston: Beacon Press, 1990.

The most up-to-date list of national organizations, books for children and adults, various support groups, movies, and videos.

For Children*

Preschool
Brown MW. *The Dead Bird*. New York: Young Scott Books, 1958.

Viorst J. *The Tenth Good Thing About Barney*. New York: Atheneum, 1972.

Young School-Aged Children
Miles M. *Annie and the Old One*. Boston: Little, Brown, 1971.

Lee V. *The Magic Moth*. New York: Seabury Press, 1972.

Rock G. *The Thanksgiving Treasure*. New York: Knopf, 1972.

Older School-Aged Children
Smith DB. *Taste of Blackberries*. New York: Crowell, 1973.

White EB. *Charlotte's Web*. New York: Harper & Row, 1952.

Stein SB. *About Dying*. New York: Walker & Co., 1974.

Young Adolescents
Alcott LM. *Little Women*. New York: Grosset & Dunlap, 1947.

For Professionals

Baker JR, Snedney MA, Gross E. Psychological tasks for bereaved children. *Amer J Orthopsychiatry* 62(1):105–116, 1992.

Committee on Psychosocial Aspects of Child and Family Health. The pediatrician and childhood bereavement. *Pediatrics* 89:516–518, 1992.

Sahler OJ (ed). *The Child and Death*. St. Louis: Mosby, 1978.

Saler L, Skolnick N. Childhood parental death and depression in adulthood: Roles of surviving parent and family environment. *Amer J Orthopsychiatry* 62(4):504–516, 1992.

Schowalter JR (ed). *The Child and Death*. New York: Columbia University Press, 1983.

Silverman PR, Warden JW. Children's reactions in the early months after the death of a parent. *Amer J Orthopsychiatry* 2(1):93–104, 1992.

*From Aradin CE. Books for children about death. *Pediatrics* 57:372–373, 1976.

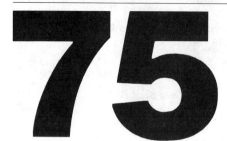

Child Care

Meg Zweiback

I. **Description of the problem.** In the past 20 years, there has been a dramatic shift in the patterns of child rearing in the United States, propelled by economic needs, increased opportunities for employment of women, and the increasing number of single-parent families. The majority of children in the United States now spend a substantial part of their days being cared for by adults other than their own parents.

A. **Epidemiology**
- In 1990, 54% of the mothers of infants younger than age 1 year were working outside the home. This percentage is expected to increase.

B. **Outcomes.** The clinician will be presented with parental concerns surrounding choice of child care. Parents will have questions about their child's behavioral response to being in child care and whether the long-term effects of child care will be detrimental or beneficial. Research in this area indicates that when children are cared for in small groups with a low ratio of children to trained and skilled child care providers, there is no impairment of children's development or behavior. Research also shows that families under stress with less than optimal child-rearing practices tend to select lower-quality child care.

C. **Types of care**

1. **Care by relatives.** This care is provided in the home of the parents or of the relatives and is the most common type of child care.

   a. **Advantages**

      (1) **This is usually the most affordable type of care.**

      (2) **Parents can often be more flexible in their work hours.**

   b. **Disadvantage**

      (1) **Conflicts may arise over differences in child care practices.**

2. **In-home care.** This care is provided by a nanny or a babysitter who may provide care for other children at the same time. Families who share the services of an in-home caregiver may rotate homes every week or month.

   a. **Advantages**

      (1) **In-home care is usually very flexible** and can be adapted to the needs of parents who work long or unusual hours.

      (2) **The child may get more individual attention than a child in group care.**

      (3) **An in-home caregiver will usually be able to care for a sick child so that the parent does not miss work.**

   b. **Disadvantages**

      (1) **This care is usually the most expensive type.**

      (2) **Parents need to be able to supervise the daily activities of an employee and take on the responsibilities of an employer,** including paying appropriate taxes and keeping records.

Table 75-1. Recommended child-to-adult ratio and group size for out-of-home programs

Age	Child-to-staff ratio	Maximum group size
Birth–24 mo	3:1	6
25–30 mo	4:1	8
31–35 mo	5:1	10
3 year olds	7:1	14
4–5 year olds	8:1	16
6–8 year olds	10:1	20
9–12 year olds	12:1	24

Source: American Public Health Association and American Academy of Pediatrics. *Caring for Our Children: Guidelines for Out-of-Home Child Care Programs,* a Collaborative Project. Copyright 1992 by the American Public Health Association and the American Academy of Pediatrics.
Note: Group size refers to number of children in a room or other well-defined space.

3. **Family day care.** This care is provided to a group of children in the caregiver's home.

   a. **Advantages**

      (1) **This care is usually reasonable in cost.**

      (2) **Family day care is licensed.** The caregiver is required by law to follow health and safety guidelines.

      (3) **The children in the group develop close relationships with each other and a strong bond with the caregiver.**

   b. **Disadvantages**

      (1) **The quality of care and skills of the caregiver vary widely.**

      (2) **Parents may have to find substitute care during vacation times or if the caregiver is ill.**

4. **Center-based care.** This care is provided by multiple adult caregivers to large groups of children in a setting designed for child care.

   a. **Advantages**

      (1) **Centers are licensed.** Supervisors and caregivers are required to have training in child development.

      (2) **The care is usually structured and predictable.**

      (3) In a well-run center, **the staff will be stable,** allowing children to form close relationships.

      (4) **Centers are usually open year-round** and can use substitute caregivers during staff vacations or illnesses.

   b. **Disadvantages**

      (1) Center-based care may be less individually oriented if groups of children are large (see Table 75-1 for recommended group sizes).

      (2) **This care is usually expensive.**

      (3) **Some centers have high staff turnover.**

5. **School-aged care.** This is provided by caregivers at or near an elementary school site for before and after school and vacation time.

   a. **Advantages**

      (1) Organized care provides **safety, adult supervision, and peer companionship.**

(2) Children in supervised after-school programs may be less at risk for social problems.

b. Disadvantages

(1) The cost is higher than that of leaving a child at home in self-care.

(2) Some older children object to being in organized programs.

II. **Role of the clinician.** The clinician's role is not to recommend specific child care but to give families the information they need to choose quality care. By providing parents with resources and written guidelines about child care, the clinician can emphasize that finding quality care is a result of a knowledgeable search, not chance.

The clinician also can help a family decide whether their child, based on factors such as temperament, behavioral patterns, family factors, and number of hours in care, can be expected to cope successfully with child care that is not of the highest quality but appears to be adequate. At times, the clinician may have to advise a family that their choice of child care seems to be inadequate for their child's needs— or perhaps for any child's needs.

The United States does not have uniform standards and regulations regarding child care. State and local regulations vary widely, and licensing mechanisms, when they exist, provide only for minimum standards. The guidelines in this chapter are those recommended by the National Association for the Education of Young Children, the American Public Health Association, and the American Academy of Pediatrics.

A. **Helping with the child care selection process.** The clinician should emphasize the importance of the careful selection of child care by providing counseling and information. Although publicity about physical and sexual abuse in child care causes anxiety to parents out of proportion to the likelihood that abuse will occur, this worry motivates parents to be more discriminating in the selection process. The clinician can advise parents that careful screening, observation, and monitoring of child care are the best method of preventing abuse.

1. **Screening.** Parents should collect the names of caregiving sites and individuals by word of mouth, advertising, or agency recommendations. An initial telephone interview can establish whether the family's needs can be met by the caregiver. The parent should request the names and telephone numbers of at least three families of children previously cared for by the caregiver. The references should be asked about any concerns about the quality of care, including the use of physical punishment and disciplinary techniques.

2. **Observation.** Parents should be encouraged to observe the caregiver for a minimum of 1–2 hours, either at the child care site or during the initial employment time at home. The parent should look for warm interactions between caregiver and children, appropriate supervision and discipline, appropriate safety and hygiene, and activities that demonstrate understanding of the developmental level of children in care.

3. **Monitoring.** After a decision is made, parents should continue to observe the caregiver by occasionally staying with the child for a period of time at the beginning or end of the day and by making unannounced visits during the day. Good child care programs never restrict parents' access to their child.

B. **Helping parents to choose age-appropriate care.** Figure 75-1 is an example of a child care checklist that parents may find useful in exploring day care.

1. **Infants.** Infants need more attention than older children and should not be expected to wait for more than a few minutes for food, comfort, changing, or holding. For this reason, a high adult-to-child ratio is essential. The plan of the day should revolve around the individual rhythm of the infant. Feeding, diapering, and playtimes should not be scheduled group activities. Infants need a small number of consistent caregivers who are responsive to their individual needs and to whom they can form attachments. The parents should be able to communicate with the caregivers openly and freely.

2. **Toddlers** (ages 1–3 years). Toddlers require more structured activities, such as group meals and nap time. Other group activities can be presented, but

General information

Name of program/caregiver _____ Telephone _____
Address _____ License _____
Hours _____ Cost _____
References (names, telephone, comments)
(1) _____
(2) _____
(3) _____

Observation (plan to spend 1–2 hours minimum)

Number of ages of children served _____
Number of caregivers working with each child _____
General atmosphere _____
Is staff warm, responsive, interactive with children? _____
Are children cheerful, active, playing happily? _____
How does staff set limits? _____
Are activities/expectations appropriate for ages of children? _____
Is there space/equipment for active play? _____
Are parents welcome at all times? _____
Does staff communicate well with parents? _____
Would my child fit into this setting? _____

Safety
Is setting clean and well maintained? _____
Are toys/equipment clean and in good repair? _____
Are children supervised at all times? _____
Is the setting completely childproofed? _____
Are smoke detectors and fire extinguishers in view? _____
Is there an emergency plan? _____

Health
Policy for caring for or excluding sick children (written is best)
_____
Are meals/snacks nutritious? Is eating atmosphere pleasant? _____
Do staff wash hands after changing diapers? _____
Do children and caregivers wash hands before handling food? ____
Is there a first aid kit? _____
Are staff members trained in CPR and first aid? _____

Figure 75-1. Checklist for parents seeking child care.

it is developmentally appropriate for 1- and 2-year-old toddlers to prefer individual activities and to be unwilling to play with a group. Toddlers are active and need ample space to run and climb. Careful childproofing and constant supervision are essential. Caregivers must understand the typical oppositional behavior of this age and the need for warm but firm limit setting that is similar in style to the parents'.

3. **Preschool** (ages 3–5 years). Preschoolers are usually very involved with peers and group activities. They are better able to verbalize their needs and understand that they must wait or defer to others. However, they still need safe, consistent supervision and warm interactions with caregivers who are skilled in helping children with sharing, cooperation, and settling disputes. Children during this age need planned, developmentally appropriate activities that encourage verbal, fine motor, and perceptual skill development.

4. **School age.** School-aged children need child care before and after school and when school is closed. Most of their time will be spent in relaxation and play with peers, so it is important to have large space for vigorous activity. Although some children are in self-care ("latchkey" care), the consensus

among professionals is that children should be under the supervision of adults until at least age 8 years.

C. **Emotional issues.** Most parents feel anxious about leaving a child in the care of others. This anxiety can interfere with their ability to make good choices of care. The clinician can provide objective and supportive counseling during the selection process to lessen anxiety and stress. It is helpful to tell parents that their concerns are normal and reflect their affection and attachment to their child.

III. Common problems in child care

A. **Communicable diseases.** Young children who play together and share toys also share viruses and bacteria. It is reasonable to advise parents that a child in group care will become ill more frequently than a child who is not. The clinician should emphasize to parents that good hygiene in the child care setting will help control the spread of most communicable diseases. Written guidelines about specific illness procedures should be provided to families at the time of enrollment. If a child needs to be given medication at child care, it is helpful to provide the parents with a chart to record dosages and to discuss plans for transporting and storing medicines.

B. **Separation problems.** The clinician can help parents prevent separation problems by letting them know that many young children need several weeks to adjust to a new child care situation. A child's adjustment can be helped by having the parent stay during the first few visits and by gradually increasing the child's hours in the new situation. Arrival and departure rituals will help lessen the stress of separation for both parent and child. If a child is consistently distressed after a parent leaves and unable to engage in the program activities for most of the day, caregivers and parents should discuss other methods for helping the child adjust. If the child's distress does not decrease or if the parents observe that the child's behavior at home has been negatively affected, parents should reconsider whether the setting is appropriate for their child.

Bibliography

For Parents

Publication

Berezin J. *The Complete Guide to Choosing Child Care.* New York: Random House, 1990.

Organization

National Association of Child Care Resource and Referral Agencies; (202) 333-4194. *This national organization can direct parents to local agencies that provide assistance in finding child care.*

For Professionals

American Academy of Pediatrics. *Child Care: What's Best for Your Family. Pamphlets for parents.*

American Academy of Pediatrics. *Health in Day Care: A Manual for Health Professionals.* 1987.

American Public Health Association and the American Academy of Pediatrics. *Caring for Our Children: National Health and Safety Performance Standards: Guidelines for Out-of-Home Child Care Programs.* 1992.
All of the above publications are available from the American Academy of Pediatrics, Department of Publications, 141 Northwest Point Boulevard, Elk Grove Village IL 60009-0927.

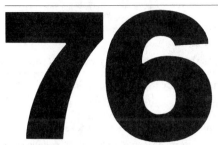

Cultural Responses to Behavioral Problems

Teresa M. Kohlenberg,
Herbert M. Joseph, Jr.,
Nicole Prudent, and
Vesta Richardson

I. **Description of the problem.** This chapter will use examples from three strong cultural traditions (African-American, Haitian, and Hispanic) to exemplify the significance of culturally based beliefs and practices about children's development. Additionally, a general framework will be offered for exploring the specific contribution of a family's culture to its response to children with behavioral or developmental differences.

   A. **Understanding cultural differences.** All families are shaped by their surrounding culture, which provides them with social norms. People from different cultures have widely differing expectations of children's behavior and development and equally differing explanations for the child who deviates from those normative expectations. For any clinician working with families from cultures other than her or his own, an understanding of these differences can play a critical role in responding accurately, sensitively, and effectively to a family's concerns. Without such an understanding, reassurance may be offered without a grasp of the family's deep concerns, and remedies may be recommended that contradict the common sense of their culture.

   B. **Sources of familial support.** The extended family and religious institutions play a central role for families from most traditional cultures. Extended family includes blood relatives as well as family friends linked by reciprocal social bonds (such as godparents) who are obligated to support the survival of its members. Religious institutions and individuals are major sources of support outside the extended family, particularly when the family is living away from its families of origin. Both the extended family and the church are more likely than the primary care clinician to be the "treatments of choice" when a problem initially presents itself.

   C. **Cultural issues in the United States.** The United States is a country of many immigrants, with new groups entering as older groups become more assimilated. The expression of a family's original culture in this multicultural setting is shaped by many intersecting factors: ethnicity, language, religion, class, number of generations in this country, experience with urban life, experience with technology and higher education, exposure to racism and prejudice, and degree of assimilation or isolation within U.S. society. Within ethnic groups, some families are strongly rooted in their original culture, while others are more assimilated to the homogeneous "American" culture. In fact, there is a great range of beliefs and practices among families from the same cultural background. This variation presents a challenge to clinicians, who must educate themselves about the cultures with which they work yet avoid stereotyping families or assuming that they know what families think because they know where they came from.

   D. **Cultural commonalities.** For all the differences among cultures and within members of the same culture, there are many commonalities in the types of questions that traditional cultures address and in the types of answers that they offer. For instance, most traditional, preindustrial cultures explain illness (physical or emotional) as an imbalance of natural and/or supernatural forces. Problems are commonly treated on both of these planes, combining special foods, massage, and herbal teas with prayers, protective medals, and prescribed interactions among family members. These practices may sound exotic, but if the reader will remember his or her own childhood experiences (whether with chicken soup, cod liver oil, holy water, or a grandmother's prayers), the universality of such remedies should be clear.

There are a core group of beliefs about health and mental health problems that are common to the majority of traditional cultures.

1. Beliefs in **prenatal influences** that mark a child in physical or temperamental ways, such as the belief that if a pregnant woman sees a person with a physical deformity, her child is likely to be born with a similar problem.

2. Concerns about **the potential of jealousy or family bad feeling to affect health and development,** as in cultures in which a baby's illness may be felt to be due to a neighbor's jealousy of the child's good looks.

3. **Strict practices for the peripartum period and for child feeding** that are expected to protect health, as in the Haitian practice of using teas and other purgatives to expel meconium from the newborn's bowel, in order to cleanse impurities from the body.

4. Worries that some form of the **"Evil Eye"** will notice and harm a child who is overly praised or cherished (which leads to the placing of protective bracelets or medals on the child).

5. Belief that **cold, wind, or exposure to the dead or to shocking sights** can set in motion physical and emotional illness (such as the Navajo and Southeast Asian beliefs in ghost sickness or possession).

6. **Concerns that the family will be shamed** or in other ways isolated because of the presence of a child with a handicap (which in many cultures may affect the child's siblings' chances of marriage).

II. **Differential cultural responses to common behavioral problems.** The following examples illustrate these different cultural patterns in the responses of three different cultures (Hispanic, African-American, and Haitian) to common behavioral problems. No single description can capture the complexity of families' responses within a given culture: these are meant as illustrative examples, not invariable stereotypes.

A. **A late-talking child**

1. **Hispanic family.** A Hispanic family may not initially worry about late talking, because it is not seen as a problem with consequences for the future or implications for the child's overall function. Therefore the clinician may become concerned before the family does.

   Late talking is often ascribed to one of three possibilities: a fright in utero or in early life, a family tendency to "laziness" in talking, or a problem with tongue function. When the family *does* become concerned, their likely responses include obtaining advice from family and friends on speech techniques, using exercises believed to strengthen the tongue, and working with the child to repeat words as part of a daily routine.

   Once it is explained that their child's hearing should be tested, they are usually eager to seek medical care and to follow up with recommended therapies.

2. **African-American family.** An African-American family would be concerned about both physical and emotional causes for late talking. They would consider a medical etiology, possibly related to prenatal influences. Parents also might view late talking as "running in the family" and seek explanations within the extended family system.

   Emotional causes are particularly relevant when language delays are encountered in school or settings other than the home or with peers. For many generations, African-Americans faced the risk of physical harm from the larger white society if they were perceived as being "uppity." This led to a pattern in which some African-American families attempted to protect their children by teaching them not to speak or to be behaviorally assertive.

   In general, an African-American family will seek advice and assistance from extended family and friends first or from institutions such as the church. A clinician might be consulted much later.

3. **Haitian family.** A Haitian family would be likely to attribute late talking to laziness, to being tongue-tied or mute (*bebe*), or being under a curse. Their first approaches might include giving the child *dlo pilon* (water that has steeped in the kitchen mortar and absorbed the taste of many spices), and

perhaps feeding the child the flesh of mockingbirds—talkative birds that imitate the songs of others.

If they suspect a mechanical difficulty, such as being tongue-tied, they would be more likely to turn to medical resources and special schools, while if they suspected a curse, they would turn to a spiritual healer for help.

B. Temper tantrums

1. **Hispanic family.** A Hispanic family would view a child with tantrums as having a nervous temperament. Such a temperament could arise from the interaction of a fragile, introverted, and "emotional" personality with stress; it could be inherited; or it could be caused by exposure to intense fear (either in utero exposure to events that frightened the mother or early infancy events that terrified the child).

   Hispanic parents worry that tantrums and head banging might leave brain damage or perhaps cause a seizure disorder. Because of these worries, they tend to acquiesce to the child's demands and turn to family members for advice.

   Typical techniques to break tantrums include applying cold water to the face, cold air pressure, or giving the child a bottle.

   If tantrums include breath-holding spells with loss of consciousness, parents would be more likely to seek medical advice.

2. **African-American family.** An African-American family would be likely to view tantrums as "acting up" and assume that the child intends to embarrass the caretaker or manipulate the situation. For some families, the tantrum may be seen as a battle of wills (the child is seen as "hardheaded" and "spoiled") and disrespectful of parental authority.

   Depending on the context and their own upbringing, African-American parents can vary widely in their response to this behavior, from time-out to physical punishment (giving the child a "whipping"), which is widely accepted in some African-American communities. The use of corporal punishment often reflects the parents' attempt to protect the child from future harm in a dangerous world by instant compliance at an early age.

   Parents may not seek professional advice until they have exhausted these options, thus giving the provider an end-stage picture of the parents' efforts to cope with the child's behavior.

3. **Haitian family.** A Haitian family would see tantrums as signs of a nervous temperament or of a hardheaded child who has not learned his or her manners. Tantrums are seen as disrespectful. Respect for elders is a highly valued trait, as exemplified by the saying, *Ti moun pa fe cole son gran moun* ("Children do not get angry at adults").

   Parents are often very embarrassed by tantrums and will intervene early. Grandparents and other adults may feel free to offer much unsolicited advice, which may further shame the parents. Attempts at control may include yelling or corporal punishment.

C. Frequent night waking

1. **Hispanic family.** For the Hispanic family, night waking is not usually seen as a problem. The child is felt to wake up because he or she is hungry or frightened. Mothers get up as many times as necessary to comfort, feed, and walk the child back to sleep. Because of the concern about hunger, overfeeding the child at bedtime is common.

2. **African-American family.** In the African-American family, persistent night waking may first be perceived as a willful, manipulative behavior. The family would consider whether the child is "spoiled" and too often gets his or her "way" with the parents. An alternative explanation would be that the child has nightmares or is fearful. Parents would then respond by providing reassurance and staying in or near the room until the child falls asleep.

   In general, parents would first turn to the extended family for help. Physical causes (e.g., potential dietary contributions or the presence of physical disease) would be sought later, in consultation with a physician.

3. **Haitian family.** For a Haitian family, the first concern would be physical illness, followed by concerns that either parental stress or a supernatural

cause (such as a curse) is causing the child to see a monster. The presence of "bad spirits" in a room can create an atmosphere that wakes the child.

The first approach would be to give the child a sweetened soporific herbal tea (guanabana leaf or coupier) or ask the clinician for a medication to make the child sleep better. The child may also be kept from napping and fed heavily to increase sleepiness at night.

If these approaches do not work and the child screams and cries during the night, the family may become concerned about a supernatural cause. Depending on their spiritual beliefs, they might consult a *vodou* priest; Christian families would ask friends to pray or bring a prayer group into the home to help get rid of the curse or bad spirit.

D. Late walking

1. **Hispanic family.** For the Hispanic family, walking by age 1 year is important, and the family will worry if this milestone is not achieved (while being less concerned about other areas of developmental lag).

   The family may come to the clinician with concerns about weakness of the bones or muscles and about spinal damage from trauma or positioning. They may be disappointed if the clinician does not share their worry and obtain x rays at a minimum.

   Other resources include *hueseros* (bone practitioners), who will massage the child and apply herbal lotions.

   Friends may recommend special shoes to encourage walking.

2. **African-American family.** The African-American family values walking as an important early skill. When a child does not walk by age 1 year, they are likely to search for a family tendency as an explanation and expect the child to "grow out of it." If they become concerned, they will turn to family and friends for advice first, then church and other community leaders, and later the medical clinician.

3. **Haitian family.** The Haitian family might be concerned about general weakness, anemia, or "anemia of bones." These are felt to come from poor nutrition or other medical conditions.

   The first treatment may be massage by family or by a folk doctor, an enriched diet with milk and vitamins, and a tonic called *bouyon pie bef,* which is made by simmering beef feet with leafy plants.

   If the late walking is part of a global developmental problem, there may be concerns about a curse, and, depending on their spiritual practices, the family may use home remedies, Christian prayers, or see a *vodou* priest.

E. Hyperactivity

1. **Hispanic family.** In the Hispanic family, hyperactivity is not recognized initially as a medical problem but as a problem in discipline or as the consequence of a prenatal event that frightened or angered the mother and left the child "nervous."

   The tasks of discipline fall first on the mother, who will withhold privileges and threaten to tell the father. Many mothers are very protective and will hide the problem rather than have the father hit the child.

   Often it is the school that requests further evaluation of hyperactive children.

2. **African-American family.** In the African-American family, hyperactivity is felt to be a temperamental tendency and/or a consequence of eating or drinking something (often sweets). The first approaches would be to make dietary changes and to seek help from family and friends on techniques for managing the child's behavior. Medical evaluation would be sought later and medication would be viewed as a last resort, used only if limit setting failed.

3. **Haitian family.** The hyperactive child in a Haitian family is viewed as "turbulent," disobedient, crazy, or hotheaded. The cause is felt to be strong emotion during pregnancy, childhood head trauma, or a curse or possession.

   The family reaction is quite negative, with a tendency to blame the child for his or her problems. Treatment may be attempted, including herbal teas and baths, special foods, special prayers and clothing, and corporal punishment.

In severe cases in older children, when the family believes that a child is possessed (*zombi*), they may use harsh corporal punishment, believing that it is the possessing spirit that suffers the pain.

III. **Assessment: Key clinical questions.** Four key clinical questions can bring cultural issues into focus for the clinician, without putting the family on the defensive about their traditional beliefs and practices. When the clinician has educated himself or herself about the beliefs and practices of the cultural groups with which he or she works, the process of delineating the role of culture in a given situation becomes more focused and comfortable and less time-consuming.

A. *When you first noticed this problem, what did you think about it? What could have caused the problem? What is the most important part of the problem for you and your family? What is most worrisome for you?* It is critical to start by assessing the family's initial reactions and nonmedical approaches to the problem.

B. *Sometimes older people in the family have very strong ideas about children and their problems. Is there anyone in your family who has different ideas from yours about this problem and what to do about it?* These questions help the clinician to determine culture-specific beliefs and generational differences about the cause and management of the problem.

C. *Did you ask anybody else in your family or in your community for advice about this problem? What did they think could have caused the problem? What did they recommend?* Traditional resource people and community institutions can be important influences on and supports for the family.

D. *Did you try anything to see if you could make the problem better? What did you try, and did it help? Are you using any remedies or special approaches now?* Culture-specific practices should be recognized and integrated with the clinician's plan; some may be benign and complement medical recommendations, while others are concerning in and of themselves, especially as they contradict what the clinician may suggest.

IV. **Management.** By the end of an interview that includes these questions, the clinician has often gathered essential information that he or she would not otherwise have had, ranging from specific family concerns about the etiology or implications of the condition, to an awareness of the other authorities in the family's life and interventions already in use. The clinician must then integrate this information in order to interpret and address the presenting problem. The clinician should be guided in this integration by several principles:

A. **Acknowledge the family's culturally based views, resources, and practices, and show respect for them where honestly possible.** The more sensitivity and respect the practitioner demonstrates, the more he or she will learn and accomplish.

B. **Support the continuation of traditional health practices and relationships with community resources that are not actively harmful or contradictory to the medical plan.** A family coping with a child's problem needs the support of familiar practices and resource people.

C. **Build common ground by explaining your understanding of the problem and the rationale for the approach you suggest.** Often the clinician's beliefs and practices are new and useful views for the family to consider.

D. **Use culturally acceptable treatment approaches whenever these are an option.** This approach will increase the patient's trust and make the physician an ally, which will make the patient more compliant.

E. **Negotiate stepwise or partial compliance when the family is uncomfortable with your views or plan.** For example, a clinician might consider obtaining a test that the family strongly desires if they will agree to discontinue a home remedy that he or she feels could be harmful.

F. **Determine a shared definition of improvement and confirm the acceptability of your plan as part of each visit.** People from traditional cultures may have a different end point for treatment than the clinician and will not directly question a professional's recommendations unless invited to do so.

G. Know thyself. Clinicians who have examined their own class and culturally based beliefs (including those of the medical culture) are best equipped to deal sensitively and effectively with families from a range of cultures.

Bibliography

Gibbs JT et al. *Children of Color: Psychological Interventions with Minority Youth.* San Francisco: Jossey-Bass, 1991.

McGoldrick M, Pearce JK, Giordano J (eds). *Ethnicity and Family Therapy.* New York: Guilford Press, 1982.

Wilson MN. Child development in the context of the black extended family. *Am Psychol* 44:380, 1989.

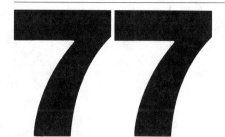

Divorce

Sharon W. Foster and
John M. Pascoe

I. Description of the problem

A. Incidence
- 40% of first children will experience the divorce of their parents before they are age 16 years.
- Children who experience divorce typically live in a single-parent household (usually the mother's) for about 5 years after the divorce.
- The majority of divorced parents will remarry, and, because the divorce rate is higher for remarriages, children who have coped with one divorce may encounter further disruption and demands for readjustment.

B. Stages of divorce.
Divorce typically represents not one event but a series of transitions for a child. There are three stages, and families proceed through them at somewhat different rates. Children's responses also vary widely and are related to their age, gender, and environmental factors.

1. **The acute phase,** involving increased conflict between the parents, separation, and a decision to divorce.

2. **The transitional phase,** in which the former spouses disengage from their relationship and focus on developing separate lives.

3. **The postdivorce phase,** in which each parent has established a relatively stable single-parent household or has remarried.

C. Emotional tasks encountered by children of divorce.
Parental divorce poses many challenges for children.

1. **They must acknowledge the fact of their parents' separation and begin to resolve unfulfillable wishes for reconciliation.** Children may respond with anger, blaming, sadness, guilt, and/or anxiety to the separation and decision to divorce. Depending on the predictability and quality of availability, they may develop negative feelings toward the noncustodial parent.

2. **Children may believe that they caused their parents' divorce** and that they can remediate the situation by becoming the "perfect" child.

3. **Children typically experience a sense of loss of the original family,** which may be compounded by other losses and changes (e.g., decreased financial resources, move to a new neighborhood with adjustment to a new school and peer group, and possible decreased availability of the custodial parent due to work demands or dating).

4. **Children need to continue to engage in activities consistent with their own developmental needs,** such as school, extracurricular activities, and friendships, to enhance their sense of competence and self-worth.

5. **A final task is to develop a sense of hope and realistic potential regarding their own future relationships.**

II. Factors affecting children's adjustment to divorce.
Early research tended to focus on differences between children in divorced families and those from intact families. More recent work has examined the diversity of children's response to divorce and identified factors that facilitate or inhibit a positive adaptation.

A. Temperament.
Investigators have found that temperamentally more difficult children may have more difficulty with challenging life events compared to

Table 77-1. Responses of child to parent's divorce within the first year

Developmental status	Child's response	Primary care clinician's role
Preschool	Regressive behavior Sleep disturbance Tantrums Aggressive behavior Bowel and bladder difficulties Clinging Fears of abandonment	Encourage stable, predictable meal and bedtime routines Develop consistent patterns of joining and separating from child Continue contact with noncustodial parent Provide reassurance
Younger school age	Sadness Fearfulness Loyalty conflicts Attempts to determine responsibility for divorce Hopes for family reconciliation Declining school performance	Empathize with child's feelings Provide regular opportunities for child to talk Support child's continuing relationship with both parents Offer reassurance
Older school age/ prepubertal	Grief, intense anger Declining school performance Disrupted peer relationships Attempts to clarify responsibility for the divorce Caretaking of a parent	Express interest in and availability to the child Support child's school and peer involvement Provide clear acknowledgment and support for child's working through feelings on the divorce
Adolescence	Depression Anger Premature emancipation Increase in adolescent acting out Sleeper effects, particularly in females	Provide opportunities for discussion Offer appropriate supports within and outside the family, including peer involvement (such as in school-based family transition groups)

Source: Adapted from Wallerstein JS. Separation, divorce, and remarriage. In MD Levine, WB Carey, AC Crocker (eds), *Developmental-Behavioral Pediatrics* (2nd ed). Philadelphia: Saunders, 1992.

temperamentally easy children. Difficult children may need more support at a time when a parent may have diminished ability to provide support. Such children may receive more negative attention for their behavior and may serve as an object for displaced frustration from their parents. Other individual characteristics, such as intelligence, independence, internal locus of control, and adaptability, can affect how a child deals with divorce.

B. **Developmental level.** Developmental level plays a key role in shaping children's concerns about and response to life transitions, including divorce (Table 77-1).

C. **Gender.** One of the most consistent findings is that males tend to exhibit more behavioral difficulties (especially externalizing difficulties and noncompliance) than do girls in female-headed households. This is particularly marked during the acute phase of the divorce. Girls may exhibit a sleeper effect, initially showing better adjustment than boys but exhibiting greater difficulty during adolescence. Some studies suggest that children may do better when living with the same-gender parent.

D. **Concomitant stress.** Children may successfully negotiate the acute or crisis phase of a divorce, only to confront changes of home, neighborhood, school, and peer group, and often a lowered standard of living. Such difficulties may be compounded if the child has witnessed parental violence or is a victim of it.

Parental dating and subsequent remarriage may also present significant challenges to a child.

E. **Family factors.** Many parents may find it challenging to cope with their emotional issues and the heightened demands of parenting. Parents may experience emotional lability, depression, emotional dependence or disengagement with the children, overindulgence, involvement in a highly active social life, or may be at risk for alcohol abuse or other health risk behaviors.

F. **Support systems.** Support systems may have a positive impact on a mother's ability to deal with a challenging child. (Fathers have been found to make less use of social support.) Children may also benefit from social support, such as structure, consistency, and emotional support in a school or day care. A consistent, supportive relationship with a friend, sibling, or adult may be especially helpful.

III. **Management.** When helping parents with a child's behavior in response to the divorce, it is useful not only to help the parents address the problem behavior but also to understand the emotional issues with which the child is struggling. For example, preschool children may fear abandonment. The feared fantasy may be compounded by infrequent visitation, emotional preoccupation of the custodial parent, and/or decreased standard of living in a one-parent household. School-aged children may be confronting changes in school, neighborhood, friends, and extent of extracurricular activities. At the same time, a parent may be less available due to increased work activities, social obligations, and/or emotional distress.

Early interventions aimed at preventing or palliating some of the adverse effects of divorce may be more successful than efforts directed toward child problem behavior *following* divorce. The primary care clinician's interventions should be organized with reference to the stages of divorce.

A. **Acute phase**

   1. **If parents raise the probability of divorce, the clinician can offer to assist them in developing a plan to tell their children.** Such disclosures ideally include both parents' meeting with the children, describing in "no-fault" language their decision to divorce, reassuring the children that the decision was not caused by them, and conveying both parents' love for them. Children may have questions, and these can be encouraged.

   2. **Conflictual interactions between the parents should be limited to times when children are not present.**

   3. As much as possible, **each parent's time with the child should be predictable.** Continuity of children's relationships with the noncustodial parent should be promoted.

   4. **Every effort should be made to foster environmental stability** (e.g., the child's neighborhood, friends, household routines).

   5. **The parents should be encouraged to seek mediation and/or divorce therapy.** Also suggest local resources for divorce support groups or those for single parents.

B. **Transitional phase**

   1. If the custodial parent increases his or her work or other time outside the home, **he or she should nevertheless have some predictable special time each day with each child.** During that time, the parent has a chance to focus on the child's positive activities that day, as well as to address the child's feelings.

   2. **A parent who has become withdrawn from, dependent on, or markedly more hostile to a child may be displacing these feelings** from the former marital relationship. The parent needs to address these issues.

   3. **Both parents should develop a strong alliance with the child's teacher,** to promote the child's mastery in school and to assist in monitoring for behavioral disruptions that may signal the need for constructive attention to the child's emotional needs.

4. The clinician can assist the family in identifying community resources that may provide some structure, warmth, and consistency for a child, such as an optimal teacher and/or day care setting.

C. Postdivorce phase

    1. Children (as well as adults) benefit from the development of a new family identity, including family traditions.

    2. The provider should provide consistent ongoing primary care, offering continuity and support.

Bibliography

For Parents
Gardner RA. *The Parents Book About Divorce* (rev ed). New York: Bantam Books, 1991.

Kalter N. *Growing up with Divorce.* New York: Free Press, 1990.

Teyber E. *Helping Children Cope with Divorce.* New York: Lexington Books, 1992.

For Children
Ives SB, Fassler D, Lash M. *The Divorce Workbook: A Guide for Kids and Families.* Burlington VT: Waterfront Books, 1985.

Kids Express, PO Box 782, Littleton CO 80160-0782.
A monthly newsletter written for children whose parents have separated or divorced.

LeShan E. *When Parents Separate or Divorce: What's Going to Happen to Me?* New York: Aladdin Books, 1978.

For Professionals
Heatherington EM. Marital transitions: A child's perspective. Special issue: Children and their development: Knowledge base, research agenda, and social policy application. *Amer Psychol* 44(2):303–312, 1989.

Krantz SE. The impact of divorce on children. In AS Skolnick, JH Skolnick (eds), *Family in Transition.* New York: Harper Collins, 1992.

Portes PR et al. Family functions and children's postdivorce adjustment. *Am J Orthopsychiatry* 62(4):613–617, 1992.

Wallerstein JS, Blakeslee S. *Second Chances: Men, Women and Children a Decade after Divorce.* New York: Ticknor & Fields, 1989.

Wallerstein JS. Separation, divorce, and remarriage. In MD Levine, WB Carey, AC Crocker (eds), *Developmental-Behavioral Pediatrics* (2nd ed). Philadelphia: Saunders, 1992.

Weitzman M, Adair R. Divorce and children. *Pediatr Clin North Amer* December: 1313–1323, 1988.

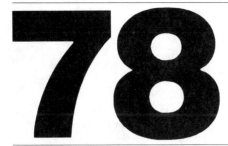

Dying Children

David J. Schonfeld and
Melvin Lewis

I. **Description of the problem.** When a child is dying, the child and the family need reassurance, support, and guidance. The primary care provider who has a supportive and ongoing relationship with the child and the family is in a unique position to provide them with that support throughout this difficult period. Some general principles to consider in providing care to dying children and their families are presented in Table 78-1.

II. **Issues in helping the dying child**

A. **Health care providers must attend to the immediate physical needs of these children.** It is crucial to relieve pain and suffering and to assure the children that adults are always available. Children should be told by both the parents and the health care providers, "We want you to tell us whenever anything is bothering you. I will always be here (or be able to be reached) anytime you want me. We will all do our best to make sure that you feel as comfortable as possible."

B. **Children at different developmental stages have different conceptual understandings of the meaning of death,** which will affect their ability to understand and adjust to their impending death (see Chapter 74). Children with a terminal illness usually do appreciate the seriousness of their illness and may develop a precocious understanding of death and their personal mortality.

C. **Many parents and clinicians are uncomfortable when children openly acknowledge an awareness of their impending death.** Children often feel that it is their task to provide emotional support to their parents and to carry on the mutual pretense that they are unaware of their health status. This conspiracy of silence isolates the child from available supports. Most children, in fact, fear the *process* of dying more than death itself.

D. **To the extent possible, children should be informed about their health status.** Children often turn to members of the health care team to ask questions, directly or indirectly, about their illness and impending death. Children who are dying may also directly ask family members and staff, "Am I going to die?" Adults should initially clarify the motivation for such questions: is the child seeking reassurance that all efforts will be made to minimize pain, that parents and family members will remain available, or that every reasonable effort will be made to treat the underlying illness? Is the child merely attempting to determine the seriousness of his or her illness? Once the motivation for the question is identified, the adult family member or health care provider can provide the necessary reassurances or information. Prohibitions on informing children about their condition force parents and professionals to lie, thereby jeopardizing a caregiving relationship built on mutual trust and respect. The principles to consider in informing children about a terminal illness or impending death are summarized in Table 78-2.

E. **Facilitating discussion about children's concerns often involves projective techniques,** such as play or picture drawing. Many children choose not to discuss their impending death directly. It is rarely necessary (or appropriate) to confront children with the reality that they are dying after they have been appropriately informed. Instead, clinicians should remain available and offer indirect outlets for addressing the child's concerns. Children will avail themselves of these opportunities when, and if, they are ready.

Table 78-1. General principles for practitioners in the care of dying children and their families

Physical context
Minimize physical discomfort and symptoms.
Optimize pain management.

Emotional context
Provide an opportunity for the expression and sharing of personal feelings and concerns for both the children and their families in an accepting atmosphere.
Tolerate unpleasant affect (e.g., sadness, anger, despair).

Social context
Facilitate communication among members of the health care team and the children and their families.
Encourage active participation of the children and their families in the treatment decisions and the management of the illness.

Personal context
Treat each child and family member as a unique individual.
Attempt to form a personal relationship with the child and the family.
Acknowledge your own feelings as a health care provider and establish a mechanism(s) to meet your personal needs.

Table 78-2. Principles involved in informing children about a terminal illness or impending death

Inform the child over time, in a series of conversations. During the initial conversation, it is important to convey that the child has a serious illness.

If the child asks directly if he or she is going to die, initially explore the reason for the question and the child's concerns (e.g., "Are you afraid that you might die?" "What are you worried about?"). Do not provide false reassurances ("No, don't worry, you're going to be O.K."), but always try to maintain hope ("Some children with your sickness have died, but we're going to do everything we can to try and help you get better").

Focus initial discussions on the immediate and near future. Young children have a limited future perspective. Dying "soon" to them may mean minutes, hours, or days, not months or years.

Answer questions directly, but do not overwhelm the child with unnecessary details.

Assess the child's understanding by asking him or her to explain back to you what you have discussed.

Reassure the child of the lack of personal responsibility or guilt. For this reason, avoid the use of the term *bad* in the description of the illness (e.g., "You have a bad sickness").

F. **Clinicians are often anxious that they will not know what to say to a child who is dying.** The goal of counseling children who are dying is not to take away their sadness or to find the "right" answers to all their questions. Rather, it is to listen to their concerns, to accept and empathize with their strong emotions, to offer support, and to assist them in finding their own coping techniques (e.g., "Some children find it helpful to talk to others about what is worrying them; other children prefer to draw pictures or keep a diary. Whatever you decide to do is fine. I'm always available to talk with you about your feelings, or just to sit and talk about something else."). In many cases, the best approach is to talk about a topic of interest to the child or merely to sit quietly and hold the child's hand.

G. **Children must be allowed, even encouraged, to continue to have hope and to go on with their lives.** These children should be regarded less as children who are dying and more as individuals living with a serious and/or life-threatening condition. The goal must be to optimize the quality of their remaining life, not merely to prolong its duration. Important routines should be continued with as little disruption as possible, such as allowing them to attend school or to do schoolwork in the hospital. Although regressive behavior may be normative and appropriate at times of stress, excessively regressive behavior (e.g., a 6 year old who begins biting staff) should be addressed supportively but firmly, often employing a behavioral management approach developed by the treatment team and family.

H. Many children and adolescents feel guilty and ashamed about their illness. Children who rely on magical thinking and egocentrism to explain the cause of illness may assume that terminal illness and death are the result of some perceived wrongdoing ("immanent justice"). Children need to be reassured frequently that they are not responsible for their illness.

I. To the extent possible, children should be informed about and participate in the decisions regarding their health care. Older children and adolescents may possess the intellectual and emotional maturity to allow them to play a significant role regarding critical and difficult decisions (e.g., whether to discontinue aggressive treatment). All children need to be aware of the nature and rationale of planned treatments and should be active participants in the treatment process, even if they are able to make only seemingly minor decisions (e.g., whether they should take the pill with juice or with soda).

III. Issues in helping the parents

A. Parents faced with the impending death of their child may demonstrate shock, denial, anxiety, depression, or anger. Almost any reaction can be seen; there is no "correct" way to deal with the death of a child. Additionally, parents may alternate among these emotional states without demonstrating any clear progression.

B. The response of family members to the death may be affected by the duration of the illness. Anticipatory grieving allows family members to experience graduated feelings of loss while the child is still alive. In the setting of open communication, many families will take advantage of this time to resolve conflicts with the dying child and to express love. Clinicians should appreciate that other families may approach this impending loss with a different coping style and may not choose to engage in this form of leave-taking behavior.

C. Members of the family may proceed with anticipatory grieving at different rates. Conflicts may result when one family member's course of grieving is not synchronous with that of another member of the family. Primary care clinicians can help families to identify when someone (either a member of the family or health care team) has abandoned the child after having prematurely reached resignation and acceptance of the child's death.

D. As part of anticipatory grieving, family members and health care professionals may wish for the death of a seriously ill or defective child. This wish may result in excessive guilt and cause the individual to compensate by becoming overly protective or indulgent with the dying child. The health care provider can assist parents with such comments as: *Many parents of children who have been critically ill for a prolonged period sometimes find themselves wishing their child would just die quickly. This is a common and normal feeling, even for parents who love their children dearly.*

E. Family members should be allowed, even encouraged, to continue to have hope and to go on with their lives. While the desire for second opinions should be honored, excessive searches for cures that compromise the health of the child or the financial well-being of the family should be discouraged. Parents must be actively assured that they have done everything reasonable to ensure the highest quality of care for their child and that they have no reason to feel guilty.

F. To the extent possible, parents should be informed about and participate actively in decisions regarding their child's care. The health care providers must provide families with clear professional recommendations and be willing to discuss alternate options, when appropriate options exist. When families are faced, for example, with the difficult decision of whether to continue aggressive therapy when little hope of cure remains, the clinician must provide information on the likelihood of success and the anticipatory morbidity associated with the treatment process. Palliative and supportive care should always remain available, even if children and their families choose a management plan that is not the preferred option of the provider. For terminal children maintained on life support at the time of death, the clinician should elicit and honor the parents' wishes about the timing of termination of life support. Care should be taken so that parents do not infer that they are being asked about whether to allow their child to die.

G. **Sudden or unexpected death requires an immediate recognition of the loss.** In this setting, families often initially use denial to cope. Family members should be allowed additional time to hold or be with the child's body in a quiet and private area of the hospital and should be given an opportunity to express their shock, disbelief, and anger before further and more detailed explanations of the cause of death are provided.

H. **Support systems for families of dying children are often hospital based and frequently withdrawn at the time of the child's death.** Providers should remain available to families after the death has occurred and should help the family establish ties, prior to the death, with community-based support systems, such as parent groups, clergy, and counseling services. Hospital support networks should not become an additional loss coincident with the death of the child.

I. **At the time of the child's death, parents and other family members should be offered assistance with immediate and pragmatic needs.** Such diverse needs include ensuring safe transportation home for grieving family members at the time of the death, making funeral and burial arrangements, and deciding how to notify family members and friends. Families should be given an appointment for a follow-up meeting (often 2–6 weeks after the death; earlier if necessary) to answer remaining questions about the illness and death (e.g., to review the autopsy report) and to inquire about adjustment of family members. Time can also be arranged to meet later with the siblings either individually or with their parents.

J. **Families in grief may feel immobilized and incapable of making even simple decisions.** Complex and emotionally laden decisions such as those regarding autopsy or organ donation may seem especially overwhelming at this time. When death is anticipated, the primary care provider may suggest that family members consider their personal feelings about such decisions before the fact. In sudden and unanticipated deaths, families may need a period of time (1–2 hours) to adjust to the reality of the loss before such questions are asked.

IV. **Issues in helping the siblings**

A. **The needs of the siblings are often neglected when a child in the family is dying.** Parents have limited reserves of energy, time, and money and strained emotional and psychological resources. Providers must ensure that outreach is provided to siblings to meet their needs.

B. **The siblings should be included in receiving information about the child's health status and treatment plan and should participate to some extent in the provision of care for the ill child.** Young children may be given simple tasks such as bringing and opening mail, watering plants in the room, or bringing toys to a child in bed. Parents must be careful not to overburden the siblings, especially the older children and adolescents, with unreasonable chores or responsibilities. Siblings should be encouraged to maintain their peer groups and continue involvement in activities outside the family.

C. **Siblings respond to the death with the same diversity of emotional responses seen in adults.** They may be angry at the child who has died or experience guilt over having survived. Primary care clinicians need to monitor how families reorganize after the death of a child, so that siblings are not scapegoated or the focus of projected defenses. For example, parents who continue to feel guilty about their child's death may overprotect the surviving siblings and interfere with normative attempts to achieve independence.

V. **Helping the health care providers**

A. **Health care providers must understand their personal feelings about death in order to be effective in providing support to others.** Often this will involve some introspection about one's own losses and an awareness of the impact of the deaths of their patients on their professional and personal lives.

B. **Providers must extend the same quality of care to themselves as they would offer to patients.** The death of a patient is one of the most stressful personal and professional experiences faced by health care providers. It triggers a similar, albeit less intense, grief response as would a personal loss. Permission and tolerance for professionals to discuss and have their personal needs met regarding bereavement (e.g., for support or reassurance of lack of personal responsibility for a patient death) is necessary. Psychosocial rounds (especially in intensive care settings), retreats, and other support services dealing directly with providers' responses to patient death are important aspects of professional development.

C. **All members of the health care team should be involved in important decisions regarding the care provided to a dying child.** Conflicts that arise when one or more members of the team disagree on the appropriateness of care being provided can seriously undermine clinical care. For example, physicians who avoid clarifying do-not-resuscitate orders with the family of a dying child may place the nursing staff in the uncomfortable position of having to initiate resuscitation efforts when the death occurs. House staff forced to continue treatment that they feel is not in the best interest of the child or family may be angry if they were not involved in the decision. Often staff differences may need to be resolved through team meetings.

D. **Primary care providers should avail themselves of the expertise and skills of members of related disciplines,** such as the clergy, child life, nursing, psychiatry, psychology, and social work when responding to the needs of the child and family members, as well as their own personal needs.

Bibliography

For Parents
Candlelighters Childhood Cancer Foundation, 7910 Woodmont Avenue, Suite 460, Bethesda MD 20814; (800) 366-2223.
For information and referral for parents, families, and professionals working with children with cancer.

Children's Hospice International, 901 North Washington Street, Suite 700, Alexandia VA 22314; (800) 24-CHILD.
For information and referral regarding local hospice care and bereavement counseling services.

Compassionate Friends, PO Box 3696, Oak Brook IL 60522-3696; (708) 990-0010.
For referral to a self-help group for parents and siblings who have experienced the death of a child.

National Sudden Infant Death Syndrome Resource Center, 8201 Greensboro Drive, Suite 600, McLean VA 22102-3810; (703) 821-8955 (ask for SIDS Resource Center).
For information and referral for parents who have lost an infant to sudden infant death syndrome.

For Professionals
Adams D, Deveau E. When a brother or sister is dying of cancer: The vulnerability of the adolescent sibling. *Death Stud* 11:279–295, 1987.

Greenham D, Lohmann R. Children facing death: Recurring patterns of adaptation. *Health Social Work* 7(2):89–94, 1982.

Krell R, Rabkin L. The effects of sibling death on the surviving child: A family perspective. *Family Process* 18(4):471–477, 1979.

Lewis M, Lewis D, Schonfeld D. Dying and death in childhood and adolescence. In M Lewis (ed), *Child and Adolescent Psychiatry: A Comprehensive Textbook*. Baltimore: Williams & Wilkins, 1991.

Sahler OJ, Friedman S. The dying child. *Pediatr Rev* 3(5):159–165, 1981.

Schonfeld D. Talking with children about death. *J Pediatr Health Care* 7:269–274, 1993.

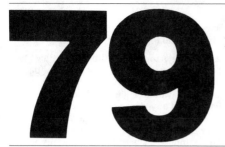

Foster Care

Howard Dubowitz

I. **Description of the problem.** Foster care refers to substitute care for children whose parents are unable or unwilling to care for them. The main types of care are family foster care, placement with relatives (kinship care), and residential group care. For brevity, the term *foster care* will be used for all three.

A. **Epidemiology.** See Table 79-1.

B. **Contributory factors.** There are many historical and current potential risks for children in foster care due to prior abuse and neglect, adverse experiences in a dysfunctional family and stressful environment, poverty, multiple separations from caregivers, inadequate services, and possible maltreatment while in care. There is a complex interplay between these risks and children's strengths, weaknesses, developmental level, and environmental buffers that influence their health and well-being.

II. **Identifying problems**

A. **General issues**

1. **Because of the vicissitudes of foster care, the periodicity schedule of the American Academy of Pediatrics for child health supervision may *not* be adequate.** More intensive support and monitoring are often needed.

2. **Discontinuous home and health care requires special efforts to gather relevant past information on a child and family** (e.g., from biologic parents, teachers, past health care providers).

3. **Over one-third of foster children have significant mental health problems.**

B. **Specific issues.** In addition to the standard care that all children need, there are specific issues concerning foster children.

1. **Primary pediatric care.** It is important that primary care clinicians address emotional and behavioral problems and functioning in school, and maintain clear communication and collaboration with the other professionals involved in the child's care. Frequent follow-up visits and a high index of suspicion for emotional and psychological problems are often necessary. Additionally, foster children may feel unloved and abandoned by their parents. It is often helpful to describe their parents as being *unable*, rather than *unwilling*, to care for them. Children who have been maltreated and placed in foster care may have great difficulty trusting others. Clinicians can play a valuable role by being a caring and consistent ally. This can be accomplished by more frequent visits to monitor the child's adjustment and by establishing a trusting relationship.

2. **Transitions from one home to another.** Foster children need special support when entering a new foster family or phasing out an old one. The primary care clinician can play an important role in advocating for appropriate preparation for the child to facilitate these transitions. A supportive foster parent is crucial. The clinician should emphasize the need for abundant patience, affection, and nurturance.

a. **Screening questions for foster parents to assess how the transition is progressing include:**

(1) *How do you think your foster child is doing?*

Table 79-1. Dimensions of foster care

Prevalence
430,000 children are in foster care (an increase of 64% since 1982)
Types of care
75% in regular (including kinship) care
16% in group or residential care
9% in other arrangements
Age of foster children
14% infants
26% ages 1–5 years
26% ages 6–12 years
33% teenagers
Race/ethnicity of foster children
56% white
26% African-American
10% Latino
8% other

    (2) *Are there some behaviors you're worried about? What's it been like for others in your home since your foster child moved in?*

    (3) *How are you coping?*

3. **The child's view of being in care.** Depending on a child's maturity and expressive abilities, it may be possible to ascertain directly how he or she perceives foster care. Useful questions, without the caregiver present, include:

    a. *What's it like for you living in this place?*

    b. *What do you like best?*

    c. *What do you like least?*

    d. *How do you get along with the people in your new home?*

    e. *What would you like changed?*

4. **Problems around children's visits with parents.** Visits to the biologic parents can evoke strong, ambivalent emotions and difficult behaviors in children. Practitioners should encourage foster parents to maintain a positive stance toward the parents. For example, foster families can help allay anxiety about a visit by anticipatory guidance and rehearsing how to manage potential difficult situations. The clinician may need to recommend a change in such visitations if they are clearly harmful to a child, such as when a parent repeatedly fails to arrive for the visit. It is advisable, however, to avoid simplistic explanations of children's responses (e.g., interpreting aggressive behavior after a visit as reflecting a child's negative feelings toward his or her parents when, it fact, it is due to the anxiety of separating from them).

5. **Discipline in substitute care.** Most agencies prohibit caregivers from hitting children placed in their care. It is useful to ask caregivers how they respond to difficult behavior (e.g., *What do you do when your foster child is driving you crazy?*). Practitioners can help explain the child's behavior and offer constructive disciplinary alternatives (e.g., time-outs, withholding privileges).

6. **Abuse and neglect in substitute care.** Abuse and neglect occasionally occur in substitute care. Primary care clinicians need to be alert to the physical and behavioral markers of maltreatment and assess whether these resulted from abuse or neglect prior to or during placement.

7. **Discontinuous health care.** Foster children often have had frequent changes in health care providers, without the necessary transfer of information. Some states have implemented medical passports, which are brief medical records with key information about each health care visit. The primary care clinician

should be mindful of gathering and maintaining medical documentation that will be useful to future clinicians.

8. **Support for substitute caregivers.** Many foster children have serious problems that their foster parents are not equipped to manage. Primary care clinicians can help with more frequent visits for education, emotional support, and counseling. Many foster parent groups have newsletters for which some practitioners write a column on health issues.

   At times, foster parents may be unfairly viewed in a negative light and their motives doubted. The clinician should show them support and respect, by saying, for example, "This child is very lucky to have you" and "I really admire you for the way you're taking care of your foster child."

9. **Involvement with biologic parents.** In some cases the biologic parents retain legal custody over their child's health care. It is important to clarify the status of such an arrangement. Since many foster children will be returned to their parents, it may be appropriate to involve them in their child's health care.

10. **Support for caseworkers.** The staff of agencies responsible for supervising foster children are often overwhelmed, undertrained, and underpaid. Clinicians should openly acknowledge the efforts of the caseworkers, for example, by saying, "You're really making a big difference in John's life by finding all the services he needs."

11. **Children preparing for independence.** Foster children are expected to assume increased responsibility for themselves as they reach age 18 years. This raises a set of complex psychological and practical issues because few of these children have the experience to manage independently. The clinician should ensure appropriate planning by asking what measures are being taken to prepare the teenager for independent living. (Materials to assist caregivers and youth in this task are available from the National Foster Care Resource Center.) Additionally, the pediatric clinician may offer to continue caring for the young adult or make a referral to another health care provider.

Bibliography

Organizations

Child Welfare League of America, 440 First Street, NW, Washington DC 20001-2085; (202) 638-2952.

Committee on Early Childhood, Adoption, and Dependent Care, American Academy of Pediatrics, 141 Northwest Point Boulevard, PO Box 927, Elk Grove Village IL 60009-0927; (800) 433-9016.

National Foster Care Resource Center, 102 King Hall, Eastern Michigan University, Ypsilanti MI 48197; (313) 487-0374.

National Foster Parent Association, 2606 Badger Lane, Madison WI 53713-2115; (608) 274-9111.

Publications

Child Welfare League of America. *Standards for Health Care Services for Children in Out-of-Home Care*. Washington DC: 1988, Child Welfare League of America.

Dubowitz H et al. The physical health of children in kinship care. *Am J Dis Child* 146:603–610, 1992.

Fahlberg V. *Child's Journey Through Care*. Indianapolis: Perspective Press, 1991.

Schor ED. Foster care. *Pediatr Clin North Am* 35:1241–1252, 1988.

Simms MD. Foster care clinic: A community program to identify treatment needs of children in foster care. *Devel Behav Pediatr* 10:121–182, 1989.

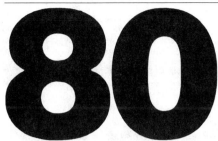

Lesbian and
Gay Parents

Tamar Gershon

I. Description of the issue

A. Epidemiology
- 8–10 million children are currently living with an estimated 3 million lesbian and gay parents.
- There has been a marked increase in the number of lesbians (either single or in a relationship) giving birth.
- Gay men are increasingly becoming parents, through adoption, foster care, surrogate mothers, or coparenting with lesbian mothers.

B. Structures of lesbian and gay families.
There is a great deal of variability in the structure of lesbian and gay families: a same-sex couple who has a child together, a single gay or lesbian parent, a lesbian mother or gay father previously in a heterosexual marriage and continuing to have joint custody of the child, or a lesbian mother raising a child with the help of a gay man who is the biologic father. There are also joint custody situations in which a same-sex couple may have separated but both parents continue to raise the child. A new same-sex partner may take on a stepparent role after a divorce or a separation.

C. Legal issues

1. **Lesbian and gay relationships are denied the legal benefits of marriage.** Some cities grant benefits to a domestic partner, but few provide significant legally mandated entitlements.

2. **Lesbian and gay parents are often denied custody and/or visitation with their children following divorce because of their sexual orientation.** Increasingly, the courts are recognizing the parenting rights of gay and lesbian parents, but this is by no means standard legal practice.

3. **Regulations governing foster care and adoption in many states make it difficult for lesbians and gay men to adopt children or to become foster parents.** Second-parent adoption is a particular type of adoption that ensures parental rights to the nonbiologic parent in a couple. Because the department of social services prohibits adoption by unmarried couples in many states, a lesbian or gay couple may obtain a second-parent adoption only at the discretion of an individual judge.

4. *Power of attorney* **is an important document to be obtained by lesbian or gay parents.** It allows a designated person, other than the biologic parent, to make decisions about the child's care in the event that the biologic parent is unavailable. *Durable* power of attorney, a specific type of power of attorney, allows the designated person to act on behalf of the biologic parent should he or she become medically incapacitated.

D. Questions about developmental and behavioral outcomes

1. **How will children's gender identity, sex roles, and sexual orientation be affected by having gay or lesbian parents?** No significant differences have been found in gender identity and sex role behaviors among children of lesbian and gay parents. Children with gay or lesbian parents are no more likely to be lesbian or gay than are children with heterosexual parents.

2. **Will children of gay or lesbian parents exhibit psychological adjustment difficulties and behavioral problems?** Existing research indicates that the

children of lesbian or gay parents have normal psychological development. No differences have been found in such areas as self-concept, locus of control, moral judgment, social competence, and intelligence.

3. Do children need adult role models of both genders? Lesbian mothers have been shown to be as concerned as divorced, heterosexual mothers that their children have opportunities for good relationships with adult men. Most lesbian and gay parents desire to raise their children with the involvement of adults of both genders.

4. Will children have psychological problems due to experiences of stigmatization and homophobia? Many issues may arise when children of gay and lesbian parents enter school. Experiences of teasing and stigmatization may lead children to be afraid to disclose information about their family to teachers, classmates, and friends. In spite of the potential for teasing and stigmatization in school, studies have shown that children of lesbian and gay parents usually develop normal social relationships with their peers.

5. Will children living with gay or lesbian parents be more likely to be sexually abused by the parent or by the parent's friends? There is no evidence that children in the care of lesbian or gay parents are at greater risk for sexual abuse.

II. Making the diagnosis

A. History: Key clinical questions. In taking the history, the clinician should create a comfortable environment in which a parent may disclose his or her sexual orientation; however, the clinician need not ask directly for a disclosure.

1. *Who makes up your family?* When dealing with parents, one should never assume heterosexuality. It is not necessary to ask a parent if he or she is lesbian or gay; rather, the clinician may make a statement to all families that he or she is accustomed to seeing all types of families including lesbian- and gay-headed families. In this way, the parent may feel comfortable enough to disclose sexual orientation.

2. *Do you share parenting responsibilities with anyone else?* For example, ask who helps with dropping off and picking up the child from school or day care.

3. *Who are the other important members of your network who share in the work of caring for your child?* There may be many different people who are mentioned here, or there may be only a parent's partner who shares in parenting responsibilities.

III. Management. Managing families with lesbian and gay parents must be individualized. The location, local support services available, and the local laws of adoption and child custody will determine whether a parent and child may be open about a parent's sexual orientation.

A. Discuss legal issues with family members. Refer the family for legal advice if they have a specific concern regarding custody, adoption, or power of attorney.

B. Discuss the child's experience of stigma in school. Ask how school is going and if the child is having any particular troubles. If there is any related specifically to stigma (e.g., teasing), the child might benefit from a support group in which he or she may meet other children with lesbian or gay parents.

C. Encourage parents to introduce lesbian and gay family issues into the school curriculum. If parents are able to be open about their sexual orientation in their child's school, the clinician might encourage them to speak to the principal and teachers and ask them to include information about lesbian and gay families in their curriculum.

D. Discuss family communication. Encourage maintaining open lines of communication between parent and child regarding issues that may arise for the child with lesbian or gay parents such as disclosure and being different from other children.

E. Revise office forms and questionnaires to be inclusive of all types of families. Change "mother/father" designations to "parent" and "family members."

F. **Provide magazines and materials in the waiting room that represent a wide range of different kinds of families, including those with lesbian and gay parents.**

G. **Ask how the child likes to refer to each parent** (e.g., "Momma Jane" and "Momma Mary" or "Daddy" and "Poppa").

H. **Include all parents involved in the child's care.** Invite coparents or other members of support system to appointments and include them in decisions.

IV. **Criteria for referral.** If a clinician does not feel comfortable dealing with gay and lesbian parents, a referral should be made to another practice. There are often clinicians in the community who are sensitive to lesbian and gay issues or are lesbian or gay themselves.

Bibliography

For Parents

Publications
Bozett FW (ed). *Gay and Lesbian Parents*. New York: Praeger, 1987.

Martin A. *The Lesbian and Gay Parenting Handbook: Creating and Raising Our Families*. New York: Harper Collins, 1993.

Rafkin L (ed). *Different Mothers: Sons and Daughters of Lesbians Talk About Their Lives*. San Francisco: Cleis Press, 1990.

Organizations
Gay and Lesbian Parents Coalition International, PO Box 50360, Washington DC 20091; (202) 583-8029.

National Center for Lesbian Rights, 1663 Mission Street, San Francisco CA 94103; (415) 621-0674.

For Children
Bosche S. *Jenny Lives with Eric and Martin*. London: Gay Men's Press, 1981.

Elwin R, Paulse M. *Asha's Mums*. Toronto: Women's Press, 1990.

Newman L. *Heather Has Two Mommies*. Boston: Alyson Publications, 1989.

For Professionals
Casper V, Schultz S, Wickens E. Breaking the silences: Lesbian and gay parents and the schools. *Teachers College Record* 94(1):109–137, 1992.

Gold M, Perrin E, Futterman D, Friedman S (in press). Children of gay or lesbian parents. *Pediatr Rev*

Patterson C. Children of lesbian and gay parents. *Child Devel* 63:1025–1042, 1992.

81

Parental Depression

Lucy Osborn

I. **Description of the problem.** Mood disorders are both widespread and debilitating. Depressed mood, the hallmark of depressive disorders, is often described as a feeling of sadness, hopelessness, or discouragement, but it may be much more severe than these words imply. Depressed adults lose interest or pleasure in all, or almost all, activities and suffer from many associated symptoms, such as irritability, appetite and sleep disturbances, decreased energy, feelings of worthlessness and guilt, psychomotor agitation or retardation, and difficulty in thinking or concentrating. In major depressive episodes, thoughts of death and suicidal ideation or attempts are common. Persons with major depression have been shown to be more functionally limited than patients with chronic physical illness, missing more work and reporting poorer physical, psychosocial, and role functioning. Parenting is difficult under the best of circumstances, so it is not surprising that children reared in an environment with a depressed adult manifest a variety of adverse outcomes reflective of their parents' illness.

A. **Epidemiology**
   - Estimates of the prevalence of diagnosable major depression among women range from 4–9%, with many more suffering from depressive symptoms.
   - There are increased rates of depression among younger women with children.
   - Higher rates (up to 45%) are associated with lower socioeconomic class, less education, poor marital relationships, immigrant status, and drug and alcohol usage.
   - Approximately 12% of women seeking pediatric care for their children in private practices also report such symptoms.
   - Postpartum depression is seen in 10% (as distinguished from normal "baby blues," seen in 80% of mothers in the first postpartum weeks).

B. **Classification of mood disorders.** Mood disorders are classified into several different syndromes. Depression can be unipolar, meaning that the patient has only depressive symptoms, or bipolar, when the depressed mood is interrupted by episodes of mania. Manic episodes are characterized by elevated mood, inflated sense of worth, and hyperactivity or irritability and can be associated with impairment in judgment. Many patients with depression also suffer from anxiety attacks.

C. **The depressed parent.** The symptoms of depression interfere with effective parenting. Depressed mothers are more negative, more irritable, and more easily annoyed than their nondepressed counterparts. They are less likely to respond positively to their children's requests and appear to be less accepting of their children's expressions of autonomy. Their discipline is often inconsistent, because setting limits for their children induces excessive guilt. They are less likely to encourage achievement. They are high users of the health care system, for both themselves and their children, and often present with psychosomatic complaints.

D. **Children of depressed parents.** The children of parents with affective mood disorders are at increased risk for learning, behavioral, and psychiatric problems. They exhibit more disruptive and oppositional behaviors and are more likely than children of normal parents to develop problems with depression and anxiety. As teenagers, they are prone to psychosomatic complaints and are likely to be rebellious and withdrawn.

Even after parental depression has been successfully treated, these children continue to function more poorly than do children whose parents have not been

---

1. In the past year, have you had 2 weeks or more during which you felt sad, blue or depressed; or when you lost all interest or pleasure in things that you usually cared about or enjoyed?

    Yes = 1
    No = 0

2a. Have you had *2 years or more in your life* when you felt depressed or sad *most days,* even if you felt okay sometimes?

    Yes = Ask 2b
    No = Skip 2b

2b. Have you felt depressed or sad much of the time in the *past year?*

    Yes = 1
    No = 0

3. How much of the time *during the past week* did you feel depressed?

    > 1 day = 0
    1–2 days = 1
    3–4 days = 2
    5–7 days = 3

The screen is considered positive if *either* Question 1 = 1 *or* Question 2a = 1 and 2b = 1 *and* Question 3 = 2 or more. Sensitivity = 81%; specificity = 95%; positive predictive value = 33%; negative predictive value = 99%.

Figure 81-1. Screening for depressive disorders. (Reprinted with permission from Rost K, Burnam MA, Smith R. Development of screeners for depressive disorders and substance disorder history. *Med Care* 31:189–200, 1993.)

depressed. The adjustment of children is related not only to their exposure to psychiatric symptomatology but also to longer-term patterns of dysfunctional parenting behaviors and aberrant social interactions.

II. **Making the diagnosis.** Pediatric clinicians should consider the diagnosis of parental depression under the following circumstances:
- All parents during the perinatal period.
- Parents who are high users of care.
- Parents with a family history of mood disorders.
- Parents who bring their children to the medical clinic with multiple vague complaints or seem overly anxious about and protective of their child.
- Parents whose children have psychosomatic illnesses.
- Parents with a chronic physical illness or a chronically ill child.
- Parents of children with behavioral disorders.

A. **Behavioral observations.** Clues to clinical depression can be gained through observing the affect of the parent and child and the interactions between them. The parent may appear to be expressionless, may speak in a monotone, or may appear restless. He or she may respond inconsistently to the demands of the child or report difficulties with setting limits.

B. **Routine screening for depression.** Because mood disorders are so pervasive and so frequently overlooked, routine use of screening instruments should be considered. Routine screening can also be helpful, both because taking a history for parental depression is time-consuming and because patients frequently are more willing to respond positively to questionnaires than to inquiries made during a face-to-face interview. Fig. 81-1 shows an instrument that can be easily administered in the waiting room. Although the negative predictive value of the screen is excellent (few depressed patients will be missed), the positive predictive value is only 33%. If the screen is positive, the clinician should take a more detailed history, inquiring about signs and symptoms.

C. **History: Key clinical questions.** The key to making the diagnosis is to keep in mind that mood disorders are very common and to consider the diagnosis in certain high-risk groups and situations, especially since parents are likely to underreport their emotional distress or family problems to their primary care provider.

There is no substitute for taking a good history: asking directly about the parents' emotional status; obtaining a family and personal history regarding psychiatric disorders and drug and alcohol use; ascertaining current and past medications taken by the parents; and inquiring about marital relationships and social support. These questions will be particularly pertinent in families who are high utilizers of care and those who present their children frequently with vague, somatic complaints. A positive response to the first question that follows or to four of the others meets the criteria for clinical depression.

1. *In the past year, have you had 2 weeks or more during which you felt sad, blue, or depressed or when you lost all interest or pleasure in things that you usually care about or enjoy?*

2. *Have you experienced changes in your eating habits, either from poor appetite or overeating?*

3. *Do you have difficulty sleeping (either with falling asleep, awakening in the middle of the night and not being able to return to sleep, or with sleeping too much)?*

4. *Have you felt fatigued or that you have little energy?*

5. *Do you feel restless or as if you have difficulty moving?*

6. *Have you had any difficulty concentrating or making decisions?*

7. *How do you feel about yourself?*

8. *Do you frequently find yourself feeling guilty about events in your life?*

9. *Do you feel hopeless?*

10. *Have you thought about suicide?*

III. Management

A. Primary goals. The primary goals of therapy for depression are to alleviate the suffering caused by the illness, to prevent recurrences, to stabilize the family and family relationships, to help the family with problematic parenting issues, and to prevent adverse psychological sequelae in the child. The immediate goal is to reduce the intensity of the dysphoria and its concomitant symptoms.

B. Initial treatment strategies. Pediatric clinicians, with their relationships and knowledge of families, are in a special position to address the needs of both the parents and the child. Options for the clinician include referral of the family for treatment elsewhere, comanagement of the disorder with a mental health provider or other primary care specialist, or assumption of primary care for the mood disorder in the parents. Even if the clinician chooses to refer the parents for psychiatric treatment, he or she should be knowledgeable enough to evaluate the efficacy of the prescribed treatment regimen and directly engage the family in counseling around the issues of parenting.

Should the clinician wish to assume care for such patients, additional education is necessary. Programs for learning to manage mood disorders are available through the American Psychiatric Association and local continuing medical education programs. Some are specifically designed for primary care clinicians. Even if the clinician does not want to undertake retraining, comanagement of patients is sometimes essential. The inertia, lethargy, and sense of hopelessness that are so much a part of depression often make referral of patients impossible, even when services are available. Some patients simply will not go elsewhere for treatment.

Excellent treatment modalities for mood disorders have been developed. Both pharmacotherapy and psychotherapy have been demonstrated to be effective, but treatment with antidepressant medications results in more rapid alleviation of symptoms. Between 65 and 75% of outpatients will respond to pharmacotherapy alone. Several classes of drugs can be used, including second-generation nontricyclic antidepressants, tricyclic antidepressants, and monoamine oxidase inhibitors. These medications appear to have similar efficacies but differ greatly in their side effects. The second-generation nontricyclics, such as bupropion (Wellbutrin) and fluoxetine (Prozac), appear to have relatively few side effects in most patients.

Counseling has been shown to be helpful, not just in the treatment of depression but also in its prevention. Postnatal depression appears to be particularly amenable to such interventions. Therapeutic listening and simple nondirective counseling have been demonstrated to be a tremendous help to women attempting to cope with their changing role as new mothers. Parent groups in pregnancy and the perinatal period provide an effective, efficient method that can easily be implemented in the pediatric office. Finally, counseling around the issues of parenting is essential.

IV. Clinical pearls and pitfalls

- The risk of suicide is significant among adults with unrecognized and untreated depression.
- About two-thirds of those who kill themselves have visited a physician within the preceding month, but physicians are generally very hesitant to ask about suicidal ideation.
- Clinicians who routinely inquire about parental emotional health will be surprised to learn how readily people will discuss their thoughts and ideas.
- If the provider is concerned about significant depression in a parent, assessing suicidal risk is essential.
- Asking a parent about his or her vision of the future may provide invaluable information regarding their overall status.
- If the likelihood of self-destructive behavior seems high, immediate referral is indicated.

Bibliography

For Parents

Depression Guideline Panel. *Depression Is a Treatable Illness: A Patient's Guide.* Rockville MD: US Department of Health and Human Services, 1993.

Jack D. *Silencing the Self: Women and Depression.* New York: Harper Collins, 1993.

Styron W. *Darkness Visible.* New York: Random House, 1990.

Woolis R. *When Someone You Love Has a Mental Illness: A Handbook for Family, Friends, and Caregivers.* New York: Putnam, 1992.

For Professionals

Organization

Agency for Health Care Policy and Research, PO Box 8547, Silver Springs MD 20907; (800) 358-9295.
The AHCPR has developed clinical practice guidelines that are available in several versions to meet differing needs. These include the Quick Reference Guide for Clinicians, Clinical Practice Guidelines, *and a* Patient's Guide *that is available in English and Spanish. Included in the* Patient's Guide *are national health care groups that can be contacted by providers or patients who need more information.*

Publications

Depression Guideline Panel. *Depression in Primary Care: Detection, Diagnosis, and Treatment.* Rockville MD: US Department of Health and Human Services, Public Health Service, Agency for Health Care Policy and Research, 1993.
*AHCPR Publication numbers 93-9552 (*Quick Reference*), 93-0550 (vol. 1, Detection and Diagnosis), 93-0551 (vol. 2, Treatment of Major Detection), and 93-0553 (Patient Guide).*

Schatzberg A, Cole J. *Manual of Psychopharmacology.* Washington DC: American Psychiatric Press, 1991.

Tollefson G. Recognition and treatment of major depression. *Am Fam Physician* 42 (suppl):59S–66S, 1990.

Elliott S et al. Parent groups in pregnancy: A preventive intervention for postnatal depression? In *Marshalling Social Support: Formats, Processes, and Effects.* Newbury Park CA: Sage, 1988.

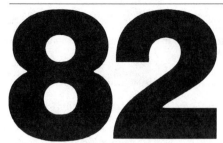

Parental Drug, Alcohol, and Cigarette Addiction

Kathi J. Kemper

I. **Description of the problem.** Addictive behaviors involving tobacco, alcohol, or other substances are characterized by:
- An individual's subjective compulsion to continue the behavior (craving) or reduced ability to exert personal control over the behavior, despite its negative impact on the person's health or well-being.
- The development of symptoms on withdrawal from the substance.
- Dependence on the use of the substance to feel "normal."
- The development of tolerance to the effects of the substance.
- The tendency to relapse into the addictive behavior following withdrawal.

An addictive experience provides a rapid and potent means of changing one's sensations and moods. The paradox of addiction is that it gives the addict a temporary sense of control at the expense of longer-term loss of self-control over the addictive behavior. Substance use and abuse represent a continuum from abstinence to social use to addiction. The point on the continuum at which parental use is hazardous to children is unknown and is strongly affected by other personal factors, such as parental mental health or chronic illness in the child, family factors such as divorce, and environmental factors such as inadequate or unstable housing.

A. **Epidemiology**

1. **Smoking**
   - In the United States, nearly 50 million adults (28% of the population) are smokers.
   - Of all current smokers, 60% began by age 14 years, and 80% became regular smokers before age 21 years.
   - Each day more than 3000 children start smoking cigarettes.
   - About 25% of pregnant women smoke, although this rate is higher among minorities, blue-collar workers, and those with less education.
   - The overall prevalence of maternal smoking is about 20%. Rates are higher among African-American (28%) and Asian (29%) mothers than among Caucasian (9%) and Hispanic (6%) mothers.
   - Married women have much lower rates of smoking than nonmarried women (14% vs. 37%).
   - Smokers are more likely to have a positive screen for drinking or drug use than nonsmokers.

2. **Alcoholism**
   - The estimated lifetime prevalence of alcohol dependence is 13.5%.
   - 18% of American adults report having lived with an alcoholic parent as a child.
   - The reported prevalence of alcohol consumption among pregnant women declined from 32% in 1985 to 20% in 1988. However, there was no decline among poorly educated women or those under age 25 years.

3. **Drug addiction**
   - The estimated lifetime prevalence of drug dependence or abuse is 6.1%.
   - The National Committee for the Prevention of Child Abuse estimates that 10 million American children are being raised by alcoholic or addicted parents.
   - It is estimated that 9000–10,000 narcotic-exposed and 300,000 cocaine-exposed infants are born each year in the United States.
   - Prenatal alcohol and drug use varies geographically (with higher rates

reported in urban areas) and across socioeconomic lines (with greater use of alcohol and marijuana reported among higher social classes and greater use of cocaine and heroin among lower social classes).

B. Etiology/contributing factors

1. **Genetic.** Children of substance abusers are three to five times more likely to develop addictions and other problem behaviors than other children. For example, the strongest predictors of initiating smoking are smoking by one's parents, peers, and/or siblings; having less educated parents; being more rebellious; and having fewer health concerns about the consequences of smoking. Evidence (largely from studies of families, twins, and adoptees) suggests a genetic predisposition to alcoholism.

2. **Environmental.** Although genetic factors may predispose toward alcoholism, a complex interaction between genetic endowment and environment leads to addiction. Excessively harsh or lax parental discipline and families with a history of behavioral problems and incarceration are at increased risk of substance abuse. Social factors associated with the development of alcoholism include a lower legal drinking age, social acceptability of drinking, availability of alcohol, and advertising and television depictions of drinking as sophisticated or sexy. Vulnerability to drug use is increased among those with low self-esteem, inadequate ties to family and community, a high need for social approval coupled with a feeling of not belonging, poor communication and coping skills, and decreased ability to delay gratification.

3. **Coexisting health problems.** There is substantial comorbidity among alcoholism, drug use, and other psychosocial pathology. Among those with an alcohol disorder, 37% have a comorbid mental disorder (especially depression). Among drug abusers, 53% have another mental disorder. Even among middle-class families, those with drinking problems often have poorer health behaviors (e.g., are more likely to be smokers and less likely to use seat belts).

II. Impact on children. Table 82-1 lists the known hazards of parental smoking, alcohol, and drug use on children. It is difficult to separate the potential teratogenic, genetic, and environmental effects of parental substance abuse on children, but it is clear that such children are at increased risk for a variety of physical, developmental, psychological, and behavioral problems.

III. Making the diagnosis

A. History: Key clinical questions

1. **Smoking**

   a. *Where might your child be exposed to tobacco smoke?* Help the parent by prompting for possible sites of exposure, such as household, day care, friends' homes, carpools, and the school. It is less threatening to start with a broad exploration of potential exposures and then focus on parental behaviors as the key factor affecting children's health.

   b. *How much do you smoke?* This is more likely to elicit a smoking history than will the question, "Do you smoke?" Many persons who smoke less than a pack a day do not consider themselves smokers.

   c. [To the mother] *How much did you smoke during pregnancy?* This is an important question to determine effects on the child's prenatal growth and potential postnatal sequelae.

   d. *How long have you smoked?* Most persons who smoke started during childhood. Asking this question provides the opportunity to discuss whether the parents have considered that their smoking might influence the child to start smoking.

   e. *Where do you smoke?* Smoking in the house or automobile poses the most intense exposure of the child to passive smoking. Parents who have already changed their smoking behavior to smoke outside the house or only when the child is not present should be praised for their efforts.

   f. *Have you considered cutting down on your smoking?* Most smokers want

Table 82-1. Impact of parental substance abuse on children

	Smoking	Alcohol	Substance abuse
Prenatal/ perinatal	Low birthweight Infant mortality Sudden infant death syndrome Lower quality and quantity of breast milk	Mental retardation Fetal alcohol syndrome Fetal alcohol effects	Neonatal abstinence syndrome Sudden infant death syndrome Prematurity Low birthweight Sexually transmitted diseases
Early childhood	Ear infections Allergies Asthma Other respiratory problems Behavioral problems	Behavioral problems (e.g., attention deficit hyperactivity disorder) Mental health problems (e.g., depression) Injuries Abuse (physical, sexual) Delayed immunizations	Behavioral problems Infectious diseases Malnutrition Neglect, abuse Unstable housing Mental health problems
Adolescence	As for early childhood, plus smoking behavior and higher low-density lipoprotein (LDL)	As for early childhood, plus: Drinking Foster care Delinquency Suicide Higher health costs	As for early childhood, plus drug use
Adulthood	Cardiovascular disease Lung cancer	Alcoholism	Substance abuse

to stop and have tried to do so. Asking this question provides the opportunity to praise the parent's intention and to explore possible plans for assisting the parent to quit smoking. If the parent has not made plans to cut down, encouragement to do so can be helpful.

    g. *How do you think your smoking affects your child?* Although most parents know that smoking is bad for their own health, many do not know about the risks that smoking poses for their child. By asking the question rather than giving a lecture, the clinician can help enable the parents to become partners in the health care of their child.

  2. Drinking. Binge drinking (defined as five or more drinks at a time) is more strongly associated with alcohol-related problems in women than are the quantity and frequency of drinking. Questions about tolerance to the effects of alcohol are also good predictors of problem drinking in women. For women, requiring three or more drinks to feel the effects of alcohol may indicate physiologic tolerance. The following questions (in a self-administered questionnaire or verbally) can be used to screen for parental drinking problems:

    a. *In the past year, have you or anyone else in your household had a problem with drinking?*

    b. *In the past year have you tried to cut down on your drinking?*

    c. *How many drinks can you hold* [or *does it take for you to feel high or get a buzz*]?

    d. *Do you ever have five or more drinks at a time?*

3. **Drug use.** Questions about drug use are a natural follow-up to questions about smoking and drinking:

   a. *In the past year, have you or anyone else in your household had a drug problem?*

   b. *In the past 24 hours, have you used any of the following drugs: marijuana, cocaine, crack, heroin, methadone, speed, LSD, amphetamines, or something else?*

   c. *Would you like to talk with other parents who are dealing with alcohol or drug problems?*

   d. *Would you like more information about alcohol or drug treatment programs in our area?*

B. **Behavioral observations.** Parents should be observed for slurred or pressured speech, flight of ideas, or level of concern inappropriate for the child's condition. Children who are brought in for evaluation of hyperactivity or poor attention span present an ideal opportunity to talk about parental health behavior such as drinking or drug use. Occasionally the symptoms of parental addiction are more subtle: missed appointments, multiple providers of child care at home, multiple providers bringing the child to health care visits, doctor shopping, an excessively happy (or unhappy) parent, or level of parental concern inappropriate to the child's health status. All clinicians should be alert to the smell of alcohol on the breath of parents. A clinician who smells alcohol on the breath of a parent must not ignore it but rather confront the parent, expressing concern about the parent's ability to drive home with this child and discussing alternative arrangements for transportation. This also is an opportune time to discuss the effect of the parent's drinking on the child's health and behavior.

IV. **Management.** Clinicians who wish to address parental addiction problems first need to address their own issues with smoking, alcohol, and drugs in themselves and family members. Judgmental attitudes are not helpful. Smoking, drinking, and drug use represent risky health behaviors, not moral failures. Parents suffering from them need assistance rather than preaching. It is helpful to explore with the parents their own ideas about ways they might quit or overcome their addiction and to explore their previous attempts at doing so. A clinician who feels uncomfortable assisting a parent in these areas should seek out experts in drug addiction. As with many other challenging issues in which the parent's behavior affects the child's health, it is helpful to keep the focus of the discussion on the impact of this behavior on the child's health rather than on the parent's behavior.

A. **Smoking**

   1. **Clinical interventions**

      a. **Advise smoking parents to stop.**

      b. **Assist smokers with quitting** (e.g., set a target date).

      c. **Assist with follow-up and referral** (e.g., to a smoking cessation program or to a clinician skilled in the use of the nicotine patch or gum as part of a smoking cessation program).

      d. **Provide anticipatory guidance about potential long-term effects of passive smoking on the child.**

      e. **Point out to the parent some of the adverse effects of smoking.** In addition to the risks of cancer and heart disease, more immediate problems include increased facial wrinkling, bad breath, increased insurance premiums, increased risk of house fires, and increased costs of cleaning clothing and upholstery. Most parents, however, are more likely to quit or reduce smoking in response to messages about the adverse effects of smoking on their child rather than on themselves.

   2. **Social interventions.** Child health professionals are in an excellent position to advocate for social changes that diminish the risk of smoking among children.

    a. **Making sales of cigarettes to minors illegal and better enforcement of existing laws.**

    b. **Banning vending machine sales of cigarettes.**

    c. **Increasing taxes on cigarettes to discourage consumption.**

    d. **Not allowing smoking in the office, hospital, or other practice settings.**

    e. **Boycotting all office magazines that contain cigarette advertising.**

B. **Alcohol and drug abuse**

  1. **Clinical interventions**

    a. **Give information to the parent** about the risks of parental behavior/addiction on the child, assistance with support, referral, and anticipatory guidance.

    b. **The child may need to be referred for individual or group counseling or to support groups,** such as Al-Anon. Interventions for children of alcoholics include providing support, giving information (e.g., on alcohol and alcoholism, the dynamics of alcoholic families, and common social and emotional reactions to having an alcoholic parent), helping to build skills (e.g., problem solving, communication, and the recognition and expression of feelings), building self-esteem and peer support, and developing coping strategies for living in an alcoholic home.

  2. **Social interventions.** Clinicians can serve as effective advocates for social change by:

    a. **Participating in community initiatives** (e.g., drunk driving campaigns).

    b. **Talking with other health professionals about the issues of substance abuse in the community and sharing strategies for problem solving.**

    c. **Participating on local school board committees or hearings and/or parent-teacher association committees related to substance abuse.**

    d. **Becoming aware of and participating in local government initiatives on alcohol and drugs.**

Bibliography

For Parents

Organizations

Alcoholics Anonymous. Refer to local telephone directory.

American Cancer Society, 1599 Clifton Road NE, Atlanta GA 30320; (404) 320-3333.

American Heart Association, 7320 Greenville Avenue, Dallas TX 75231; (214) 750-5300.

American Lung Association, 1740 Broadway, New York NY 10019.

Families Anonymous, PO Box 528, Van Nuys CA 91408; (818) 989-7841 or local telephone directory.

Mothers Against Drunk Driving, 699 Airport Freeway, Suite 310, Hurst TX 76053; (817) 268-MADD.

Narcotics Anonymous, 16155 Wyandotte Street, Van Nuys CA 91406; (818) 780-3951 or local telephone directory.

National Clearinghouse for Alcohol and Drug Information, PO Box 2345, Rockville MD 20852; (301) 468-2600.

National Federation of Parents for Drug-Free Youth, 8730 Georgia Avenue, #200, Silver Springs MD 20910; (301) 585-5437.

Publications

US Dept of Health and Human Services. *The Health Consequences of Involuntary Smoking: A Report of the Surgeon General.* DHHS Pub. no. (CDC) 87-8398, 1986.

For Professionals

Donovan DM, Marlatt GA (eds). *Assessment of Addictive Behaviors.* New York: Guilford Press, 1988.

Epps RP, Manley MW. A physician's guide to preventing tobacco use during childhood and adolescence. *Pediatrics* 88:140–144, 1991.

Galanter M (ed). *Recent Developments in Alcoholism,* vol 9, *Children of Alcoholics.* New York: Plenum, 1991.

Glynn TJ, Manley MW. *How to Help Your Parents Stop Smoking: A National Cancer Institute Manual for Physicians.* National Cancer Institute, NIH Pub. no. 89-3064, 1991 (revised).
Obtained by calling (800) 4CANCER.

Schonberg SK. *Substance Abuse: A Guide for Health Professionals.* Elk Grove IL: American Academy of Pediatrics, 1988.

83

Sibling Rivalry

Robert Needlman

I. **Description of the problem.** The child psychiatrist Winnicott has said that with the birth of a younger sibling, the child "discovers hatred." Parental concerns about sibling rivalry often arise soon after the birth of a second child, when the older sibling manifests behavioral regression or aggressive behaviors toward the baby. Later, school-aged siblings who seldom fight with peers regularly wage war, physically and psychologically, within the home. Seemingly endless battles between siblings irritate, drain, and worry many parents. On the other hand, sibling rivalries offer children some of their earliest lessons in conflict resolution and the concept of sharing, and the relationship often evolves into one of extraordinary closeness and depth.

A. **Epidemiology and other characteristics**
- Some degree of distress over the birth of a younger sibling is probably universal, as is transient behavioral regression.
- One-third of older siblings show developmental *gains* after the birth of a sibling. For example, a child who starts wetting the bed again might also start dressing himself, picking up his room, and referring to himself as a "big boy."
- The degree of upset following the birth of a sibling does not predict the quality of the sibling relationship. However, if the older child's initial response is to become withdrawn, the risk of longstanding animosity between siblings is increased.
- The prevalence of conflicts between older siblings severe enough to cause parental distress has not been reported; 35–40% of school-aged siblings engage in physical fights at home, although significant injury is rare.

B. **Etiology/contributing factors**

1. **Environmental**

   a. **Relationship with parents.** Children with the closest relationships to their mothers may show the greatest upset after the birth of a sibling. In contrast, a close relationship with the father may be protective. When parents regularly become involved in intersibling conflicts (as do about 60%), the number of incidents increases, but so does the degree of verbal negotiation between the siblings. In the absence of parental refereeing, conflicts tend to be resolved by force, and younger children learn to submit if they cannot win.

   b. **Parental favoritism.** Parental favoritism exacerbates conflicts, as does type-casting of children into roles, such as "my stubborn one; my messy one." Even positive roles, such as "my good listener" or "my little helper," can lead the child to misbehave in order to escape from the label or can imply to the other children that they are *not* expected to listen or help.

   c. **Spacing of siblings.** Siblings spaced about 2 years apart may experience the most intense rivalries, perhaps because the older child must deal with increased separation from the mother at a time when separation is particularly difficult. Additionally, many 2-year-old children lack the verbal and cognitive sophistication to understand explanations or to express complex emotions. Twins, by contrast, seem less prone to rivalry, as do children born 3 or more years apart.

II. Recognizing the issue

A. Signs and symptoms. Sibling conflicts may be brought up as the chief complaint, or they may be unmentioned causes or complicating factors in other clinical situations, such as when a sibling has a chronic illness or developmental disability.

B. History: Key clinical questions

1. *How did this child respond to the birth of the next child?* The clinician must go back to the beginning to establish a pattern of jealousy or rivalry. Rivalry may not have arisen until after several weeks, when it became clear that the new baby was staying, or until the baby became more interactive (around age 4 months) or began to walk and take the older child's toys. The clinician should inquire about each of these developmental stages.

2. *How was this child as a baby, compared to his or her sibling(s)?* Differential parental responses to siblings can exacerbate rivalry and may be due to temperamental differences in early infancy or to family differences at that time. For example, the parent may recall that the sibling was "always cranky" or born at a time of unusual stress in the family, such as marital conflict or job loss.

3. *Tell me about your other children.* The clinician should listen for type-casting ("my touchy one; my peacemaker"), stereotyping ("She's *always* the first to get into an argument"), and siblings with special problems or accomplishments.

4. [To the child] *Tell me about your brother(s) and sister(s).* It is important to ask verbal children directly about their sibling(s), as these perceptions may vary greatly from the parent's and may be the key to the child's behavior. For example, if the child responds that his sister is "always perfect," he may have decided that he can never hope to compete and has stopped trying to comply.

5. *Do the children have separate bedrooms, separate places for personal belongings, and individual time with parents?* Conflicts may be greater in families in which privacy and personal possessions are not respected. Individual special time is another highly valued commodity that can become a focus of contention.

6. *Tell me exactly what happened the last time you had a fight with your brother or sister. Start at the beginning, and give me a play-by-play account.* Analysis of the chain of events can sometimes reveal how seeming victims are actually provocateurs and how parental interventions may actually exacerbate the conflicts. For example, if one child is always seen as the wrongdoer, the other child may be encouraged to provoke more fights. Such analysis can also reveal the adaptive value of sibling rivalry for the family system. For example, siblings may collude in creating a disturbance in order to deflect interparental tensions or to attract the attention of an otherwise distant parent.

III. Management

A. Primary goals. Parents need to have reasonable expectations. They cannot ensure that their children will not be rivals, particularly if the children are temperamentally incompatible. Parents can, however, insist on civil behavior and can avoid parenting practices (such as comparisons and labeling) that exacerbate the problem.

B. Treatment strategies

1. **Increase parental understanding.** Parent counseling around the birth of a second or subsequent child should begin before delivery. Tell parents the following parable to increase their empathy with the displaced sibling:

   Imagine that your spouse came home one day and announced, "I have decided to bring home another beautiful, young wife [husband]. She will live with us and I will now spend most of my time with her. I want you to be nice to her. But I still love you as much as I always have." How would you feel?

2. **Support the older child.** Parents can expect that the older child will need additional support during this time of crisis. Toddlers, both male and female, may benefit from a baby doll to take care of. Involving the older child in the care of the new infant encourages him or her to take on the role of protective older sibling. It may be helpful to model ways for the parent to involve the older child, such as saying: "The baby is crying! What do you think? Should we try getting him a new diaper?"

A second crisis may occur when the younger sibling begins to walk and compete for toys. Parents need to be careful not to assume that the larger child is always the aggressor. Some degree of sharing is desirable, but it is also important for each child to have some things that are his or hers alone.

3. **Explain differential treatment.** Children who have reached the cognitive stage of concrete operations may become upset by what they perceive to be unfair treatment (e.g., "Johnny gets to stay up until 9, but I have to go to bed at 8. It's not fair!"). Parents should explain that everyone in the family gets what he or she needs; since everyone is different, those needs are different too.

4. **Teach civil behaviors.** With older children, strategies include reinforcing ownership and property rights (communal property must be shared, but individual property must be respected), clarifying household responsibilities, restricting physical or verbal attacks according to the principle of not harming one another, and holding older siblings responsible for settling their own disputes.

5. **Avoid comparisons and labeling.** Comparisons between children, even when complimentary, increase competition. Similarly, parents should avoid labeling children, such as, "Jane's my smart one. You're my little athlete." Even though couched in positive terms, the implication of this statement is, "You're dumb." The better alternative is for parents to comment on *behaviors* but avoid passing judgment on *character*.

C. **Follow-up/backup strategies.** Following the initial consultation, several brief visits at monthly intervals may be helpful to reinforce the parent training and encourage compliance with recommendations. The frequency of sibling conflicts may actually increase for a time after the parent announces that the children are to settle their own disputes. One or two well-timed follow-up visits can help the parent avoid being drawn back into the fray. It is also helpful to have the parent role-play management strategies (e.g., praising the child's behavior while avoiding comment on the child and comparison with siblings).

If problems persist unchanged, consider a family interview with all members present. The role of sibling conflicts in the overall dynamic of the family must be considered. In some cases, a referral for family counseling will be helpful.

Bibliography

For Parents
Faber A, Mazlish E. *Siblings Without Rivalry: How to Help Your Children Live Together So You Can Live Too.* New York: Avon Books, 1988.
An excellent guide designed to help parents understand their children's behavior and make the necessary changes in their own. It presents sound principles using wonderfully clear examples. The cartoon scenarios are particularly helpful. For some parents, "prescribing" this book may be of great assistance.

Reit S. *Sibling Rivalry.* New York: Ballantine Books, 1985.
Good review of the subject, written for parents, full of useful information.

For Professionals
Dunn, J. *Sisters and Brothers.* Cambridge MA: Harvard University Press, 1985.
Dunn has carried out some of the best and most relevant longitudinal research on siblings, well summarized here. The book is peppered with dialogues and other examples, making it particularly clear and enjoyable reading.

Dunn J, Kendrick C. *Siblings: Love, Envy and Understanding.* Cambridge MA: Harvard University Press, 1982.
Describes a longitudinal study in rich detail.

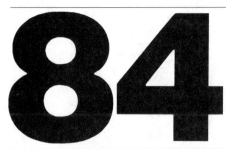

Single Parents

J. Lane Tanner

I. **Description of the problem.** While a variety of family reconfigurations have become prevalent over the past two decades, none have been more dramatic than the shift toward families headed by a single parent. While single parent status does not represent a problem in itself, single parent families as a group are significantly more strapped for personal, social, and economic resources, and are more likely to have experienced significant losses and change. This chapter is intended to alert the clinician to the stressors and special needs that commonly confront the single parent family.

A. **Epidemiology**
   - At least 50% of American children born in the 1980s and 1990s will spend a substantial period of time living in a home headed by a single parent or guardian.
   - Between 1970 and 1992, the numbers of children of all races living in single-parent homes has more than doubled (from 12 to 27% of all American children).
   - For African-American children, only 36% live with both parents (down from 59% in 1970).
   - 88% of children in one-parent families live with the mother.
   - Single-parent status is the result of parental divorce (37%), a never-married single parent (34%), parental separation (24%), and parental death (5%).

B. **Problems of single-parent families**

   1. **Limitations of available resources**

      a. **Money.** With 61% of children in mother-only households living below national poverty levels, the clinician is increasingly obliged to inquire regarding the family's financial resources, the parent's employment status, and the family's dependency on contributions from others (Table 84-1).

      b. **Time.** Single parents who are employed are likely to feel that they are continually in a race to provide adequate time to the family, the job, and the endless details of daily life, from groceries to taxes. Unpredictable events, such as an important school activity or a household emergency, or a child's illness, further intrude on this tightly stretched schedule.

      c. **Physical and emotional energy.** In addition to providing the tangible goods and supplies needed by the family, the single parent is called on to provide almost 100% of the emotional support and sustenance for her or his children. Alone, this parent must shoulder the responsibility for decisions, great and small, that shape their lives.

   2. **Network of social support.** Mapping the sources of social support for the single parent requires an awareness of the availability of those sources and the frequency with which the parent actually uses them. Are there other adults (relatives, friend, lover) living in the home? Are they emotionally or responsibly involved with the family? Who is dependent on whom? Are there other people who are emotionally close to the parent who can offer understanding and support? What about institutions (such as the school, workplace, church, or clinic) that can provide support for both parent and child?

   3. **Major life events, losses, or transitions.** Single-parent status is often born out of crisis (e.g., separation or divorce or the partner's death). These events

Table 84-1. Financial status in two-parent vs. one-parent families

	% of children under age 18 living with:	
	Two parents	One parent
Parent employed	85	55
Family income > $40,000	53	11
Own their own home	72	34
One parent with 4 or more years of college	26	8

Source: US Bureau of the Census. *Marital Status and Living Arrangements*. Current Population Reports, ser. P20, no. 468. Washington DC: US Government Printing Office, 1992.

may also bring a cascade of secondary losses, which may include changes in the family home, the child's school, friends, or community. Grief, anger, guilt, and depression regularly follow the trauma of such changes. The subsequent transitional period is likely to be disorganized and tumultuous until a realignment of schedule, roles, expectations, and feelings can permit a new and stabilized family life.

Such events may have very different meanings for the child than for the parent. For example, divorce and the loss of the family home may bring desired independence and relief for the parent but an unmitigated sense of loss for the child. The clinician must assess these differential meanings and be aware of the time course of adaptation displayed by each family member.

4. **Shifts in relational dynamics.** Family dynamics are substantially different when children are oriented to a single parent as the sole authority and provider and when the parent has only the children as her or his companions at home.

C. **Common clinical issues.** As with other risk factors, single-parent status by itself confers no predictable condition on the child. The following clinical issues are thus presented as common concerns and in no way specifically or universally apply to single-parent families.

1. **The single parent who feels off-balance and uncertain regarding parenting and child management.** While self-doubt is surely universal for all parents, single parents are even more susceptible. The parent seeks advice but also "reality testing" and reassurances that her or his efforts, responses, and feelings (especially negative feelings) are warranted, or at least understood.

2. **The helpless, overwhelmed single parent.** The clinician becomes aware that this parent is not simply looking for good advice but for someone else to lean on, to make the hard decisions and to take over the responsibility that has become incapacitating. Parental isolation and depression are especially common concomitants.

3. **Child behavioral disorders.** These are particularly likely to emerge when the child is pushing the parent to provide unmet needs or when the parent's sense of concern, guilt, or exhaustion regarding the child renders behavioral management ineffective.

4. **The child who takes on a parentified helper role.** This may be necessary and adaptive for the family. The payoff for the child may be the closeness that such a partnership with the parent provides. The clinical question is whether this parental role infringes on the sociodevelopmental needs of the child.

5. **The child who becomes the parent's companion and confidant.** The key issue concerns the boundaries between parent and child—whether each has his or her own friends, activities, rights of privacy, and freedom to disagree or express anger with the other.

6. **Issues related to the absent parent.** Children must come to terms with developmentally staged personal dilemmas regarding who the absent parent was, is, and will be to them. Additionally, they must adapt to what it means, within their own community norms, to grow up in a single-parent home.

7. **The adolescent single parent and the three-generation household.** This "kinship family" provides crucial social support, shared child rearing, and other resources. There are, however, likely to be intrinsic tensions between the grandparent(s) and the teenage parent. These most predictably center on issues of parental authority for the young child and personal autonomy for the adolescent. The nature of the grandparents' support for their daughter or son and whether they realistically and flexibly encourage the growth of her or his competencies is an important question to address.

8. **The introduction of a new adult into the household.** Whether a friend, relative, or potential future mate, the arrival of a new adult into an established single-parent household is a major event. Its meaning to the child is shaped by his or her own developmental stage and past events and patterns. The potential for the child to feel displaced, intruded on, or disregarded is substantial. Long-term adaptation requires that the parent display her or his intention to remain the head of the household, in charge not only of the children but also in overseeing the authority and responsibilities that are delegated to the new adult.

II. Management

A. **Empathy with the issues.** The primary care clinician is often called on to hear, understand, and validate the concerns and responses of the single parent. Most common to these parents is the sense of aloneness in the consuming and awesome task of child rearing. It is an attitude of respect for this experience that becomes the clinician's first and most important tool.

The clinician's direct inquiry of the parent (e.g., *You have a lot to juggle. How is it going?* or *How are you doing balancing everybody's needs? How about your own?*) opens the door to establishing this basis of understanding and respect.

B. **Monitoring the needs of the child.** In order to monitor the needs of the child in the single-parent family, the clinician must remain mindful of the challenges confronting the child and assess his or her adaptation to them. As always, behavioral patterns, school performance, social functioning, and overall sense of happiness and confidence are the best indicators of the child's adaptation to stress. However, in some children signs of difficulty may not be obvious. For example, the child's anxious loyalty to a single parent or the parent's own urgent or unmet needs may keep either from acknowledging the stressful influences that impinge on the child. The child's needs may come into direct conflict with those of his or her parent (e.g., a parent's new adult relationship that takes away time with the child). Thus, it falls to the clinician to initiate, with the child as well as the parent, an exploration of the potential problems and issues. Directly asking the child about daily routines such as sleep patterns, home responsibilities, daily schedule, and school achievement will often open the door to an exploration of stress and poor adaptation.

C. **Supporting the parent.** With rare exceptions, support for the child requires support for the parent. The clinician can encourage and support a parent by simply valuing her or his efforts. Advocacy for clearly established generational boundaries and effective parental authority may help clear away some of the hesitancy and doubt the parent is experiencing. Concern for the parent as a person, with individual needs and goals, may encourage her or him to seek an effective network of social support.

For the single parent who comes across as helpless and overwhelmed and seems to be pushing for a truly dependent relationship, simple empathy, validation, and good advice are not enough. The clinician may experience the urge to rescue the parent in some way or, alternatively, to run away from such expressed neediness. Advice and helpful ideas offered by the clinician may be met with a disparaging "yes, but" response from the parent.

For such parents, redescribing expressions of helplessness in terms of particular dilemmas introduces the possibility of choice and action (e.g., *It sounds as if you are dealing with a lot, and your child's behavior sounds particularly difficult right now, for both of you. Tell me your ideas for handling it.*). By resisting the impulse to provide the answers and by encouraging and organizing the parent's own efforts at problem solving (e.g., *What will be the effect on your child of such a plan? How about on you and on your goals for yourself as a parent in the short term and in the long term?*), the clinician's role shifts from that of the fantasized rescuer to that of an understanding yet realistic coach. Additionally, reminding the parent of her or his demonstrated competencies, especially those that contradict the current perceptions of helplessness, may bolster self-efficacy and hopefulness.

Bibliography

For Parents
Parents Without Partners International, 8807 Colesville Road, Silver Springs MD 20910-4346; (301) 588-9354.

For Children
Horner CT. *The Single-Parent Family in Children's Books: An Annotated Bibliography* (2nd ed). Metuchen NJ: Scarecrow Press, 1988.

For Professionals
Allmond B, Buckman W, Gofman H. The single parent family. In *The Family Is the Patient: An Approach to Behavioral Pediatrics for the Clinician*. St. Louis: Mosby, 1979.

Carter B, McGoldrick M. *The Changing Family Life Cycle: A Framework for Family Therapy* (2nd ed). Boston: Allyn and Bacon, 1989.

Lindblad-Goldberg M. *Clinical Issues in Single-Parent Households*. Rockville MD: Aspen, 1987.

Weltner JS. A structural approach to the single parent family. *Family Process* 21:203–210, 1982.

Stepfamilies

John S. Visher and
Emily B. Visher

I. Description of the problem

A. Epidemiology
- Of all children born in the 1980s, 45% will experience the divorce of their parents and 35% will live with a stepparent before they are age 18 years.
- By the year 2000, the stepfamily will be the most common type of American family.

B. Stresses for children

1. **Loss.** Stepchildren come into the remarried family with a history of many losses, including loss of the full-time presence of one of their parents and loss of familiar surroundings. The remarriage may bring a new set of losses. Some obvious ones include leaving a familiar house, neighborhood, and school and losing a best friend. More subtle losses include the new status of being the eldest or youngest child in the family, of not being an only child, and of sharing time, attention, and intimacy with a parent who previously had no competing emotional ties. The newly remarried parents, often caught up in their own personal happiness, may not be fully aware of their children's sense of loss.

2. **Loyalty conflicts.** Loyalty conflicts are inevitable. An emotional connection to a stepparent may be experienced as a betrayal of the parent who is no longer present.

3. **Loss of control.** Loss of control is at the root of much of the anger and depression in children from remarried families. The adults have chosen to make major changes in their lives; the children have had those changes imposed on them.

4. **Stepsiblings.** The presence of stepsiblings can exacerbate the stresses that accompany a remarriage. Feelings of sibling rivalry—jealousy, insecurity, and the fear that a sibling is more loved—are more intense in a remarried family. Visiting stepsiblings may be offered special treats or exempted from the house rules that resident children must follow. Grandparents may give their biologic grandchildren more lavish gifts than their stepgrandchildren. If a baby is born into the stepfamily, sibling jealousy can be magnified by the fear that the "mutual child" will be more loved by the adults. At the same time, the birth may help to solidify the stepfamily because the new baby is biologically related to all of the children and adults. It is certainly true that many stepsiblings develop close bonds, united by their common experience of a disrupted family.

C. Children's responses

1. **Preschool.** The stress of a remarriage often causes preschoolers to cling to parents and to regress behaviorally. In the stage of magical thinking, they may believe that their angry thoughts already have led to or will lead to family disruption. Conversely, they may harbor thoughts that they can magically reunite the divorced parents.

2. **School age.** School-aged children are often angry about their powerlessness

Condensed and adapted, with permission, from "Why stepfamilies need your help," by Emily B. Visher, Ph.D., and John S. Visher, M.D., *Contemporary Pediatrics,* March 1992, pages 146–164.

to halt the disruption of their lives. They may counter these feelings of helplessness by imagining that they caused the breakup of the marriage, a fantasy that at least offers some influence over a situation they cannot control. They may still wish that their parents were together and fantasize that if they are "good," their parents will be reunited, or that if they are "bad" or "sick," their parents will come together to help.

Children at this stage are rarely able to express these feelings verbally and are likely to act out their anger and guilt. They may have tantrums at home, fight with siblings or classmates, develop psychosomatic symptoms, become accident prone, start failing in their schoolwork, or even try to break up the new marriage. Conversely, they may respond by behaving with an angelic virtue, following all the rules and making no obvious waves, so that their inner turmoil remains concealed.

3. **Adolescence.** Adolescents present special difficulties for the remarried family. They are caught up in their own issues of identity and autonomy, making the new relationships even more difficult to accept. Their own sexuality is burgeoning at the very time they enter a household that is, inevitably, more sexualized than their biologic family had been. The presence of stepsiblings or a stepparent of the opposite sex can also create sexual tensions.

Often an independent teenage child of a single parent is pressured, after a remarriage, to return to a more childish stage of dependency. Teenagers who are used to being the "man" or "woman" of the house find themselves losing that favored status as they are asked to become "kids" again. This may accelerate their drive to separate from the parents or to return to the home of the other biologic parent.

D. **Stress for remarried parents.** Remarried parents must also deal with many strong emotions. Their loyalty to their children predates the remarriage and may create conflicts with the new spouse. They may attempt to please the children at all costs in order to make up to them what they have lost. They may also be unable to form a solid bond with a new spouse because to do so would be experienced as a betrayal of their relationships with their children. This, in turn, frequently conflicts with the needs of the new spouse, who may feel like an outsider in an established household.

II. **Helping children**

A. **General principles**

1. **Accept the child's feelings.** Do not attempt to force the child to understand the perspectives of adults.

2. **Reassure the child (repeatedly, if necessary) that he or she is not responsible for the dissolution of the parents' marriage.**

3. **Stress that the child is a worthwhile, special person, no matter what decisions parents have made about their own lives.**

4. **Help the child put feelings into words rather than into negative behaviors.** Encourage verbal expression (e.g., *A lot of children feel very angry when they have to share a room with stepbrothers or stepsisters. Maybe you feel that way sometimes*).

5. **Encourage the child to communicate with parents and stepparents.** The clinician can do this by talking to the family as a group or by asking a child privately for permission to communicate specific information to the adults (e.g., his or her feeling that a stepsibling is being favored or distress over parents' fighting).

6. **Provide support to the parents and stepparents.** The psychological well-being of children depends more on the functioning of the family than the *type* of family.

B. **Teenagers**

1. **The acting out of sexual attraction between stepsiblings can be minimized by having the family adopt a dress code and by making appropriate bedroom arrangements.** Adults also need to be aware of and deal with their

sexual feelings toward a stepchild who may appear to be a younger version of their spouse.

2. **Adolescents are often reluctant to become part of the stepfamily because of their developmental drive for independence and autonomy and the primacy of their peer relationships.** The adults need to allow them to maintain their independence from the stepfamily and to integrate at their own pace. In some cases, the teenager chooses to move out in order to find his or her identity.

3. **Divided loyalties may make the adolescent act out in a negative way toward the stepparent.** It is important to emphasize to the adolescent the need to act in a respectful, if not warm, manner toward the stepparent.

4. **The stepparent may never be able to serve as a parent to the adolescent.** However, other types of relationships, such as adult friend or confidant, can play equally important and rewarding roles for both adolescent and stepparent.

III. Helping adults

A. The couple

1. **The adults almost always have unrealistically high expectations of what their new family will be like.** Such misconceptions can be avoided by anticipatory guidance and by directing them to sources of information that provide realistic information about stepfamily life, especially in the early phases. They can also talk with other, more experienced remarried parents and stepparents.

2. **Communicate to remarried parents acceptance of their family as a valid entity, not a flawed version of the nuclear family norm.** Reassure them that their struggles are not unique but are an expected part of the complex task of creating a remarried family.

3. **Remind the parents that a strong relationship with one another is not a betrayal of their biologic children.** All children need a solid bond between the adults in the household, especially to allay fears that the stepfamily will dissolve in the way that their previous family did. They also need a model of a couple working well together, to help them when they grow up and form successful relationships on their own.

B. Stepparenting

1. **The best advice is, "Don't try to be an instant parent."** The foundation of good relationships is a supply of positive, shared memories. Parental relationships need time to build; with older children, they may *never* fully materialize.

2. **The stepparent should make clear to the children that he or she is not a replacement for a dead or absent parent.** Instead, a stepparent is another person who can fill some of the child's needs for closeness and love. Stepparents may be relieved to learn that there are many different yet satisfactory roles they can play in their stepchildren's lives, roles that depend on the ages and needs of the children as well as the desires of the stepparent. For example, a stepparent can be a parent to a young child, a friend to an older child, or a confidant to a teenager.

3. **Adults may come into a new marriage with very dissimilar parenting experiences.** It is helpful to supply information about child development, correct misconceptions, and, in some cases, recommend that the couple take a parenting course together.

IV. Questions frequently asked by stepfamily adults

A. What should children call a new stepparent? "Mother" and "father" (or variations on these) are more than just names; they describe relationships. It is not helpful to insist on such terms when a relationship has not yet developed or when the child feels uncomfortable using the name. All but the youngest children may initially feel that by calling the stepparent "Mommy" or "Daddy," they are forsaking the absent parent.

What children call their stepparents often progresses through different stages. At first, the child may call the stepparent by his or her first name. Later, it might become "daddy John" or "mommy Mary." The important point is that the name feel comfortable for both child and adult and not imply a rejection of the absent parent.

B. **What can stepparents do about discipline?** Discipline is a major source of tension in most remarried families. Frequently a remarried parent unrealistically expects a new spouse to discipline the children effectively. Children, however, do not view a new stepparent as someone with the instant authority to set limits on their behavior. The best approach is for the two adults to work out house rules together and, at least initially, leave the enforcement of those rules to each child's biologic parent. It may take 1½–2 years with young children (longer with older children) for the stepparent to have sufficient emotional authority to discipline the child effectively.

C. **How should the absent parent be dealt with?** The adults should not criticize a child's other parent and should not use children as messengers or spies in unresolved hostilities. Children feel that criticism and anger toward any parent are also directed at them. It hurts them to hear negative comments about a parent they love. The clinician can help by showing parents how this behavior harms children and by supporting the children's desire not to be involved in conflicts between their parents. Encourage parents to give children permission to care about *all* of the adults in their lives, with no need to choose sides or take part in a battle.

D. **How long does it take to feel like a family?** Adults and children feel like a family when they identify themselves as part of a system to which they all belong, where they feel comfortable, and where their basic needs are met. The time it takes to feel that way varies but is almost always much longer than the adults expect. With young children, the process of settling down takes at least 18–24 months; with older children, it may take 5–7 years.

E. **Should children continue to see the noncustodial parent?** Children in remarried families usually do better if they can maintain ties to both of their biologic parents, as long as no physical or emotional risk is involved. If children move back and forth between households, the adults should collaborate as a parenting coalition. A parenting coalition is a *limited* alliance, formed to promote the welfare of the children. It is a cooperative rather than a competitive relationship and is based on an understanding that all the adults are important to the children.

F. **What can make the children's "dual citizenship" easier?** When children have just returned from visiting their other household, they need some time to adjust. It usually works better if the adults inform children about what happened while they were away, rather than interrogating them about what happened in the other household. Children should have a space of their own: a separate room or part of a room, a closet where special belongings are kept, or even a drawer. What matters is a house rule that nothing in a child's own place can be touched without that child's permission.

Children may be disturbed over the differences in rules between the two households, and they may use those differences as a weapon to play one household against the other. Nevertheless, children do eventually learn that codes of acceptable behavior differ between households (just as they differ between home and school). What matters is to know what the rules are in each place and to abide by them. Children accept this most readily if they have some input into establishing the rules in the newly formed household and if the parents are not defensive about the rules they have established. Finally, it is important to keep the consequences for misbehavior within the household where it occurred. An infringement of one household's rules should not affect time spent in the other household.

Bibliography

For Parents

Organization
Stepfamily Association of America, 215 Centennial Mall South, Suite 212, Lincoln NE 68508; (800) 735-0329.

Publications
Burns C. *Stepmotherhood: How to Survive Without Feeling Frustrated, Left Out, or Wicked.* New York: Harper Collins, 1986.

Gorman T. *Stepfather.* Boulder CO: Gentle Touch Press, 1985.

Roosevelt R, Lofas J. *Living in Step.* New York: Stein & Day, 1977.

Stepfamily Association of America. *Stepfamilies Stepping Ahead.* Lincoln NE: Stepfamily Association of America, 1989.

Visher E, Visher J. *How to Win as a Stepfamily* (2nd ed). New York: Brunner/Mazel, 1991.

For Children
Berman C. *What Am I Doing in a Stepfamily?* Secaucus NJ: Lyle Stuart, 1982.

Evans M. *This Is Me and My Two Families.* New York: Magination Press, 1989.

Vigna J. *She's Not My Real Mother.* Chicago: Albert Whitman, 1980.

For Teenagers
Getzoff A, McClenahan C. *Stepkids: A Survival Guide for Teenagers in Stepfamilies.* New York: Walker, 1984.

Wesson C. *Teen Troubles: How to Keep Them from Becoming Tragedies.* New York: Walker, 1988.

For Professionals
Papernow P. *Becoming a Stepfamily: Patterns of Development in Remarried Families.* San Francisco: Jossey Bass, 1993.

Visher E, Visher J. *Stepfamilies: A Guide to Working with Stepparents and Stepchildren.* New York: Brunner/Mazel, 1979.
Also available in paperback under a different title: Stepfamilies: Myths and Realities. *Secaucus NJ: Carol Publishing.*

Visher E, Visher J. *Old Loyalties, New Ties: Therapeutic Strategies with Stepfamilies.* New York: Brunner/ Mazel, 1988.

86

Teen Mothers

Teresa M. Kohlenberg

I. **Description of the problem.** For most of human history it has been normal for a young woman to bear her first child in her teens, and this continues to be the norm in most of the Third World. In such settings, teen mothers make good parents, supported by extended families and intact child-rearing traditions. Yet in industrialized, Western societies teens are viewed as inherently inadequate parents, and stigmatized as "children having children." Many studies have shown that early childbearing in the United States places mother and child at psychosocial risk, but it is clear that it is not primarily maternal age that determines the outcomes. Rather the outcomes appear to relate to pre-existing family and individual factors that lead some young women to become mothers before they have completed the educational and developmental processes necessary for adult function in this society. This chapter reviews what is known about the correlates of teen parenting in the United States, and suggests a framework for approaching the pregnant teen and her family to enhance their strengths and resources for the tasks ahead.

A. **Epidemiology.** Several factors may account for the increase in single-teen parenting: a decrease in the stigma attached to early sexual activity and unwed motherhood, a decrease in marriage as a response to pregnancy, and perhaps a lessening of hope or ambition for further education and higher-status jobs. By comparison, many Western European countries that also underwent the sexual revolution have teenage birthrates much lower than in the United States.
   - Each year, 11% of all U.S. females ages 15–19 years become pregnant, and about half of them (over 500,000) give birth.
   - 25% of all young women in the United States become pregnant by age 18 years.
   - While the overall teenage birthrate is stabilizing, the rate of births to very young teenagers continues to rise.

B. **Problems of teen motherhood.** Longitudinal studies of the outcomes of teen parenting demonstrate a worrisome spectrum of developmental and behavioral difficulties affecting both mother and child (Table 86-1). Overall, about two-thirds of teen mothers and their children appear to suffer from at least one of the problems documented by such studies. These studies focused largely on young mothers of color raising their children in poverty in big cities, in spite of the fact that 60% of teen mothers are white and teen mothers come from a wide variety of economic backgrounds. Consequently, we need to be cautious in assuming that the findings of such studies apply universally, especially since early parenthood is common and accepted in many subcultures of U.S. society. In these settings early parenthood is not necessarily viewed with alarm and may not lead to the problems encountered by teen mothers in cultures in which this choice is not as common or acceptable. In general, very young teens (under age 16 years) are the most likely to have trouble, while those ages 18–19 years, who are more mature and better accepted and supported by their families, often cope well with parenthood.

C. **Environmental risks.** There is a high prevalence among teen mothers of risk factors that can affect the mental health and ability to function of any parent. Over 75% of teen mothers in the United States report at least one (and usually several) significant psychosocial risk factors, including:
   1. **Sexual molestation in childhood.**
   2. **Abuse or neglect in childhood.**

Table 86-1. Problems for teen mothers and their children

Mother
  Poor prenatal care
  Lower status jobs
  Less marriage or partner support
  Lower educational achievement
  More time on welfare
  Higher stress and depression
Child
  More injuries
  More behavioral problems
  More delinquency
  Lower IQ on standard tests
  More grade failure and dropout
  Daughters more likely to become teen mothers themselves

3. **Being a child of an addicted parent.**

4. **Loss of a parent to death or separation from parents by placement in foster care.**

5. **Family mental health problems.**

6. **Poor school function with grade failure and low self-esteem.**

7. **Chronic depression and/or anxiety disorders.**

8. **Abuse by partners (domestic violence).**

D. **Strengths of teen mothers.** Despite the risks, a significant minority of teen mothers and their children lead healthy, independent, and successful lives. Some of the ways that teen mothers differ from older mothers can actually be adaptive strengths in their lives as parents, including:

1. **Physical health, energy, and stamina.**

2. **Optimism and idealism.**

3. **Ability to use peers for support.**

4. **Extended family network.**

5. **Developmental readiness for growth and change.**

II. **Working with the teen mother.** Teen mothers and their children come from a variety of backgrounds, bringing both risks and strengths to their lives. To work effectively with them requires an awareness of the social context of early parenting for each teen and her family and of the particular crises and vulnerabilities that accompany different developmental stages in the lives of mother and child. At each stage the provider must be aware of:
• The teen's progress toward her own life goals.
• The child's developmental status.
• The impact of the child's behavior on the teen.
• The social supports available to the mother.
• The conflicts between her needs and those of the child.
    By making explicit to the teen and her family the challenges that these dual developmental processes present and by providing consistent and empathic guidance, the primary care clinician can play a critical role in preventing developmental and behavioral problems for both mother and child.

A. **During pregnancy**

1. **Issues**

a. **Only 25% of teens say they planned their pregnancy.** Thus, the first crisis for most is acceptance of the pregnancy and the decision of whether to continue it.

    b. Disclosure to the baby's father, their families, and peers may be stressful.

    c. Grappling with the physical and role changes of pregnancy is challenging. Younger teens have the most difficulty adapting to pregnancy.

    d. Many families are thrown into turmoil during a teen's pregnancy, sometimes leading to the teen's moving out to live with friends or with her baby's father's family. Often a reconciliation occurs after the child is born.

2. Key clinical questions

    a. *How are you feeling about being pregnant? Is being pregnant like you expected it would be?* Teens need information about the normal course of pregnancy and fetal development to make healthy choices and to attach to their growing baby.

    b. *How is this pregnancy changing your life? What are the best parts, and what are the hardest parts?* Many teens are angry, anxious, or depressed in early pregnancy. The clinician must identify those who need mental health referral.

    c. *Who are the most important people in your life now, and how are they reacting to your pregnancy?* Teens sometimes lose important support people when they reveal their pregnancy.

    d. *What are your plans for after the baby is born?* It is natural for teens to focus on the present; the clinician can lay the groundwork for realistic future planning.

    e. *Would you or anybody else in your family like to talk with other teen mothers and their families?* Peer support groups are an effective way to convey information to pregnant teens and their families.

3. Management strategies. The primary care clinician can aid the entire family during this adjustment, particularly by helping the teen to define and balance her role as mother-to-be with her roles as a child in her family and an adolescent in society. The first step toward providing this help is to maintain regular contact during the pregnancy, even if the young mother's obstetric care is provided at another site. It is critical that the provider become comfortable and competent in asking questions about risk factors and be prepared to provide support, information, and appropriate referral for the teen who reveals trauma, loss, and chronic distress.

B. Birth and the postpartum period

1. Issues

    a. As with older parents, **this is a time of pride and major adjustment** to the demands of caring for an infant.

    b. Young fathers often are not living with the mother and baby and have much less opportunity to develop as parents.

    c. Teens of both sexes may be more surprised and confused by infant behavior and more ambivalent about their ability to parent than older parents. This makes them particularly vulnerable to being displaced by their own parents as primary caregivers for their baby.

    d. Many school systems demand that teen mothers return to classes within 1–2 months of delivery, which leaves little time to establish a solid mother-child relationship.

    e. Teen mothers may react to their changed bodies and the demands of parenting with a drive to reestablish their adolescent life-style, to get out of the house, and to spend time with their peers and boyfriends. Some family members respond angrily to this adolescent behavior, taking a position typified by, "You had this baby. Now you take care of it." This can be the first of many struggles over the teen's conflicting roles and responsibilities.

2. **Key clinical questions**

   a. *How did your delivery go? How do you feel about your body now?* Many teens had unrealistic expectations about delivery and the postpartum recovery.

   b. *Who's helping you at home? Do you get enough help?* These questions may uncover early power struggles over the teen's adequacy as a caregiver.

   c. *Is there anything about the baby that you are worried about?* In addition to addressing any concerns, the provider can establish herself or himself as a resource for questions about normal development and child rearing.

   d. *Is being this baby's mother like you expected being a mother would be? Are you having enough room for the other parts of your life?*

3. **Management.** At this early stage, the primary care clinician can reinforce the teen's shaky confidence while helping the grandparents and others to find a balance between support and intrusion. Teens may accept advice and guidance from the provider that they will not take from their parents. The clinician should help the family to develop conflict resolution strategies around child-rearing disagreements.

C. **Infancy**

1. **Issues**

   a. **The first year of the baby's life is usually marked by the teen's growing sense of competence and pride in herself and her baby** and by the teen's idealistic and optimistic expectations of parenting and child development.

   b. **The baby's father's role is usually set during this first year** and often enhanced by his parents' investment in their new grandchild.

   c. **The great majority of teen mothers live with their families of origin for at least the first year.** Flexible families allow the teen independence in certain areas, while providing ongoing support for her development in others. In less adaptable families, however, the teen can be isolated, punished, or mistrusted in a situation of escalating tension and unhappiness.

   d. **Issues for the baby** include the presence of multiple caregivers (who may have quite different caretaking styles) and the impact of less competent parenting by some teen mothers (marked by less verbal interaction, more punitive attitudes, and less ability to facilitate the infant's emerging skills).

   e. **When the teen mother is very limited in her ability or willingness to parent, the baby's care may revert to the grandparents.** When this is an adaptive response, the clinician should commend the family on their responsible decision and give the teen permission to attend to her own developmental tasks.

2. **Key clinical questions**

   a. *How is it feeling, being a mother and a teen at the same time?*

   b. *What questions or worries do you have about your child?*

   c. *How is your support network? Do you have any conflicts with people in that network?*

   d. *What are your plans for the future? For school? For work? Living on your own? What are you doing about birth control?*

3. **Management.** The prevention of early repeat pregnancy is a critical intervention during this year. When teen mothers can focus on one baby and on their own development for at least 2 years, outcomes are improved.

   Parenting attitudes and skills are another focus of the first year. Since teens accept information and advice better from peers than professionals, this is a time to promote support groups and play groups.

D. Toddlerhood

1. Issues

a. **With younger, less insightful parents and parents who are survivors of abusive or neglectful parenting, the toddler period is a dangerous one.**

b. **The loss of the lovable, cuddly infant** (who may have fulfilled fantasies and unmet needs for unconditional love) **may leave a vulnerable young mother feeling rejected and abandoned.** This loss and distance can stress the relationship between mother and child and lead to the mother's "replacing" her lost infant by having another baby.

c. **The normal provocative behaviors of a toddler can overwhelm an immature or impulsive mother's self-control,** particularly when her child's behaviors resonate with her own autonomy struggles. This can foster inconsistent and harsh discipline, alternating with poor supervision, that makes injury more likely. The grandparents and other caregivers may undercut the mother by being overcontrolling or overindulgent.

d. **The toddler period is typically when a teen who has been living with her family moves out on her own or with a partner.** Although this independence may represent cherished freedom and a sense of maturity, both the teen and her child lose the buffering support of the extended family. Additionally, the child may have to adapt to new caregivers with different styles and expectations.

2. Key clinical questions

a. *Are you enjoying your child? Do you have questions about behavior and how to manage it? Who gives you advice, and how useful is it? Do you agree with the other people who take care of your child?* The focus during the toddler years should be on developmental challenges for both mother and child, particularly on the intersection of their parallel struggles for autonomy.

b. *How is your support network? Is the baby's father helping out?*

c. *Are you enjoying your own life? Do you have plans that you need help to carry out? What are your thoughts about family planning? Education? Work? Child care?*

3. Management. Mature, well-supported teen mothers will benefit from anticipatory guidance and child management suggestions, just as older parents do. For teens in conflict with their own parents over parenting, the primary care clinician can help by anticipating these struggles and presenting them as common experiences for many parents. When teens move out and separate their babies from their grandparents, the provider can help make the teen mother aware of the elements of loss or stress in the situation and suggest ways to ease the transition (such as visits and good-bye rituals).

Repeat pregnancy is not always a red flag. Some young women who have their families in their teens and early twenties do a good job of parenting and then resume school or work when their children are a little older. It is very important that the clinician not communicate frustration or hopelessness when the teen becomes pregnant again or chooses to remain at home with her first child. Rather, the provider should continue to explore with the teen how well her choices are working out for her and what she needs in order to be effective in whatever roles she chooses.

E. The school years and beyond

1. Issues

a. **Studies of the children of teen mothers in urban poverty show them to be more likely than their peers to have behavioral or learning problems in school.** These problems are multifactorial, with poverty and frequent changes of caregivers playing as much of a role as teen parenting style and heritable learning disabilities.

b. **The two strongest predictors of school and behavioral problems in children of teen parents are the mother's prolonged dependence on public assistance and unstable parental relationships.**

c. **By the time a teen's child is in school, she is no longer in her teens, yet she still faces issues related to early parenthood.** Some teen mothers can be overcontrolling in their efforts to make sure that their children do not follow in their own footsteps, and many are deeply disappointed and bitter if they do.

d. **Teen mothers often find their own children's adolescent struggles particularly difficult.**

e. **When children of teen mothers bear children as teens, they turn their mothers into 30-year-old grandmothers.** For a mother who looks forward to being an independent adult for the first time, the responsibility (for her grandchild) and sense of failure (as a parent) can be very stressful.

2. **Key clinical questions**

   a. *How is your child doing in school? What are your hopes and fears for him or her?*

   b. *How are you coming in reaching your goals for yourself?*

3. **Management.** The clinician can help the teen parent to support the child's school readiness (such as regular bedtime and practice in turn-taking), and suggest ways to build school-related skills (such as reading together and learning about books). The provider should advocate for early assessment and treatment of school difficulties, before they consolidate into failure cycles. For the parent who herself experienced school failure, the provider's support and partnership in working with the school can be critical.

   The primary care clinician can help the parent to recognize and prepare the child for the impact of changes in her life (such as where and with whom she lives, how much she is away from the child at school or work, and the birth of siblings). The provider should also begin to talk about adolescent issues well before puberty begins and help the "grown-up" teen mother to recognize her own hopes and fears as they are projected onto her child.

   Teen mothers and their children can be successful in every domain. Each intervention that helps the adolescent to parent and the child to succeed in school helps to prevent the repetition of teen parenthood in the next generation.

Bibliography

For Parents
Lindsay JW. *Your Pregnancy and Newborn Journey; Your Baby's First Year; Discipline from Birth to Three; The Challenge of Toddlers; School-Age Parents: The Challenge of Three-Generation Living.* Buena Park CA: Morning Glory Press. *These excellent resources include books for teens, their parents, and teachers.*

Maternal and Child Health Bureau. National Center for Education in Maternal and Child Health. *Comprehensive Adolescent Pregnancy Services.* McLean VA, 1993.

For Professionals
Francis J, Marx F. *Learning Together: A National Directory of Teen Parenting and Child Care Programs.* Wellesley MA: Center for Research of Women, 1989.

Hayes CD, ed. *Risking the Future: Adolescent Sexuality, Pregnancy and Childbearing.* Washington DC: National Academy Press, 1987.

Sander J. *Before Their Time: Four Generations of Teenage Mothers.* San Diego: Harcourt Brace Jovanovich, 1991.

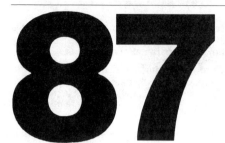

Television

Victor C. Strasburger

I. **Description of the problem.** Young people spend more time watching television than any other activity except sleeping—an average of 21–23 hours/week. By the time today's children reach age 70 years, they will have spent 7–10 years of their lives watching television.

Children are especially vulnerable to the influence of television. According to social learning theory, children and adolescents learn from watching their parents and other adults model certain behaviors. Certainly there are no more attractive models than on television, discussing everything from sex and alcohol to food and careers. Television gives young people secret glimpses into the adult world and serves as a powerful teacher, shaping attitudes and influencing behavior.

According to the cultivation effect, heavy viewers of television tend to believe that the television world is real, and people in everyday life should behave accordingly. The medium also exerts a powerful displacement effect: 23 hours a week spent viewing television is 23 hours lost from schoolwork, reading, and exercise.

II. **Areas of concern.** Television can be both good and bad. Unfortunately, most of current American network television (which is then exported to the rest of the world) is unhealthy for children and adolescents. Practitioners should familiarize themselves with the specific areas of concern.

A. **Violence.** Children view an average of 10,000 television murders, assaults, and rapes per year. Violence is frequently portrayed as an acceptable solution to a complex problem, particularly for the "good guy." Hundreds of studies have demonstrated a link between viewing a heavy diet of television violence and aggressive behavior in certain children and adolescents. Children in single-parent households and lower socioeconomic groups are at particular risk. In one study, children became more violent in their play after television was introduced into the community. They also exercised less and were less creative in their play. In a remarkable 22-year study, a heavy diet of violent programming at age 8 years correlated significantly with more aggressive behavior at ages 19 and 30 years.

B. **Commercialism.** Children view 20,000 commercials per year. Currently, Saturday morning television has become inundated with toy-based, program-length commercials—programs created by toy companies to sell more product. This is especially problematic for young children under age 8 years, who do not understand the difference between programming and commercials or that commercials do not always tell the truth.

C. **Obesity.** New studies demonstrate a link between the amount of television viewed and the prevalence of obesity in children. Television displaces more active activities and gives children unhealthy ideas about nutrition (e.g., many of the advertisements on Saturday morning programs are for heavily sugared breakfast cereals). Recent data also indicate that the metabolic rate during television viewing may actually be lower than during rest.

D. **Sexuality.** Since less than one-third of parents discuss sex or birth control with their children, and most schools do not offer comprehensive sex education programs, television has become the leading sex educator in America. Although children and adolescents view nearly 15,000 sexual situations and innuendoes per year on American television, fewer than 175 of these involve birth control, self-control, or abstinence. At the same time that programming represents one large invitation for teenagers to begin early sexual activity, the networks have refused to air birth control advertising. The 1985 Guttmacher Report attributed the high teenage pregnancy rate in the United States to inadequate access to birth control, ineffective sex education in school, and inappropriate media portrayals of human sexuality.

E. **Alcohol.** American children view 1000–2000 beer and wine commercials per year, most of them creating the illusion that people are more successful, sexier, and happier if they consume alcohol. Children will view 25–50 beer and wine commercials for every antidrug public service announcement (PSA) they see. And, unfortunately, these PSAs deal only with marijuana or cocaine, not alcohol, the leading killer of American teenagers today. An estimated 15,000 young people ages 15–24 years die each year in alcohol-related accidents or homicides.

F. **Rock music and music videos.** Despite the fact that rock music lyrics have become sexier and more violent since the 1950s, there are no data to show that such lyrics have a negative behavioral impact. Indeed, only 30% of young people even know the lyrics to their favorite songs, and their ability to decipher the meaning of the lyrics is age dependent.

Music videos, on the other hand, have become extremely popular and are more likely to have a demonstrable impact. Although many music videos are harmless "performance videos" (of the band playing), others are concept videos that often tell a story replete with sexual imagery, violence, and sexism.

III. **Advice and guidance for families**

A. **The American Academy of Pediatrics (AAP) recommends that parents limit their children's television viewing time to no more than 1–2 hours per day.** The easiest way to limit television viewing is not to allow children to establish a pattern of 3–4 hours of viewing per day (the current norm). That means counseling parents of 6–12-month-old babies about the potential harmful effects of television on the children and advising them to set strict limits from the outset.

B. **The AAP recommends that parents control which shows their children watch and that they watch television with their children.** Studies show that parents can override any potentially harmful effects of television programming by discussing objectionable scenes with their children.

C. **Advising parents not to use the television as an "electronic babysitter" is probably unrealistic. Rather, parents should be counseled to use the videocassette recorder to control what their child views during those times.** An easy way to put the issue into perspective for parents is through the following analogy: No parent would allow a stranger into his or her home to teach his or her child for 3–4 hours per day (especially a stranger who is obsessed with sex and violence). Yet that is precisely what television is doing.

D. **Primary care clinicians should periodically take a detailed television history** (how many hours watched per week, what shows, is there a television in the child's room, etc.).

E. **Clinicians and parents need to familiarize themselves with the high-quality, low-cost videotapes that are available.** For preschoolers, the Rabbit Ears series of classic childhood stories, narrated by Hollywood stars, with music by well-known performers, is an outstanding alternative to the usual network fare. Also, an excellent nonprofit newsletter for parents, *Parents' Choice,* is available, which reviews children's videos, television programming magazines, and books. The Coalition for Quality Children's Videos is another nonprofit organization that focuses exclusively on videos and produces a quarterly newsletter.

F. Since increased media literacy helps to mitigate the negative effects of television, **clinicians need to stress the importance of parents' discussing television content with their children.** The Center for Media Values has several excellent publications that can help parents develop their children's critical viewing skills. The Yale Television Research Center also has an excellent curriculum for younger children and a health curriculum for older children adapted from the Degrassi Junior High series.

G. **Feedback to the networks, both negative and positive, is critically important in trying to improve the quality of programming for children.** The networks estimate that one letter represents 10,000 viewers. Following are addresses for the networks:

ABC, Entertainment President, 2040 Avenue of the Stars, Fifth Floor, Los Angeles CA 90067.
CBS, Entertainment President, 7800 Beverly Boulevard, Los Angeles CA 90036.
NBC, Entertainment President, 3000 West Alameda, Burbank CA 91523.
Fox, President, Fox Broadcasting, PO Box 900, Los Angeles CA 90213.

The following organizations are also important:

Action for Children's Television, 20 University Road, Cambridge MA 02138; (617) 876-6620.
American Academy of Pediatrics, Committee on Communications, 141 Northwest Point Boulevard, PO Box 927, Elk Grove Village IL 60009-0927; (708) 228-5005.
Federal Communications Commission, Mass Media Bureau, Enforcement Division, Room 8210, 2025 M Street, Washington DC 20554.

Bibliography

For Parents
Center for Population Options: *Talking with TV* (booklet). 1025 Vermont Avenue, NW, Suite 210, Washington DC 20005; (202) 347-5700; $4.00.

Coalition for Quality Children's Videos, 535 Cordova Road, Suite 456, Santa Fe NM 97501; (505) 989-8076 ($25/year).

Listening Library (Rabbit Ears), 1 Park Avenue, Old Greenwich CT 06870-1727; (800) 243-4504.

Parents' Choice, Box 185, Waban MA 02168; (617) 965-5913 ($18/year).

TV Alert: A Wakeup Guide to Television Literacy, Center for Media Values, 1962 South Shenandoah, Los Angeles CA 90034; (310) 559-2944 ($27.95).

Yale Television Research Center, 405 Temple Street, New Haven CT 06511; (203) 432-4565.

For Professionals
Dietz WH, Strasburger, VC. Children, adolescents, and television. *Curr Probl Pediatr* 21(1):8–31, 1991.

Liebert RM, Sprafkin J. *The Early Window—Effects of Television on Children and Youth* (3rd ed). New York: Pergamon Press, 1988.

Singer DC, Singer JL, Zuckerman DM. *Using TV to Your Child's Advantage.* Reston VA: Acropolis Books, 1990.

Strasburger VC. Children, adolescents and television. *Pediatr Rev* 13:144–151, 1992.

Strasburger VC, Comstock G (eds). *Adolescents and the Media. Adolescent Medicine: State of the Art Reviews.* Philadelphia: Hanley & Belfus, 1993.

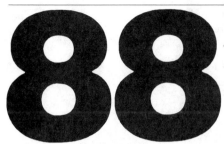

Twins

Jessie R. Groothuis

I. Description of the problem

A. Epidemiology
- Twins occur in approximately 1 in 80 pregnancies.
- Monozygotic twins occur with uniform frequency (3.5/1000 births) and are not appreciably influenced by race, maternal age, or other known factors.
- The incidence of dizygotic twins (the result of multiple ovulation) increases with maternal age, greater parity, in African populations, and with the use of fertility drugs. Dizygotic twins are genetically no more alike than nontwin siblings.
- The increased perinatal mortality observed in twins appears to be primarily due to the incidence (over 40%) of prematurity. Monozygotic twins are at a greater disadvantage for perinatal morbidity and death than are dizygotic twins because of a higher incidence of lethal anomalies and an increased risk for twin-to-twin transfusions.

II. Advice to parents of twins

A. Infant twins.
Parents of infant twins need support and advice regarding organization, feeding, individualization and separation issues, and stress management (Table 88-1). Ideally, discussion of these issues should begin *before* the birth of the twins. It is an excellent idea to refer expectant parents to a local Mother of Twins Club for advice and support both before and after delivery.

1. **Organization.** Efficient organization of the household and anticipatory preparation for caregiving tasks are essential for twin families. Parents should try to enlist outside help in the first weeks after the birth.

   Parents should have enough essentials such as bottles, baby clothes, and diapers. A diaper service may be less expensive than disposable diapers for two babies.

   Parents can buy either a twin stroller or two less expensive umbrella folding-type strollers, which can be clamped together. Two infant car seats will be necessary. Parents do not need to buy double sets of infant clothing. Infant twins can sleep in bassinets or even in a bed with bolsters rather than in two expensive cribs.

   Organizing daily activities is very important to reduce stress. It may be helpful to make charts for feeding and other essential daily activities (a daily bath for the babies is not essential). Time alone and time spent with other family members should be planned.

2. **Feeding.** Feeding infant twins can be very stressful. This may be due to specific feeding problems with premature or small-for-gestational-age twins or simply because it takes so long to feed two babies.

   Twins may be breast-fed simultaneously, which will cut down on feeding time, or the parents can awaken the second twin to feed after the first is fed. Many mothers will elect to bottle-feed their twins at least some of the time. Whenever possible, two adults should be enlisted so that both twins are held for feedings. When this is not possible, the mother or other caregiver should prop one twin up against a leg or across the lap while holding the second infant so that both may be fed simultaneously. Individualized demand feedings should be discouraged.

   When babies advance to solid foods, freezing large quantities of food at one time will cut down on the work of preparation.

Table 88-1. Concerns of twin parents

Infant twins
  Organization
  Feeding strategies
  Separation
  Individualization
  Stress management
  Financial concerns
  Siblings
Preschool twins
  Verbal/motor development
  Discipline
  Toilet training
  Siblings
School-aged twins
  Classroom separation
  Learning issues
  Independent peer relationships
  Independent activities, goals

Table 88-2. Parental behavior promoting individualization of twins

Choose different-sounding names.
Do not dress twins alike all the time.
Use individual names when referring to twins.
Take twins on separate excursions.
Spend quality time alone with each twin.
Refer to other twin as "your brother/sister" or by his or her name.
Provide separate bedrooms as space allows.
Praise individually.
Discipline individually.
Do not leave twins to entertain each other for extended time periods.
Encourage frequent opportunities for individualized contact with other adults, siblings, and peers.
Provide toys according to individual preferences, needs, and interests.
Expect that twins' behavior should differ most of the time, and approve of differences.
Expect twins to think differently, and approve of differences.
Encourage relatives and friends to treat twins as two individuals (e.g., individualize gifts and social activities).

3. **Separation and individuation.** Facilitating separation and individuation of twins is important. Whereas a single infant bonds primarily to his or her mother, a twin also develops a strong tie to his or her twin. Problems with separation and individuation may be compounded if twin children are always treated as a unit by family and friends. Table 88-2 outlines parental behaviors that will promote successful individualization of twins, and Table 88-3 presents questions for assessing the level of individualization of each twin.

4. **Stress.** Stress is a particular problem for families with young twins, evidenced by the fact that child abuse and neglect are significantly higher in families with twins. While it is tempting to shuttle the family with two crying infants out of the office as quickly as possible, it is important to allow sufficient time to question parents carefully about stress and their coping ability. This may require having someone take the twins out of the examining room to provide a quiet environment to discuss parental needs.

Table 88-3. Assessment of twins' level of individualization

Infant twins
  Does he or she cry if the other twin cries?
  Who is his or her main source of comfort? (It should be the parents.)
  Does he or she think his or her mirror image is the twin (after age 15–18 months)?
  Does he or she engage in excessive imitation games with the twin?
  Does he or she only respond to his or her own name (not the twin's) when called?
  Is he or she frequently upset when the other twin is disciplined or upset?
  Is there a "twin language"? Do the twins speak at an appropriate developmental level?
  Is the developmental level appropriate for each twin?
  Is he or she excessively upset when separated from the twin?
School-aged twins
  Are the twins afraid to be separated (e.g., at school, overnight stay)?
  Do the twins enjoy dressing differently?
  Are the twins excessively jealous of the co-twin's friends?
  Do the twins exhibit either excessive competition or total lack of competition with each other?
  Do the twins have age-appropriate peer relationships and social activities?
  Does each twin have individual interests, hobbies, and goals?

5. **Acute illness.** Common childhood infectious illnesses frequently occur in both twins. It is advisable to warn the family of the inevitability of the other twin's becoming ill should one develop an infectious disease. Consequently, caregivers should give instructions for both twins even if only one is ill. The clinician can minimize additional stress by counseling against the use of separation measures (such as separate feeding utensils), which are extra work and do not prevent disease spread.

B. **Preschool twins**

1. **Developmental issues.** Monozygotic twins (in the absence of perinatal risks) should achieve developmental milestones at about the same time. Verbal and motor delays are common in preschool twins. While much of this is due to perinatal factors, some delays may occur if excessive time is spent together, with little adult stimulation.

2. **Discipline.** Disciplining twins poses a unique challenge. It is important to remind parents to discipline each twin appropriately and separately. There is a temptation to discipline both twins even when only one misbehaves, increased by the fact that the "good" twin will often attempt to do what the "bad" twin just got punished for. Biting is a particularly common problem in twins. The type of discipline used should be no different from that suggested for singleton children. Twins should not be compared to each other in terms of behavior (e.g., "Why aren't you good like your twin?").

3. **Toilet training.** Twins may toilet train at a somewhat later age than singleton children. Parents should delay toilet training until the twins are truly interested and can verbalize this interest. Parents should be sensitive to individual twin preference and not compare their twins or encourage excessive competition. Some twins will prefer to train together; others will do better when trained separately.

4. **Siblings.** Twins attract a great deal of attention, and siblings should not be neglected. Twins may also actively exclude nontwin siblings from their activities. Health care providers should encourage parents to set up outings that include only one twin and the nontwin sibling(s) or siblings alone. Activities should be planned where all siblings can interact equally together (e.g., music, sport activities, etc.).

C. School-aged twins

1. **School entry.** Entry into school is a major step in separation from family, and it may be the first time that twins are separated from each other. Parents, teachers, and school administrators need to anticipate the particular difficulties twins may encounter when they first enter school.

2. **Classroom placement.** It is usually advisable to have twins assigned to different classrooms to decrease intertwin dependency; accelerate individual independent, academic, and social growth; and discourage excessive comparison by teachers and peers. Emotional or psychological problems may occur when one twin performs better than the other. If twins seem anxious about classroom separation, having them carry a picture of their twin or permitting occasional visits to their twin's classroom may be helpful. If twins experience significant academic and emotional problems because of classroom separation, placement in one classroom for a period of time may be necessary. Within a single classroom, placement into separate work groups may encourage independence.

3. **Social relationships.** School is an important place for social growth and peer relationships. The initiation of separate social relationships may be particularly difficult for twins and for their parents. Twins should be encouraged to have their own friends and develop individual and separate social experiences. Decisions about individual dress and hair styles should be left to the twins themselves. It must be emphasized to parents and to schools that the social and educational process must be individualized for each twin. Comparisons should be actively discouraged.

Bibliography

For Parents

Organization
National Organization Mother of Twins Club, PO Box 23188, Albuquerque NM 87192-1188; (505) 275-0955.

Publications
Double Talk (published bimonthly), PO Box 412, Amelia OH 45102; (513) 231-8946.

Leigh. *All About Twins,* Boston: Routledge and Kegan Paul, 1983.

Theroux, Tingley. *The Care of Twin Children: A Common Sense Guide for Parents.* Albuquerque NM: National Organization Mother of Twins Club.

Triplet Connection (published bimonthly), PO Box 99571; Stockton CA 95209; (209) 474-0885.

Twins Magazine (published bimonthly), PO Box 12045, Overland Park KS 66212; (913) 722-1090.

For Professionals

Groothuis JG et al. Increased child abuse in families with twins. *Pediatrics* 70:771–773, 1982.

Scheinfield A. *Twins and Supertwins.* Baltimore: Penguin Books, 1979.

Siegel SJ, Siegel MM. Practical aspects of pediatric management of families with twins. *Pediatr Rev* 4:8–12, 1982.

Vulnerable Children

Brian W. C. Forsyth

I. **Description of the problem.** The term *vulnerable child* is used to refer to any instance in which parents, because of earlier events, perceive their children to be abnormally susceptible to illness or death. The term *vulnerable child syndrome* was coined by Green and Solnit to describe children with severe behavioral and learning problems who had experienced serious illnesses or accidents early in childhood. Although these children had recovered fully, their parents continued to view them as especially prone to illnesses and death. It was the continuing, overprotective, enmeshed relationship between parent and child that adversely affected the child's psychological development.

This classic description represents the extreme end of a spectrum. Less severe experiences can also heighten parents' anxieties and cause them to perceive their children to be at increased risk for illness or death. Similarly, there is a wide spectrum of developmental and behavioral outcomes: some children have severe problems, and other have few apparent ill effects. The term *vulnerable child syndrome* should be reserved only for cases meeting the criteria in Table 89-1.

A. **Epidemiology.** It is unknown to what extent the vulnerable child syndrome accounts for psychopathology among children.
  • In a community-wide study of 1095 children ages 4–8 years, 10% of children were categorized as "perceived vulnerable." In that study, 21% of all the mothers reported that they had had prior fears that their child might die.
  • A number of studies have demonstrated an increased sense of vulnerability among mothers who are unmarried, less educated, and of lower socioeconomic status.

B. **Etiology.** A number of different factors have been reported to contribute to parental perceptions of vulnerability (Table 89-2). In general, the earlier in a child's life that an event occurs, the more likely it is to enhance the parent's perception of the child as vulnerable. The translation of parental fears into childhood behavioral problems is a complex process. Most are believed to result from distortions in the normal development of a sense of separateness, independence, and self-esteem.

II. **Making the diagnosis**

A. **Presentation.** The most important factor in managing the vulnerable child is early identification. This should be a consideration in a child with any of the following:

1. **A child who is brought frequently to the clinician with minor medical complaints.**

2. **Recurring symptoms that may be psychosomatic,** such as headaches or stomachaches.

3. **Behavioral problems or school learning difficulties.**

4. **Parents who are having difficulty separating from their children.**

B. **History: Key clinical questions.** Sensitive history taking begins the therapeutic process by conveying to the parent a sense of understanding and empathy. The clinician should ask questions that lead to an understanding of the parent's sense of vulnerability.

1. *To understand your child better, I need to know more. Let's go right back*

Table 89-1. Diagnostic criteria for the vulnerable child syndrome

1. An event early in the child's life that the parent considered to be life-threatening.
2. The parent's continuing unrealistic belief that the child is especially susceptible to illness or death (often associated with frequent telephone calls and visits to the clinician for trivial symptoms).
3. The presence of a behavioral or learning problem in the child.

Table 89-2. Antecedents of the vulnerable child

Preexisting
    Death of a relative or previous child early in life
    Prior miscarriage or stillbirth
Pregnancy related
    Pregnancy complications (e.g., vaginal bleeding)
    Abnormal screening results (e.g., abnormal alpha-feto protein)
    Delivery complications
Newborn period
    Prematurity
    Neonatal illness or complications
    Congenital abnormalities
    Hyperbilirubinemia
    False-positive results of screening (e.g., phenylketonuria)
Early childhood
    Excessive crying, colic, spitting up
    Any serious illness
    Admission to hospital for such things as "to rule out sepsis"
    Self-limited infectious illnesses (e.g., croup, gastroenteritis)

to the beginning. Let's start with your pregnancy. This allows a more complete history that can focus on factors contributing to perceptions of vulnerability.

2. *What did the doctors tell you might happen? Did you at any time fear that the child might not make it?* This type of question should be asked whenever a parent reports a problem, particularly during the pregnancy, delivery, and early childhood, no matter how minor it might appear.

3. *That must have been very frightening for you.* Whenever parents report something that might have been particularly worrisome to them, an empathic response will encourage them to talk further about their fears.

4. *How often do you leave him or her with a babysitter?* Try to assess the parents' level of comfort in separating from their child by asking questions about the use of babysitters and their level of worry when apart from the child. Other questions should include information about other separation difficulties (e.g., when the child first started day care or school).

III. **Management**

    A. **Prevention.** The clinician must realize that any event or illness, even one considered to be medically insignificant, may have a very different meaning and implications for the parent. The clinician needs to take time to understand parents' beliefs and fears and address these appropriately. This may occur, for example, when a colicky infant's formula is changed. Some parents might interpret the change as implying that the child has a gastrointestinal abnormality. By explaining that colic is a self-limited condition affecting normal infants and by reinforcing this concept by changing back to the original formula within a few weeks, the clinician should be able to prevent the development of perceptions of vulnerability. When a child who is hospitalized for an acute illness is ready for discharge, the clinician should emphasize to the parents that recovery is or will be complete, that no special precautions will be necessary after a certain time, and that the child is no more vulnerable to illness than other children.

B. Treatment. Once it is recognized that parental perceptions of vulnerability are affecting a child's behavior or development, the following approach should be taken:

1. **After taking a complete history and performing a conspicuously meticulous physical examination, the clinician should give a clear statement that the child is absolutely physically sound.** He or she should not use equivocal comments such as, "He doesn't look too bad" or "I can't find anything wrong."

2. **Help the parents to understand and accept the notion that the child is considered special by the family and that this derives from their response to earlier events.** It may be helpful to explain the vulnerable child syndrome and describe it as a known entity. However, the clinician should be careful about labeling it as a "syndrome," which might have a stigmatizing implication for some parents.

3. **Support the parents in dealing with the child more appropriately** by setting consistent limits, discontinuing patterns of infantilization and overprotectiveness, dealing more effectively with problems of separation, and being less panicked about the child's somatic complaints.

4. Although these problems can usually be managed by the primary care clinician, **a mental health referral may be necessary if the parents are unable to accept this approach.**

Bibliography

Carey WB. Psychological sequelae of early infancy health crises. In JL Swartz, LH Swartz (eds), *Vulnerable Infants*. New York: McGraw-Hill, 1977.

Forsyth BWC, Canny PF. Perceptions of vulnerability 3½ years after problems of feeding and crying behavior in early infancy. *Pediatrics* 88:757–763, 1991.

Green M. Vulnerable child syndrome and its variants. *Pediatr Rev* 8:75–80, 1986.

Green M, Solnit AJ. Reactions to the threatened loss of a child: A vulnerable child syndrome. *Pediatrics* 34:58–66, 1964.

Appendixes

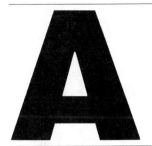

Preschool Children's
Behavior Checklist

Child's name: _____ Birth date: _____

Your relationship to child: _____ Child's doctor: _____

A. Are you concerned about any of these behaviors your child may have? Circle Yes or No.

1. Bed-wetting	Yes	No
2. Wetting during the day	Yes	No
3. Restless sleep	Yes	No
4. Getting him/her to go to sleep at night	Yes	No
5. Thumb sucking	Yes	No
6. Nervous habits	Yes	No
7. Being high-strung or easily upset	Yes	No
8. Being hyperactive	Yes	No
9. Being shy	Yes	No
10. Getting feelings hurt too easily	Yes	No
11. Wanting too much attention	Yes	No
12. Contrary or stubborn	Yes	No
13. Disobedient	Yes	No
14. Discipline problems	Yes	No
15. Selfish, not wanting to share	Yes	No
16. Fighting with other children	Yes	No
17. Destroying things on purpose	Yes	No
18. Appetite (too much or too little)	Yes	No
19. Problems at meals	Yes	No
20. Sad, unhappy	Yes	No
21. Hearing problems	Yes	No
22. Speech problems	Yes	No
23. General development	Yes	No
24. Poor attention span	Yes	No
25. Frequent stomachache/headaches	Yes	No
26. Temper tantrums	Yes	No
27. Problems with toilet training	Yes	No

28. Other problems _____

B. Below are listed some situations often troubling to many families. Circle those that are of concern to you.

1. Day care or preschool   Yes   No
2. Divorce, separation, or other marital problems   Yes   No
3. Death or illness of family member   Yes   No
4. Adjustment to a new brother or sister   Yes   No
5. Moving   Yes   No
6. Effects of both parents' working   Yes   No
7. Other problems (financial, drug or alcohol, etc.)   Yes   No

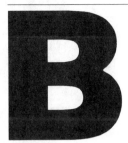

Please mark under the heading that best fits your child:

	Never	Sometimes	Often
1. Complains of aches or pains	_____	_____	_____
2. Spends more time alone	_____	_____	_____
3. Tires easily, little energy	_____	_____	_____
4. Fidgety, unable to sit still	_____	_____	_____
5. Has trouble with a teacher	_____	_____	_____
6. Less interested in school	_____	_____	_____
7. Acts as if driven by a motor	_____	_____	_____
8. Daydreams too much	_____	_____	_____
9. Distracted easily	_____	_____	_____
10. Is afraid of new situations	_____	_____	_____
11. Feels sad, unhappy	_____	_____	_____
12. Is irritable, angry	_____	_____	_____
13. Feels hopeless	_____	_____	_____
14. Has trouble concentrating	_____	_____	_____
15. Less interest in friends	_____	_____	_____
16. Fights with other children	_____	_____	_____
17. Absent from school	_____	_____	_____
18. School grades dropping	_____	_____	_____
19. Is down on himself or herself	_____	_____	_____
20. Visits doctor with doctor finding nothing wrong	_____	_____	_____
21. Has trouble with sleeping	_____	_____	_____
22. Worries a lot	_____	_____	_____
23. Wants to be with you more than before	_____	_____	_____

24. Feels he or she is bad   _____   _____   _____

25. Takes unnecessary risks   _____   _____   _____

26. Gets hurt frequently   _____   _____   _____

27. Seems to be having less fun   _____   _____   _____

28. Acts younger than other children his or her age   _____   _____   _____

29. Does not listen to rules   _____   _____   _____

30. Does not show feelings   _____   _____   _____

31. Does not understand other people's feelings   _____   _____   _____

32. Teases others   _____   _____   _____

33. Blames others for his or her troubles   _____   _____   _____

34. Takes things that do not belong to him or her   _____   _____   _____

35. Refuses to share   _____   _____   _____

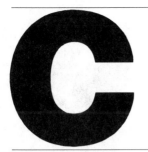

Child Development in the First 5 Years

Reprinted with permission from Harold Ireton, Ph.D. Behavior Science Systems, Inc., Box 580274, Minneapolis MN 55440.

Age	SOCIAL	SELF-HELP	GROSS MOTOR	FINE MOTOR	LANGUAGE
5-0 yrs.	Shows leadership among children	Goes to the toilet without help	Swings on swing, pumping by self	Prints first name (four letters)	Tells meaning of familiar words
4-6	Follows simple game rules in board games or card games	Usually looks both ways before crossing street	Skips or makes running "broad jumps"	Draws a person that has at least three parts - head, eyes, nose, mouth, etc.	Reads a few letters (five+)
4-0 yrs.	Protective toward younger children	Buttons one or more buttons	Hops around on one foot, without support	Draws recognizable pictures	Follows a series of three simple instructions
		Dresses and undresses without help, except for tying shoelaces			Understands concepts - size, number, shape
3-6	Plays cooperatively, with minimum conflict and supervision	Washes face without help	Hops on one foot, without support	Cuts across paper with small scissors	Counts five or more objects when asked "How many?"
				Draws or copies a complete circle	Identifies four colors correctly
3-0 yrs.	Gives directions to other children	Toilet trained	Rides around on a tricycle, using pedals		Combines sentences with the words "and," "or," or "but"
	Plays a role in "pretend" games - mom-dad, teacher, space pilot	Dresses self with help	Walks up and down stairs - one foot per step	Cuts with small scissors	Understands four prepositions - in, on, under, beside
2-6	Plays with other children - cars, dolls, building	Washes and dries hands	Stands on one foot without support	Draws or copies vertical (	) lines	Talks clearly - is understandable most of the time
	"Helps" with simple household tasks	Opens door by turning knob	Climbs on play equipment - ladders, slides	Scribbles with circular motion	Talks in two-three word phrases or sentences

Child Development Milestones (Birth to 2 Years)

Age	Social	Self-Help / Feeding	Gross Motor	Fine Motor / Vision	Language
2-0 yrs	Usually responds to correction - stops; Shows sympathy to other children, tries to comfort them	Takes off open coat or shirt without help	Walks up and down stairs alone	Turns pages of picture books, one at a time	Follows two-part instructions
18 mos	Sometimes says "No" when interfered with; Greets people with "Hi" or similar; Gives kisses or hugs	Eats with spoon, spilling little; Eats with fork; Insists on doing things by self such as feeding	Runs well, seldom falls; Kicks a ball forward; Runs	Builds towers of four or more blocks; Scribbles with crayon; Stacks two or more blocks	Uses at least ten words; Follows simple instructions; Asks for food or drink with words; Talks in single words
12 mos	Wants stuffed animal, doll or blanket in bed; Plays patty-cake	Feeds self with spoon; Lifts cup to mouth and drinks; Picks up a spoon by the handle	Walks without help; Stands without support; Walks around furniture or crib while holding on	Picks up two small toys in one hand; Picks up small objects - precise thumb and finger grasp	Uses one or two words as names of things or actions; Understands words like "No," "Stop," or "All gone"
9 mos	Plays social games, peek-a-boo, bye-bye; Pushes things away he/she doesn't want	Feeds self cracker	Crawls around on hands and knees; Sits alone . . . steady, without support	Picks up object with thumb and finger grasp	Word sounds - says "Ma-ma" or "Da-da" as name for parent; Wide range of vocalizations (vowel sounds, consonant-vowel combinations)
6 mos	Reaches for familiar persons; Distinguishes mother from others	Comforts self with thumb or pacifier	Rolls over from back to stomach; Turns around when lying on stomach	Transfers toy from one hand to the other; Picks up toy with one hand	Responds to name - turns and looks; Vocalizes spontaneously, social
Birth	Social smile	Reacts to sight of bottle or breast	Lifts head and chest when lying on stomach	Looks at and reaches for faces and toys	Reacts to voices; Vocalizes, coos, chuckles

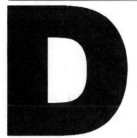

Child Development in the First 21 Months

	Social	Self-Help	Gross motor	Fine motor	Language
Birth	Responds positively to feeding and comforting.	Alert: interested in sights and sounds.	Kicks legs and thrashes arms.	Looks at objects or faces.	Cries.
1 mo.	Social smile.	Responds to voices: turns head toward a voice.	Raises head and chest when lying on stomach.	Follows moving objects with eyes.	Cries in a special way when hungry.
2 mos.	Recognizes mother.	Reacts to sight of bottle or breast.	Holds head steady when held sitting.	Holds objects put in hand.	Makes sounds—ah, eh, ugh. Laughs.
3 mos.	Recognizes most familiar adults.	Increases activity when shown toy.	Makes crawling movements.	Shakes rattle.	
4 mos.	Interested in his or her image in mirror, smiles, playful.	Reaches for objects.	Turns around when lying on stomach.	Puts toys or other objects in mouth.	Squeals. Ah-goo.
5 mos.	Reacts differently to strangers.		Rolls over from stomach to back.	Picks up objects with one hand.	Makes razzing sounds—gives you the "raspberry."
6 mos.	Reaches for familiar persons.	Looks for object after it disappears from sight—for example, looks for toy after it falls off tray.	Rolls over from back to stomach.	Transfers objects from one hand to the other.	Babbles. Responds to his/her name, turns and looks.
7 mos.	Gets upset and afraid if left alone.	Anticipates being lifted by raising arms.	Sits without support.	Holds two objects, one in each hand, at the same time.	Makes sounds like da, ba, ga, ka, ma.
8 mos.	Plays "peek-a-boo."	Feeds self cracker or cookie.	Crawls on hands and knees.	Uses forefinger to poke, push, or roll small objects.	Makes sounds like ma-ma, da-da, ba-ba.
9 mos.	Resists having a toy taken away.		Pulls self to standing position.	Picks up small objects using only finger and thumb.	Imitates speech sounds that you make.

Age	Social	Self-Help	Gross Motor	Fine Motor	Language
10 mos.		Plays "patty-cake."	Sidesteps around playpen or furniture while holding on. Or walks.	Picks up two small objects in one hand.	Understands single words like bye-bye and nite-nite.
11 mos.	Shows or offers toy to adult.	Picks up spoon by handle.	Stands alone well.	Puts small objects in cup or other container.	Uses Mama or Dada specifically for parent.
12 mos.	Imitates simple acts such as hugging or loving a doll.	Removes socks.	Climbs up on chairs or other furniture.	Turns pages of books a few at a time.	Says one word clearly.
13 mos.	Plays with other children.	Lifts cup to mouth and drinks.	Walks without help.	Builds tower of 2 or more blocks.	Shakes head to express "No." Hands object to you when asked.
14 mos.	Gives kisses.	Insists on feeding self.	Stoops and recovers.	Marks with pencil or crayon.	Asks for food or drink with sounds or words.
15 mos.	Greets people with "Hi" or similar.	Feeds self with a spoon.	Runs.	Scribbles with pencil or crayon.	Says 2 words besides Mama or Dada. Makes sounds in sequences that sound like sentences.
18 mos.	Sometimes says "No" when interfered with.	Eats with a fork.	Kicks a ball. Good balance and coordination.	Builds tower of 4 or more blocks.	
21 mos.					Uses 5 or more words as names of things. Follows a few simple instructions.

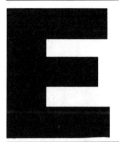

Early Language Milestone Scale

James Coplan

The Early Language Milestone Scale, second edition (ELM Scale-2) is designed primarily as a structured history of speech and language development, to be used by clinicians with varying degrees of expertise in early child development. The scale may be administered by either a pass-fail or a point-scoring method. The pass-fail method separates children into two groups: the slowest 10% with respect to speech and language development ("fail") and everyone else ("pass"). The point-scoring method yields age-, percentile-, and standard score equivalents for all possible point scores. The pass-fail method is recommended when screening large numbers of low-risk subjects; the point-scoring method is recommended when examining children who are at high risk for the presence of developmental delay or when evaluating a child with a known developmental disability. Complete instructions and pads of scoring forms are available from PRO-ED, 8700 Shoal Creek Boulevard, Austin TX 78758.

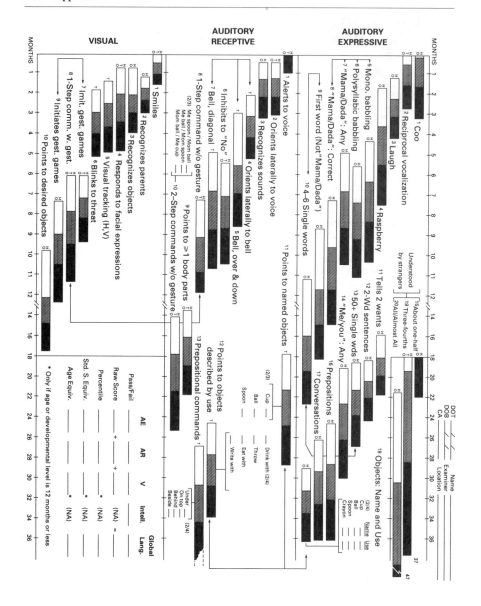

I. General Instructions

25% 50% 75% 90%   Percentage of Children Passing Item

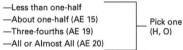

Item may be elicited by
- H = History
- T = Direct Testing
- O = Incidental Observation

- Always start with H, where allowed.
- Child passes item if passed by any of the allowable means of elicitation for that item.
- Basal = 3 consecutive items passed (work down from age line).
- Ceiling = 3 consecutive items failed (work up from age line).

II. Auditory Expressive (AE)

A. Content

AE 1. Prolonged musical vowel sounds in a sing-song fashion (ooo, aaa, etc.), <u>not</u> just grunts or squeaks.

AE 2. H: Does baby watch speaker's face and appear to listen intently, then vocalize when the speaker is quiet? Can you "have a conversation" with your baby?

AE 4. H: Blow bubbles or give "bronx cheer"?

AE 5. H: Makes isolated sounds such as "ba," "da," "ga," "goo," etc.

AE 6. H: Makes repetitive string of sounds: "babababa," or "lalalalala," etc.

AE 7. H: Says "mama" or "dada" but uses them at other times besides just labelling parents.

AE 8. H: Child <u>spontaneously, consistently,</u> and <u>correctly</u> uses "mama" or "dada," <u>just</u> to label the <u>appropriate</u> parent.

AE 9, AE 10, AE 13. H: Child <u>spontaneously, consistently,</u> and <u>correctly</u> uses words. Do not count "mama," "dada," or the names of other family members or pets.

AE 11. H: Uses single words to tell you what he/she wants. "Milk!" "Cookie!" "More!" etc. Pass = 2 or more wants. List specific words.

AE 12. H: Spontaneously, novel 2-word combinations ("Want cookie" "No bed" "See daddy" etc.) <u>Not</u> rotely learned phrases that have been specifically taught to the child or combinations that are really single thoughts (e.g., "hot dog").

AE 14. H: Child uses "me" or "you" but may reverse them ("you want cookie" instead of "me want cookie," etc.)

AE 17. H: "Can child put 2 or 3 sentences together to hold brief conversations?"

AE 18. T: Put out cup, ball, crayon, & spoon. Pick up cup & say "What is this? What do we do with it? (What is it for?)" Child must <u>name</u> the object and give its use. Pass = "drink with," etc., <u>not</u> "milk" or "juice." Ball: Pass = "throw," "play with," etc. Spoon: Pass = "Eat" or "Eat with," etc., <u>not</u> "Food," "Lunch." Crayon: Pass = "Write (with)," "Color (with)," etc. Pass item if child gives <u>name and use</u> for 2 objects.

B. Intelligibility

AE 15, AE 19, AE 20. "How clear is your child's speech? That is, how much of your child's speech can a stranger understand?"

—Less than one-half
—About one-half (AE 15)
—Three-fourths (AE 19)   Pick one (H, O)
—All or Almost All (AE 20)

To score:
If less than one-half: Fail all 3 items in cluster.
If about one-half: Pass AE 15 only.
If three-fourths: Pass AE 19 and AE 15.
If all or almost all: Pass all 3 items in cluster.

III. Auditory Receptive (AR)

AR 1. H, T: Any behavioral change in response to noise (eye blink, startle, change in movements or respiration, etc.)

AR 2. H, T: What does baby do when parent starts talking while out of baby's line of sight? Pass if any shift of head or eyes to voice.

AR 3. H: Does baby seem to respond in a specific way to certain sounds (becomes excited at hearing parents' voices, etc.)?

AR 4. T: Sit facing baby, with baby in parent's lap. Extend both arms so that your hands are behind baby's field of vision and at the level of baby's waist. Ring a 2"-diameter bell, first with 1 hand, then the other. Repeat 2 or 3 times if necessary. Pass if baby turns head to the side at least once.

AR 5. T: See note for AR 4. Pass if baby turns head first to the side, then down, to localize bell, at least once. (Automatically passes AR 4.)

AR 6. H: Does baby understand the command "no" (even though he may not always obey)? T: Test by commanding "(Baby's name), no!" while baby is playing with any test object. Pass if baby temporarily inhibits his actions.

AR 7. T: See note for AR 4. Pass if baby turns directly down on diagonal to localize bell, at least once. (Automatically passes AR 5 and AR 4.)

AR 8. H: Will your baby follow any verbal commands without you indicating by gestures what it is you want him to do ("Stop" "Come here" "Give me" etc.)? T: Wait until baby is playing with any test object, then say "(Baby's name), give it to me." Pass if baby extends object to you, even if baby seems to change his mind and take the object back. May repeat command 1 or 2 times. If failed, repeat the command but this time hold out your hand for the object. If baby responds, then pass item, V 8 (1-step command with gesture).

AR 9. H: Does your child point to at least 1 body part on command? T: Have mother command baby "Show me your..." or "Where's your..." without pointing to the desired part herself.

AR 10. H: "Can child do 2 things in a row if asked? For example 'First go get your shoes, then sit down'?" T: Set out ball, cup, and spoon, and say "(Child's name), give me the spoon, then give the ball to mommy." Use slow, steady voice but do not break command into 2 separate sentences. If no response, then give each half of command separately to see if child understands separate components. If child succeeds on at least half of command, then give each of the following: "(Child's name), give me the ball and give mommy the spoon." May repeat once but do not break into 2 commands. Then "Give mommy the ball, then give the cup to me." Pass if at least two 2-step commands executed correctly. (Note: Child is credited even if the order of execution of a command is reversed.)

AR 11. H: Place a cup, ball, and spoon on the table. Command child "Show me/where is/give me... the cup/ball/spoon." (If command is "Give me," be sure to replace each object before asking about the next object.) Pass = 2 items correctly identified.

AR 12. T: Put cup, ball, spoon, and crayon on table and give command "Show me/where is/give me... the one we drink with/eat with/draw (color, write) with/throw (play with)." If the command "Give me" is used, be sure to replace each object before asking about the next object. Pass = 2 or more objects correctly identified.

AR 13. Put out cup (upside down) and a 1" cube. Command the child "Put the block under the cup." Repeat 1 or 2 times if necessary. If no attempt, or incorrect response, then demonstrate correct response, saying, "See, now the block is under the cup." Remove the block and hand it to the child. Then give command "Put the block on top of the cup." If child makes no response, then repeat command 1 time but do not demonstrate. Then command "Put the block behind the cup," then "Put the block beside the cup." Pass = 2 or more commands correctly executed (prior to demonstration by examiner, if "underneath" is scored).

IV. Visual

V 1. H: "Does your baby smile—not just a gas bubble or a burp but a real smile?" T: Have parent attempt to elicit smile by any means.

V 2. H: "Does your baby seem to recognize you, reacting differently to you than to the sight of other people? For example, does your baby smile more quickly for you than for other people?"

V 3. H: "Does your baby seem to recognize any common objects by sight? For example, if bottle or spoon fed, what happens when bottle or spoon is brought into view before it touches baby's lips?" Pass if baby gets visibly excited, or opens mouth in anticipation of feeding.

V 4. H: "Does your baby respond to your facial expressions?" T: Engage baby's gaze and attempt to elicit a smile by smiling and talking to baby. Then scowl at baby. Pass if any change in baby's facial expression.

V 5. T: Horizontal (H): Engage child's gaze with yours at a distance of 18". Move slowly back and forth. Pass if child turns 60° to left and right from midline. Vertical (V): Move slowly up and down. Pass if child elevates eyes 30° from horizontal. Must pass both H & V to pass item.

V 6. T: Flick your fingers rapidly towards child's face, ending with fingertips 1–2" from face. Do not touch face or eyelashes. Pass if child blinks.

V 7. H: Does child play pat-a-cake, peek-a-boo, etc., in response to parents?

V 8. T: See note for AR 8 (always try AR 8 first; if AR 8 is passed, then automatically give credit for V 8).

V 9. H: Does child spontaneously initiate gesture games?

V 10. H: "Does your child ever point with index finger to something he/she wants? For example, if child is sitting at the dinner table and wants something that is out of reach, how does child let you know what he/she wants?" Pass only index finger pointing not reaching with whole hand.

Index

Index